EXERCISE
for
FRAIL ELDERS

Second Edition

Elizabeth Best-Martini, MS, CTRS

Kim A. Jones-DiGenova, MA

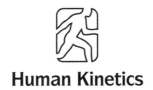

Human Kinetics

Library of Congress Cataloging-in-Publication Data

Best-Martini, Elizabeth, 1948-
  Exercise for frail elders / Elizabeth Best-Martini, Kim A. Jones-DiGenova. -- 2nd ed.
    p. ; cm.
  Includes bibliographical references and index.
  I. Botenhagen-DiGenova, Kim A., 1957- II. Title.
  [DNLM: 1. Exercise Therapy. 2. Frail Elderly. 3. Aged. WB 541]
  RC953.8.E93
  613.7'0446--dc23

                         2013003909

  ISBN-10: 1-4504-1609-8
  ISBN-13: 978-1-4504-1609-2

The web addresses cited in this text were current as of August 2013, unless otherwise noted.

Acquisitions Editor: Amy N. Tocco; **Developmental Editor:** Christine M. Drews; **Assistant Editors:** Casey A. Gentis and Amy Akin; **Copyeditor:** Bob Replinger; **Indexer:** Bobbi Swanson; **Permissions Manager:** Dalene Reeder; **Graphic Designer:** Fred Starbird; **Graphic Artist:** Dawn Sills; **Cover Designer:** Keith Blomberg; **Photograph (cover):** Neil Bernstein; photograph © Human Kinetics; **Photographs (interior):** Neil Bernstein; photographs © Human Kinetics; **Visual Production Assistant:** Joyce Brumfield; **Photo Production Manager:** Jason Allen; **Art Manager:** Kelly Hendren; **Associate Art Manager:** Alan L. Wilborn; **Illustrations:** © Human Kinetics, unless otherwise noted; **Printer:** Sheridan Books

We thank Long Life Living in San Rafael, California, for assistance in providing the location for the photo shoot for this book.

On the cover: Bill Bromley, age 92, demonstrating balance and core work with a ball.

Printed in the United States of America   10 9 8 7 6 5 4 3 2 1

The paper in this book is certified under a sustainable forestry program.

Human Kinetics
Website: www.HumanKinetics.com

United States: Human Kinetics
P.O. Box 5076
Champaign, IL 61825-5076
800-747-4457
e-mail: humank@hkusa.com

Canada: Human Kinetics
475 Devonshire Road Unit 100
Windsor, ON N8Y 2L5
800-465-7301 (in Canada only)
e-mail: info@hkcanada.com

Europe: Human Kinetics
107 Bradford Road
Stanningley
Leeds LS28 6AT, United Kingdom
+44 (0) 113 255 5665
e-mail: hk@hkeurope.com

Australia: Human Kinetics
57A Price Avenue
Lower Mitcham, South Australia 5062
08 8372 0999
e-mail: info@hkaustralia.com

New Zealand: Human Kinetics
P.O. Box 80
Torrens Park, South Australia 5062
0800 222 062
e-mail: info@hknewzealand.com

E5545

To my dearest husband, John A. Martini, whose love for me and recognition of the importance of my work have been immeasurable gifts. As a well-known author yourself, you understand this process, and you have helped me with editing, photography, graphics, and most of all, support. Thank you for being you and loving me.

To my mom, Peggy. Every time I look at your smiling face in one of the exercise photographs, I can hear your laugh and feel your love and presence.

And a special dedication to all the elderly people who have touched my life and work. You are at the heart of this book.

Betsy Best-Martini

In honor of John R. Jones, my beloved husband; my father, Alfred; my mother, Anna; and Auntie Mary, whose unconditional love and support give me time to follow my heart and passions, such as writing this book.

To my students of many years, my best teachers, who give joy and meaning to my life.

And to you, the teachers, who are dedicated to helping our frail elders and those with special needs.

Kim A. Jones-DiGenova

List of Important Topics

Preface

The concept for this book, *Exercise for Frail Elders*, originated from our relationships with elderly participants in our exercise classes. They mentored and showed us the profound effect that physical activity has in each of our lives—regardless of age or situation. Today's fitness leader needs an understanding of the limitations and special needs of those with illnesses, disabilities, chronic disorders, and sedentary lifestyles. There is a direct link between losing fitness and function and losing independence. Some of the simple movements and tasks that we take for granted can slip away through inactivity. Any person, no matter how out of shape, can improve his or her fitness and function through proper exercise. The authors of this second-edition text aspire to help you improve your students' functional fitness (the ability to perform activities of daily living such as pushing, pulling, lifting, squatting, balancing, and sitting and standing erect that enhance well-being and quality of life) through proper exercise. The terms *exercise program*, *fitness program*, and *functional fitness program* are interchangeable in the context of this book.

The need for qualified fitness leaders increases with the growing population of older adults. This field is an exciting one in which to work. You can see the benefits of your exercise program in your participants' increased functional fitness and independence.

Exercise for Frail Elders is a training manual for beginning as well as experienced fitness professionals. Professionals in this field include activity directors, recreation directors, wellness directors, recreational therapists, occupational therapists, physical therapists, dance therapists, physical education teachers, adaptive physical education specialists, exercise physiologists, personal trainers, certified and noncertified fitness instructors, aerobics instructors, gerontologists, adult education instructors, college instructors, and students in specialties related to older adults. Whether you are an experienced or a beginning fitness instructor, or one who is required to follow federal or state regulations for physical exercise instruction, you will find this book to be of great value as a manual that takes you through every step of the process in teaching safe and effective exercise.

This book also stands out from other exercise books for older adults in its thorough and user-friendly presentation of special needs, including Alzheimer's disease and related dementias, arthritis, cerebrovascular accident, chronic obstructive pulmonary disease, coronary artery disease, depression, diabetes, hip fracture or replacement and knee replacement, hypertension, multiple sclerosis, osteoporosis, Parkinson's disease, sensory losses, and traumatic head injury. Regular physical activity is recommended as a therapeutic intervention for the treatment and management of numerous chronic diseases and conditions, including dementia, depression, pain, and so on (ACSM 2009b, USDHHS 2008b). This book will prepare you to meet the challenge of leading exercise for adults with one or more special needs.

Exercise for Frail Elders gives you the tools to plan and implement a successful functional fitness program. At the opening of each chapter you'll find a quotation, an example of one way to open (or even close) a class with a relevant inspirational, motivational, or even humorous saying. You'll also find the addition of learning objectives at the beginning and review questions at the end of each chapter to facilitate your learning. Answers to the review questions can be found in appendix C2. Part I, "Planning a Successful Exercise Program for Frail Elders and Adults With Special Needs," covers the participants, the exercise program, and the leader. In chapter 1 you will learn about participants' individual and special needs. In chapter 2 you will learn about the exercise program and how you can make it motivating, safe, and effective according to industry standards. You

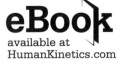

eBook available at HumanKinetics.com

will also learn about the wellness model, which includes physical activity. This chapter provides a foundation for integrating balance, core, and agility exercises into your program. Chapter 3 walks you through steps and strategies needed to be a successful leader. Part II, "Implementing an Exercise Program for Frail Elders and Adults With Special Needs," provides warm-up (good posture, deep breathing, joint range of motion, and light stretching), resistance training, aerobic and dynamic balance (chapter 6, by Janie Clark), and cool-down exercises (comprehensive stretching and relaxation). Each exercise component in chapters 4 through 7 has an easy-reference chart and photographs of the exercises. Each chapter also includes safety precautions, guidelines, seated and standing exercises, and variations and progression options for the exercises to meet the diverse needs of this population through the years. Although part II of the book is geared toward class or group instruction, the information is also applicable when working one on one with this population. Thus, the terms *student*, *resident*, *client*, and *patient* can be used interchangeably with *participant*, and *session* and *appointment* can be used interchangeably with *class*, which is used throughout part II.

Start with the basic seated exercises in chapters 4 through 7, which are intended to help frail elders and those with special needs have a successful experience in your class. Throughout chapters 4 through 7 you'll learn tools for adapting the exercises for your participants' individual needs, particularly in the sections "Specific Safety Precautions for Those With Special Needs" and "Illustrated Instruction," which includes exercise and safety tips and variations and progression options (VPOs) for each exercise. Carefully progress to the basic standing exercises with participants who are able to stand safely. The seated and standing exercises are designed to be taught at the same time, which allows you to accommodate people with a wide variety of special needs.

The second edition of *Exercise for Frail Elders* provides a broader focus on balance, a critical component of a functional fitness program for reducing risk of falling and improving quality of life for older adults. Chapter 2 includes a new section on balance, core, and agility training, including user-friendly tables for balance and core (a key contributor of balance ability) exercises. Many of the exercises included in part II of this book provide balance benefits by increasing joint range of motion with ROM and stretching exercises (chapters 4), by strengthening the muscles with resistance training (chapter 5), by increasing flexibility with stretching (chapter 7), and by improving posture (chapter 4). Seated exercises can give frail and deconditioned participants the strength and flexibility to stand to gain further balance benefits. Also, the standing exercises that involve a one-legged stand for static balance benefits are now indicated in the variation and progression sections in chapters 4 through 7. Lastly, in chapter 6, you will find additional fun and functional dynamic balance exercises.

 The exercises in part II that provide more significant balance benefits are indicated with a balance symbol.

In chapter 8 you will learn about putting it all together to implement an exercise session or program that incorporates one or more components—warm-up, resistance, aerobic and dynamic balance, and cool-down exercises—from chapters 4 through 7. You will also learn how to design, schedule, modify, progress, maintain, and monitor a functional fitness program for frail elders and adults with special needs. Chapter 8 also has a new section on the balance component to aid you in designing an exercise class that includes or focuses on balance.

In the back of the book are appendices that provide you with necessary and useful forms, educational handouts, answers to the review questions, and other information to help make your role as fitness leader easier. In "Suggested Resources" you will find a new section, "Balance," that lists books and supplies for developing a class that includes or concentrates on balance. We encourage you to use "Suggested Resources" to enhance your knowledge base and embrace life-long learning.

It is our sincere hope that this book will enhance your competence and confidence in meeting the special needs of people in your exercise classes.

Acknowledgments

Thank you to the residents of Long Life Living Assisted Living, who continue to exercise with our routine twice weekly. They participated in our photo shoots and named some of the exercises. Thanks to Faye Chang, administrator and owner of this beautiful residential setting, who strongly supports this program and appreciates its importance in enhancing quality of life and independence.

Thank you to the members of the Millennium Movers exercise class, the first strength-training class to be offered in a convalescent setting in Marin County. You taught us about resiliency, determination, and fun with "attitude."

Thanks to our models:

College of Marin—Lucian Wernick, Dolores Cuerva, Beatrice Ross

Long Life Living Assisted Living: Doris M.,Tanya B., Shirley B., Joanne G., Kathy G., Bill B., Henry W., Beverly O., Ratu, M., Glenn F., Suzanne S., Nancy B., Marge G.

Parnow Friendship House—Ali Rostambeik

Many people helped us bring this book to life. We thank each of you for your contributions: the Marin Commission on Aging Strength Training Task Force, Liz Rottger in particular, who introduced the authors to one another; the Marin Association of Senior Strength Trainers (MASST) for their enthusiastic support of our book and us as cofounders of MASST; Janie Clark, MA, for writing chapter 6; and (in alphabetical order) Myles Babcock; Tom Beek, BS; Bryan A. Duff, DC; Terri Fennelly, MSW, LCSW; Randy Gibson, MA, MS, LAc; Jacqui Gillis, PT; Vicki Jackson, MLS; Jon Kakleas, DC, PT; Mary Lockett, PT; Shay McKelvey, RN, MS; Stephen P. Mongiello, PT; Kaylin Mordock, PT; Martin Rossman, MD; Nicolas T. Roth, PT; Mary Dale Scheller, MSW; Kathy M. Schmidt (lead trainer for the Arthritis Foundation Exercise Program, Northern California chapter); Robert Teasdale, MD; Frank Verducci, PhD; and Lucian Wernick, MA, for helping to create and fine-tune the exercise protocols and for offering other valuable contributions; and Kelly Sturgeon, a lawyer and elder advocate who reviewed our medical clearance forms.

Many thanks to Amy Tocco, our acquisitions editor and coach; Chris Drews, our developmental editor; Bob Replinger, our copyeditor; Amy Akin and Casey Gentis, our assistant editors; Neil Bernstein, our photographer; Fred Starbird, our graphic designer; and Dawn Sills, our graphic artist. We appreciate your guidance and commitment to excellence.

On a personal note of acknowledgment, we thank one another for the time, dedication, friendship, and focus on fun during our second "working on the book" journey. Here is to more fun and fitness ahead.

Planning a Successful Exercise Program for Frail Elders and Adults With Special Needs

In chapters 1 through 3 you will learn about the participants in your exercise program, the exercise program itself, and the leader of the program. The first part of this book covers general characteristics and guidelines for these three important areas. To this framework you will add the program specifics in part II.

Part I is designed to help you plan a successful exercise program. Each chapter offers you easy-to-use forms, reference charts, charts of special needs, and much more. These resources help you to plan a safe and effective program that addresses the needs of your participants.

Chapters 1 through 3 cover the following topics:

- Special needs of elderly participants
- Assessing the needs of individual participants
- Setting realistic goals with each participant
- Programming guidelines (including industry curriculum guidelines) to increase motivation, safety, and effectiveness
- Balance, core stability, agility, and fall prevention
- Leadership strategies and teaching skills
- Group dynamics and behavioral interventions

Chapter 1 introduces you to frail elders and adults with special needs. Addressing the needs of this audience is what makes this book unique. Each exercise class is as diverse as the participants participating in it. The more you understand about medical disorders and special needs and the way in which they affect your participants' ability to perform activities of daily living, independence, and lives, the more successful your exercise class will be. Many of these disorders and special needs can be invisible to the leader (such as cardiac issues, osteoporosis, and hypertension). Additionally, these invisible conditions may be undiagnosed and unknown by the participant. Because of this, you will want to adhere to all recommended safety precautions while getting to know the

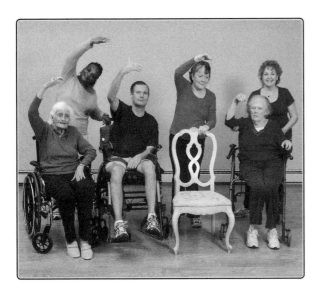

individual needs of your participants. You will also learn about specific medications and how they can affect participation. The charts in chapter 1 identify characteristics of people with common medical disorders and special needs and give you easy-to-use teaching tips for exercise and safety.

Chapter 2 explains ways to make the exercise program motivating, safe, and effective with current industry standards. Your initial goal as the fitness leader is to keep participants coming to class and becoming more physically active, so we start by addressing wellness and motivation. The focus then moves from motivation to safety issues (including medical clearance, assessments, and safety guidelines), as well as physical function levels. Responding to a participant's needs such as relieving pain and ensuring safety while teaching a large group are addressed. The emphasis then moves to effectiveness. In addition, we focus on balance,

core stability, agility, and fall prevention with corresponding exercises and references. Careful attention to exercise program components helps the fitness leader design a motivating, safe, and effective program.

Chapter 3 is about you, the fitness leader, and the leadership and strategies that you can use to lead a motivating, safe, and effective (fun and functional) program. We start by addressing the social environment and mood of the class (including challenging behaviors) and some typical group goals. The next sections of the chapter take you through opening, leading, and closing the exercise class. Included in this chapter are successful strategies for teaching participants who are experiencing communication, cognitive, and sensory losses. The finishing touches of the exercise class, beyond leading the class, include your feedback to participants and all aspects of organizing supplies and space.

CHAPTER 1

The Participants: Know Their Individual Needs

People say that what we're all seeking is a meaning to life. I think what we're seeking is an experience of being alive, so that our life experiences on the purely physical plane will have resonances within our own innermost being and reality, so that we actually feel the rapture of being alive.

—*Joseph Campbell*

LEARNING OBJECTIVES

After completing this chapter, you will have the tools to

- recognize characteristics and exercise and safety tips for 15 common medical disorders and special needs in the frail elderly as well as all adults,
- define gerokinesiology,
- identify the nine modules of the international curriculum guidelines for preparing physical activity instructors with older adults,
- understand main side effects of specific medications commonly used by older adults, and
- modify specific exercises to address individual special needs.

The most important factor in teaching exercise to frail elders and adults with special needs is knowing your audience. Each group can be as varied as the entire population of older adults. We hope to inspire you to get to know each of your participant's strengths and limitations. With this information, you can tailor exercise to an individual participant and to the group as a whole.

This chapter is designed to help you better understand and recognize symptoms and characteristics of frailty and other common special needs including Alzheimer's disease and related dementias, arthritis, cerebrovascular accident (stroke), chronic obstructive pulmonary disease, coronary artery disease, depression, diabetes, hip fracture or replacement and knee replacement, hypertension, multiple sclerosis, osteoporosis, Parkinson's disease, sensory losses, and traumatic head injury. The primary focus is to work safely and effectively with both frail elders and adults who have special needs.

To meet this challenge, you need to understand common medical disorders and their implications. This chapter covers specific diagnostic areas that are relevant to your work with frail elders and adults with special needs. With an understanding of these medical issues, you will be prepared to teach exercise to participants with diverse medical needs. In addition, you will be able to recommend safe exercise techniques for individual participants according to their medical conditions and needs.

Gerokinesiology is a term that was coined in 2004 by Ecclestone and Jones in the *Journal of Aging and Physical Activity*. This definition was part of the move to identify specific content areas thought significant to include in standardizing entry-level training for the specialty of fitness programs for older adults:

> Gerokinesiology is a specialized area of study within the larger discipline of kinesiology that focuses on understanding how physical activity influences all aspects of health and well-being in the older adult population and the aging process in general.

The International Curriculum Guidelines for Preparing Physical Activity Instructors of Older Adults comprises nine recommended training modules:

1. Overview of aging and physical activity
2. Psychological, sociocultural, and physiological aspects of physical activity and older adults
3. Screening, assessment, and goal setting
4. Program design and management
5. Program design for older adults with stable medical conditions
6. Teaching skills
7. Leadership, communication, and marketing skills
8. Client safety and first aid
9. Ethics and professional conduct

The complete guidelines can be found at www.tinyurl.com/HKolderadultsguidelines or www.tinyurl.com/ASFAcurriculumguidelines.

Exercise for Frail Elders meets all recommended areas.

Before we identify the specific special needs areas and their implications for exercise, let's start with an examination of the terms *frail* and *special needs*.

FRAILTY AND SPECIAL NEEDS IN OLDER ADULTS

What age is "old" to you? We each answer this question according to our own experience with family members and with older people and the way in which we see ourselves physically. In past years, "old" was defined by chronological age. Chronological age used to be more relevant because life expectancies were far shorter than they are today. A man of 40 in the 1800s may have been considered old. Today, an 80-year-old man may water-ski and be physically active.

Many of us will probably live into our 70s, 80s, 90s, or 100s. In 2008, an estimated 39 million people—13 percent of the population—were age 65 or older. By 2030, 20 percent of Americans—about 72 million people—will have passed their 65th birthday. The fastest growing segment of the older population is people aged 85 and older (Ecclestone and Jones 2004).

Have you ever heard the term *old-old* or *older-old*? These terms were created to differentiate between younger and older old people. We need this distinction because people are living much longer. If a 65-year-old is old, then what should we call an 80-year-old? Old-old refers to the older segment of the older generation, but it really comes down to the individual. Many 80-year-olds today bicycle, play tennis, or engage in other demanding activities. Many of them are still quite active.

Thus, what is important is how we *feel* at an older chronological age and how well we can function physically, mentally, and emotionally (referred to as functional status). A direct relationship is usually found between an individual's functional status, health and wellness, and quality of life. However, the World Health Organization (WHO 2013) defines health as "the state of complete mental, physical and social well-being, and not merely the absence of disease or infirmity." This definition is important because it addresses the fact that health and well-being can be experienced even while living with chronic disorders and other health issues.

An individual's functional status is a major determinant of successful aging. As physical function declines, a person can begin to become frail. Let's look more closely at the term *frail*.

What Is Frailty?

Frail is a term that can describe anyone, young or old. Refer to table 1.1 for common medical disorders and special needs that contribute to frailty. Frailty is not as much a definition as it is a syndrome of signs and symptoms. Some of the factors creating and affecting this frailty syndrome can include physical inactivity, nutritional status, cognitive and psychological conditions, preexisting chronic disorders, and aging (Signorile 2011).

The causes of frailty vary among people. Commonly identified causes of frailty include the following:

- A medical condition
- A loss of one or more senses
- A chronic disorder
- A chronic disorder along with a new medical diagnosis
- Adverse changes in the musculoskeletal system
- Psychological issues
- Sarcopenia (loss of muscle mass)
- Very old age
- Nutritional imbalances
- Intellectual disabilities
- Physical inactivity

Frailty is normally related to a combination of circumstances that leaves a person unable to accomplish normal activities of independent daily living. Some people in your exercise group who are quite elderly may appear physically frail but are not. Looks can be deceiving. Function is what determines level of frailty. The possibility that you may misidentify an elderly person who is not frail as frail is one of the many challenges in leading exercise programs for older adults.

The term *frail elders* combines the ideas of advanced age and frailty. Normally, the term refers to very old people who have difficulties performing activities of daily living without assistance from others. This term includes added complexities. A person with a chronic disorder such as arthritis might be considered frail because of another complicating factor, such as emphysema. The combined limitations from the two disorders may contribute to the frail condition.

You should know that not all frailty is chronic or long term. Some people find themselves in a frail state because of surgery or illness. When they recover, the frailty may decrease or disappear.

People may also decrease frailty by increasing their physical activity. Research has verified that exercise improves muscle strength, balance, coordination, and cardiovascular fitness in even the most frail and elderly participants (Fiatarone et al. 1994). Resistance training in particular has proven to be especially beneficial with deconditioned (not in strong or good physical condition caused by a sedentary lifestyle) elderly people (American College of Sports Medicine 2009b). Skeletal muscle weakness places a person at higher risk of falls. These falls can lead to fractured bones and hospitalization. Strengthening and stretching exercises (particularly specific balance exercises) help maintain balance and range of motion and are recommended in many fall-prevention studies.

Fatigue is another area that may contribute to the perception of a person as frail. Older adults tell us often that they are fatigued and do not have the energy to exercise or complete specific activities of daily living. In assessing an individual, you should consider all these factors and then go through a process of elimination (all the things that are not affecting function and energy level). Many of the common disorders reviewed in this chapter can affect energy and create a sense of fatigue.

The 2010 *Surgeon General's Vision for a Healthy and Fit Nation* encourages even moderate exercise to help frail people recapture lost function, functional independence, health, and well-being (USDHHS 2010b). Your exercise class is profoundly important to this group.

What Are Special Needs?

A participant may have one or more special needs that, when combined, create a frail state. For example, a participant in your group may be frail because of her age of 98 years and her poor overall physical condition. Seated next to her may be a man in his 60s with special needs related to a diagnosis of Parkinson's disease. He is an older adult with special needs, but he is 30 years younger than the frail 98-year-old is. You could not call this man frail, even though he has some special needs. Seated next to these two people may be a younger woman who is frail and has special needs, both related to a diagnosis of multiple sclerosis. Figure 1.1 helps visually distinguish these conditions and individual needs.

Anyone, young or old, can have special needs. A special need can be temporary or permanent. The term *special* indicates that the fitness leader needs to know what an individual's disorder or limitation is before initiating an exercise program for that person. This large category of special needs includes a vast array of individual needs from a variety of causes.

Some special needs are related to

- a medical disorder,
- sensory losses (vision loss, loss of hearing, loss of touch),
- communication difficulties (including aphasia [the loss of or decline in the ability to speak, understand, read, or write] and language barriers [not speaking the language of the predominant culture]),
- cognitive losses,
- a sedentary lifestyle, or
- sarcopenia.

A special need may be for

- specific medical equipment (e.g., oxygen, IV),

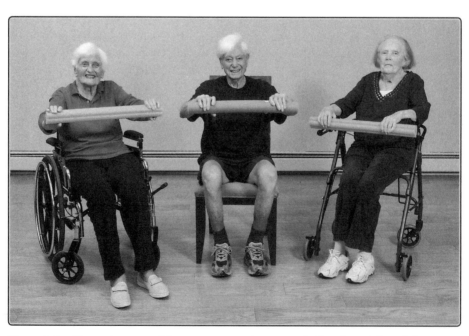

Figure 1.1 These three participants capture the terms *frail* and *special needs* because of advanced age, mobility issues, declining physical function, Parkinson's disease, diabetes, hypertension, cancer, and cardiac issues.

- emotional support caused by mental health issues (e.g., depression),
- specific medications,
- adaptive equipment, or
- physical assistance with movement.

As you lead a class, be sure to keep these needs and their combinations in mind. For example, a client who has COPD may need to have space near the door for an easy exit if he or she begins to feel claustrophobic and may need space for oxygen equipment. Or, a client who has had a stroke and is aphasic should be placed close to you so that you can communicate easily with visual and verbal cues.

Effects of Medications

All medications have side effects that could affect a participant's ability to participate fully or safely in exercise. Here are some things to know about medications, frail elders, and adults with special needs:

Older adults and frail elders take more medications than those in any other age group. Many take 6 to 8 medications. Although vitamins are not medications, they are counted as medications in skilled nursing settings, so the number of medications could reach 10 to 12 daily.

- Some medications are taken short term, such as antibiotics. But other medications may be taken long term for chronic disorders such as diabetes, arthritis, and cardiac issues.
- All medications have the potential for side effects, and taking daily multiple medications together can place a participant at higher risk for adverse reactions.
- Older adults and frail elders have slower metabolisms, so medications stay in their systems for a longer time. In addition, a large percentage of medications have side effects of dizziness, light-headedness, and confusion (Best-Martini et al. 2011). These medications and side effects affect their ability to exercise, balance, walk

safely, and at times, understand the directions.

The fitness leader needs to know what medications or what type of medications a participant may be taking. For example, the category of psychotropic medications (mind-, mood-, and behavior-altering medications) has significant side effects that need to be closely monitored. There are four types of psychotropic medications:

1. Antidepressants
2. Antipsychotics
3. Antianxiety
4. Sedatives

The risk of falling increases when a person is taking more than one of these psychotropic medications (Rose 2010). A good source and reference for psychotropic medications can be found at www.psyd-fx.com. This chart was created by John Preston, PsyD, and is updated frequently. Refer to appendix A4, "Medical History and Risk Factor Questionnaire," for obtaining a list of medications for each participant.

COMMON MEDICAL DISORDERS AND SPECIAL NEEDS

Some of the common medical disorders or special needs that can contribute to frailty are listed in table 1.1. This section describes the disorders that are most important for leading exercises classes for adults with special needs. In addition, a table for each disorder gives characteristics related to the disorder and identifies relevant safety and exercise tips (see tables 1.2 through 1.15). The tables and descriptions are grouped together at the end of the chapter and are intended to be a brief review and a hands-on resource for the fitness instructor.

In addition, refer to "Specific Safety Precautions for Those With Special Needs" for warm-up (chapter 4), resistance training (chapter 5), aerobics (chapter 6), and cool-down (chapter 7). *ACSM's Exercise Management for Persons With*

Table 1.1 Common Medical Disorders That Contribute to Frailty in Elderly Individuals

System	Medical disorders
Cardiovascular	Hypertension, hypotension, coronary artery disease, valvular heart disease, heart failure, dysrhythmias, peripheral arterial disease
Pulmonary	Asthma, chronic obstructive pulmonary disease, pneumonia
Musculoskeletal	Arthritis, degenerative disc disease, polymyalgia rheumatica, osteoporosis
Metabolic and endocrine	Diabetes, hypercholesterolemia
Gastrointestinal	Dental disorder, malnutrition, incontinence, diarrhea
Genitourinary	Urinary tract infection, cancer
Hematologic and immunologic	Anemia, leukemia, cancer
Neurologic	Dementia, Alzheimer's disease, cerebrovascular disease, Parkinson's disease
Eye and ear	Cataracts, glaucoma, hearing disorders
Psychiatric	Anxiety disorders, hypochondria, depression, alcoholism

Adapted, by permission, from American College of Sport Medicine, 1997, *ACSM's exercise management for persons with chronic diseases and disabilities* (Champaign, IL: Human Kinetics), 114.

From E. Best-Martini and K.A. Jones-DiGenova, 2014, *Exercise for frail elders*, 2nd ed. (Champaign, IL: Human Kinetics).

Chronic Diseases and Disabilities, Third Edition (2009a) is highly recommended as a comprehensive resource. That book takes the reader through the medical disorder; effects on the exercise response; training, management, and medications; testing and programming; and evidence-based guideline recommendations.

According to the American College of Sports Medicine (2009b, p. 1515) position stand "Exercise and Physical Activity for Older Adults," "There is growing evidence that regular physical activity reduces risk of developing numerous chronic conditions and diseases including cardiovascular disease, stroke, hypertension, type 2 diabetes mellitus, osteoporosis, obesity, colon cancer, breast cancer, cognitive impairment, anxiety, and depression."

You now have a clearer concept of frailty and special needs. Some of the causes of frailty and special needs may be related to one or a few chronic disorders in addition to sensory deficits. Before we begin to look more closely at the 14 common special need areas, remember that the participants in your group may not appear to have multiple medical disorders and special needs. Many of these are what we call invisible or silent disorders such as osteoporosis,

cardiac issues, diabetes, depression, previous hip or knee replacement, hypertension, and so on. Because we do not know the complexity of issues for each participant when we are starting a class, the recommended approach is always to follow the safety precautions for special needs just to be on the safe side.

Alzheimer's Disease and Related Dementias

Dementia is a neurologic disorder that is progressive and degenerative. The common definition of dementia is the progressive loss of intellectual functioning. Dementia is not a disease itself but a cluster of symptoms. Alzheimer's disease is one of the largest classifications of dementia. The disease begins with signs and symptoms of memory loss that begin to increase and worsen. Besides having memory loss, a person with Alzheimer's disease can experience anxiety, because he or she loses the ability to function independently in day-to-day life. Depression is prevalent as the losses become more profound. The combination of these psychological difficulties, compounded by the inability to express oneself or understand others, is often the reason for problematic behaviors associated with dementia.

Some common behaviors that you may see in adults with Alzheimer's disease are restlessness, wandering, crying, aggression, withdrawal, and apathy. These behaviors are all a form of communication for the person lacking the verbal language to share his or her feelings and concerns. Do your best to communicate clearly, patiently, and compassionately with people who have Alzheimer's disease and related dementias. Try to look beyond the behaviors and limitations and more at the person.

Other dementias are related to traumatic brain damage, cerebrovascular accidents (strokes), AIDS, Parkinson's disease, and substance abuse. The most important fact to remember about dementia is that certain parts of the brain are injured from either trauma or lack of blood flow to the brain, not because of normal aging patterns as previously believed. The symptoms and behaviors are all related to the part of the brain that has lost normal function. The person remains. Even people with advanced dementia retain strengths and ability. Regardless of the level of dementia, these people feel the respect and care that they receive from others emotionally if not intellectually.

Although people with dementia struggle with intellectual functions, they usually are ambulatory (in the early and middle stages of the disease) and can be interested in physical activity. They retain this strength. Physical exercise is vitally important to their well-being because it helps maintain their physical functioning as long as possible and enhances their self-esteem. Functional fitness can make the difference in maintaining these skills as the disease progresses and affects fine and gross motor skills, strength, power, and balance.

Music and dance or movement is successful with this group of participants. The focus of the physical activity program is in the moment. Plan to have fun with movements and exercises that promote success. If the movements portray life skills such as sweeping, reaching up, looking at the toes, breathing into a pinwheel that each person is holding, and singing older familiar songs, the level of participation will increase. In an exercise class, participants with dementia may have difficulty staying focused and following directions. By adding colorful props to hold and move with, the participant who lacks self-initiation skills is able to participate actively at a higher level. Some ideas can be found in appendix B4, "Exercise Equipment." Other ideas include using gymnastic ribbons on a stick, large and small balls with color and sound inside, handheld plastic tubes to stretch in and out for range of motion, and colorful discs or plates on the floor to place feet on during seated exercise routines. The leadership skills for working with participants with cognitive losses are discussed in chapter 3. Refer to table 1.2, Alzheimer's Disease and Related Dementia Disorders: Teaching Tips, at the end of the chapter.

Arthritis

Arthritis is a general term under the broader category of rheumatic diseases that cause pain, stiffness, and swelling in joints and connective tissues. More than 46 million people in the United States have some type of rheumatic disease. Twenty-seven million of these people have osteoarthritis (National Institutes of Health, Arthritis and Musculoskeletal and Skin Diseases 2011). The most common types of arthritis are osteoarthritis and rheumatoid arthritis. Many of the symptoms of these two types of arthritis are similar. A less common type of arthritis is fibromyalgia.

Osteoarthritis, also known as DJD, or degenerative joint disease, is characterized by joint pain. The pain is caused by the breakdown of the articular cartilage (tissue that covers and protects the end of the bones). Without this cartilage, the bone edges become rough and do not move smoothly on one another. In addition, bone spurs (osteophytes) may develop. Osteoarthritis does not always cause the symptom of inflammation, but it usually causes pain.

Rheumatoid arthritis is an inflammatory, multijoint, multisystem disease. It is defined as an autoimmune disorder (an immune or allergic reaction of the body against itself) because it affects not only the lining of the joint but also other organs and systems (the cardiac and pulmonary systems). Swelling, along with pain and stiffness, occurs with rheumatoid arthritis. Rheumatoid arthritis causes acute episodes of joint pain and inflammation. The duration of these flare-ups varies. People may experience periods of few or no flare-ups, referred to as remissions. Participants with rheumatoid arthritis have a greater tendency toward fatigue. Because of this, remind them to pace themselves and go slowly.

Fibromyalgia is a chronic pain in the soft tissue (ligaments and tendons) and muscles surrounding the joints. The pain is often experienced in the shoulder and hip regions. Treatment for this disorder is multidisciplinary and uses physical therapy, relaxation techniques, and lifestyle changes to eliminate the triggers (such as stress, inactivity, and lack of sleep). One of the most important components of treatment for fibromyalgia is a safe exercise program. Refer to table 1.3, Arthritis: Teaching Tips, at the end of the chapter.

Cerebrovascular Accident (Stroke)

A cerebrovascular accident (CVA), or stroke, is a circulatory accident that results in neurologic impairment. A stroke occurs when blood flow to the brain is interrupted. This can occur in two ways.

1. Ischemic stroke occurs when an artery is blocked and no blood can get through to a portion of the brain. This is the most prevalent type of stroke. Ischemic strokes are of two types. One is caused by a fixed blood clot, or thrombosis. The other is caused by a wandering blood clot, or embolism. Both of these strokes occur because of a buildup of fatty deposits, referred to as atherosclerotic plaques, in the blood vessels of the neck and head. A stroke is sometimes referred to as a brain attack because of its similarity to a heart attack, which is caused by the buildup of atherosclerotic plaque in the coronary arteries of the heart (Levine 2009).

2. Hemorrhagic stroke occurs when an artery leading to the brain ruptures. This rupture, known as a cerebral hemorrhage, spills blood into the brain or a surrounding area between the outer surface of the brain and the skull. In some instances, a congenital weak spot called an aneurysm may cause this type of stroke.

A stroke affects the area of the brain where the blood flow ceased (ischemic) or from the intracranial pressure created from the ruptured blood vessel. In addition, it may cause pressure to the brain that may result in swelling. Stroke victims' symptoms and limitations vary depending on the location of the stroke and the extent of the damage to brain tissue. If the right side of the brain is affected, the left side of the body exhibits weakness or paralysis and vice versa.

Here are some problems specific to the location of a CVA:

Right-side CVA	*Left-side CVA*
Spatial or perceptual deficits	Speech and language problems
Memory deficits	Memory deficits
Impulsive behavior and overestimated abilities	Difficulty with new tasks
Left field of vision restricted	Slow and cautious behavior
Unawareness (neglect) of left side of body	Right field of vision restricted
Weakness or paralysis on left side	Problems knowing left from right
	Weakness or paralysis on right side

Commonly, the most significant benefits of rehabilitation and exercise can be achieved in the first 2 years from the time of the initial stroke. People differ in their injuries and rehabilitation, and many individuals will experience some level of functional improvement with continued exercises after this initial 2-year period. Frontera, Slovik, and Dawson (2006) state, "The therapeutic program typically incorporates instruction in compensatory techniques to improve functional abilities. . . . Performance is improved when the training occurs with actual rather than simulated functional tasks" (pp. 211–212). This recommendation is a reminder to the fitness leader that the program should promote daily functional tasks. This approach assists the participant in learning new ways and strategies to compensate for losses associated with the stroke. We do know that exercise enhances circulation, builds endurance, and strengthens the body, all of which contribute to better quality of life and support recovery to the greatest extent. The American Heart Association (AHA) recommends stretching, flexibility, balance, and coordination exercises two or three times per week for people who have had a stroke. In addition, resistance training and aerobics may become part of their prescribed program.

The first week after a stroke is the most crucial in determining its extent, severity, and potential recovery. During this time, the medical team analyzes and assesses what damage has occurred. The rehabilitation and exercise aspects of stroke recovery begin immediately after this assessment has been made. Recovery is slow for many stroke victims, and their prognoses for complete recovery are guarded. Regardless of the prognosis for a full recovery, range-of-motion movements (see chapter 4) and basic fine and gross motor skill progressions are extremely important.

Fine motor skills are small, precise, coordinated movements that require integrating muscular skeletal and neurological functions in perfect timing. These exercises and movements could be anything from shooting marbles, stretching the hands and fingers, moving individual fingers, and moving the affected hand with the other hand. All these movements can be incorporated into the exercise program.

As we can see, all components of the exercise program have benefits for the participant who has had a stroke. For example, aerobic exercise is important as prevention in keeping the fatty deposits from building up again in the blood. Sitting balance helps strengthen core stability. In addition, exercises that focus on seated reaching tasks appear to help improve sitting balance because these movements require activating the core muscles to reach forward. Most stroke patients will move into a cardiac rehabilitation program before they join your exercise program. Be sure to ask for their prescribed exercises so that you can reinforce individualized therapy goals. Participants in an exercise class who have had a CVA (as well as all participants) should be discouraged from any fast movements of the head and neck. Remind them to move slowly through the head and neck ROM and flexibility exercises.

As a fitness leader, you need to become familiar with the signs and symptoms of a stroke so that you can act quickly. A recent 5-year study conducted by the National Institute of Neurological Disorders and Stroke (NINDS 2011) found that patients who got to the hospital within 60 minutes and started receiving medication to dissolve blood clots because of an ischemic stroke had a 30 percent better chance of recovery with little or no disability after 3 months.

If a participant has any of the following signs and symptoms of a stroke, follow the emergency protocol for the setting in which you are teaching (refer to the section "Emergencies" in chapter 2). The Stroke Association identified these signs and symptoms in 2011:

- Any sudden numbness or weakness of the face, arm or leg (especially all on one side of the body)
- Problems speaking or understanding, or experiencing sudden confusion
- Problems not being able to see out of one or both eyes

- Sudden severe headache with no known cause
- Sudden loss of balance, dizziness, lack of coordination or trouble walking

Refer to table 1.4, Cerebrovascular Accident (CVA, Stroke): Teaching Tips, at the end of this chapter.

Chronic Obstructive Pulmonary Disease

Chronic obstructive pulmonary disease (COPD) is a category of pulmonary disorders that includes emphysema, chronic bronchitis, and asthma. In each of these disorders, the lungs are inefficient and ventilation (the passage of air into and out of the respiratory tract) is compromised. Many people have only one type of COPD, but others may have more than one if the initial disorder was not diagnosed for a long time and progressed to further lung damage.

COPD, the fourth-leading cause of death in the United States, affects the lives of 30 million Americans. Smokers are at higher risk of developing COPD. The primary cause of COPD is cigarette smoking; an estimated 80 percent of people with COPD are current or former smokers (ACSM 2009a). COPD can also be caused by working or living in an environment that has toxins that damage the lungs. Asthma can sometimes be reversed if it originated from environmental triggers. If reversal is not possible, avoiding the environmental triggers may lessen asthmatic symptoms.

COPD does not occur overnight. It is gradual and progressive. Because ventilation is compromised, a person with COPD finds himself or herself breathing ineffectively, wheezing, coughing, and gasping for air. This difficulty in breathing is called dyspnea.

Breaths may be short, shallow, and too rapid to provide the needed level of oxygen. This lack of oxygen seriously compromises physical endurance and stamina. Dyspnea worsens if a person becomes fearful of physical activity.

Besides having difficulty breathing, many people with COPD experience frequent peri-ods of anxiety. Not being able to breathe can be extremely stressful. A person with COPD may avoid situations that cause an emotional response such as laughing or crying. Laughing and crying both place additional demands on the already compromised breathing function. People with COPD do not normally feel comfortable in small spaces or large groups. They need to pay attention to any toxins that might exacerbate their condition. Lifestyle changes associated with COPD may also cause depression. Individuals with COPD commonly experience some level of depression (AACVPR 2011, 53).

With all these issues to consider, you may wonder whether exercise is a good prescription for people with COPD. In fact, exercise can improve efficiency in ventilation, increase cardiovascular function, and increase muscle strength. All these benefits enhance breathing function and help to decrease the anxiety related to dyspnea. Exercise is a required component in almost all pulmonary rehabilitation programs. Exercises that strengthen the arm and shoulder muscles not only make breathing easier but also promote functional independence. Exercise needs to be safe and customized to the individual's current level of COPD. See *Guidelines for Pulmonary Rehabilitation Programs, Fourth Edition* (AACVPR 2011) in "Suggested Resources" to further your understanding of and effectiveness for participants with this disease. Refer to table 1.5, Chronic Obstructive Pulmonary Disease (COPD): Teaching Tips, at the end of this chapter.

Coronary Artery Disease

Coronary artery disease (CAD) occurs when the coronary arteries that supply blood to the heart muscle (myocardium) become progressively narrower. This narrowing of arteries is referred to as atherosclerosis. The narrowing is caused by atherosclerotic plaques (made up of fat, cholesterol, calcium, and other substances found in the blood) that form on the sides of the coronary artery wall, similar to those that cause ischemic stroke, and eventually cut off blood flow to the heart muscle.

The portion of the heart that is deprived of blood, and therefore oxygen, is said to be ischemic (deficient of blood). Myocardial ischemia accompanied by effort or excitement can cause chest pain (often radiating to the arms, particularly the left), known as angina pectoris. Myocardial ischemia can progress and eventually cut off all blood flow to the heart muscle, causing a myocardial infarction, or heart attack. The damage can be mild, moderate, or severe, depending on the location and severity of the infarct (tissue death).

Coronary artery disease is greatly influenced by both genetics and lifestyle factors, such as diet, level of physical activity, stress, and smoking history. Atherosclerosis is a preventable and treatable condition. Anything that decreases atherosclerotic buildup decreases the risk of CAD. Among other risk factors, high blood pressure, high cholesterol, and diabetes can increase the risk of CAD.

Cardiac rehabilitation is offered after a myocardial infarction. Typically, cardiac rehabilitation takes place in three stages. Stage 1 begins in the hospital. The rehabilitation team works on basic skills of daily living. Stage 2 is done on an outpatient basis; the patient has returned home but goes to the hospital to participate in the rehabilitation program. Stage 3 is an individual program that the patient follows independently at home. In this important stage the client learns how to create a lifestyle that improves cardiovascular health and learns how all the dimensions of the wellness model significantly enhance quality of life and reduce the risk of subsequent heart attacks.

As a fitness leader you need to be familiar with the first signs or symptoms of overexertion or cardiac complications, particularly dizziness, abnormal heart rhythm, unusual shortness of breath, or chest discomfort.

A mnemonic to remember this vital information is ABCD:

Abnormal heart rate

Breath—unusual shortness

Chest discomfort

Dizziness

Teach participants to recognize the ABCD symptoms of overexertion or cardiac complications and to stop exercise and let you know if they experience any of them. Refer to the section "Emergencies" in chapter 2 for guidelines about when to seek immediate medical attention. Also, *AACVPR Cardiac Rehabilitation Resource Manual* (AACVPR 2006) and *Guidelines for Cardiac Rehabilitation and Secondary Prevention Programs* (AACVPR 2004) are good resources (see "Suggested Resources"). Refer to table 1.6, Coronary Artery Disease (CAD): Teaching Tips, at the end of this chapter.

Depression

Depression is not a normal part of the aging process. It is classified as a mood disorder in the *Diagnostic and Statistical Manual of Mental Disorders* (*DSM-5*) (APA 2013). This manual defines all currently recognized categories of mental disorders.

Mood is best described as emotional content, or how someone feels, and it is influenced by various situations that a person encounters in everyday life. A mood disorder occurs when the cause of the mood is no longer as relevant as the effect of the mood on one's work, relationships, coping skills, and potential for happiness.

Depression falls into four diagnostic categories: major depression (the most severe type), dysthymic disorder (milder depression with symptoms lasting over 2 years), adjustment disorder with depressed mood (a depressed mood resulting from a stressful event that exceeds the normal reaction to such an event), and bipolar disorder (also known as manic–depressive illness, which is characterized by extreme mood swings). Healthy and noninstitutionalized older adults in the United States account for 1 percent of elderly with depression. Although this number appears low, many other elderly people in the community, about 15 percent of older adults, are living with depression that exhibits symptoms that are under the threshold of the current *DSM-5*. In the United States, one-third of nursing home residents suffer from depression at some point during their stay in a nursing home. Newly admitted nursing home residents have greater functional impairment and are 1.5 times more likely to die within 12 months of admission than long-term residents (Wagenaar, Colenda, Kreft et al. 2003).

Depression is the second most common mental disorder in long-term care settings, after dementia. For many older people, the losses associated with age, illness, and change can bring about one of these types of depression. In general, depression has clearly defined symptoms, but these vary among individuals. Depression must be diagnosed by a physician who has tested the individual. Many people experience the blues from a specific sad or traumatic event or even as a side effect from some medications. Others may not recognize that they are in a depression because they do not associate memory loss, lack of appetite, and especially sleep disturbances as symptoms. Depression is a complex illness.

Most depressions are treatable. The good news is that exercise is an excellent intervention for all types of depression. Exercise is beneficial for those living with depression because it helps reduce the symptoms of depression, which then enhances quality of life on a daily basis. Depression is often masked behind anger and other behaviors. Because physical activity can reduce some of the symptoms of depression, it opens up the possibility for more social interaction for the affected person. Refer to table 1.7, Depression: Teaching Tips, at the end of this chapter.

Diabetes

Diabetes is a chronic metabolic disease in which an absolute or relative deficiency of insulin results in hyperglycemia (an increase in blood sugar). Hyperglycemia can cause undue stress and damage to the kidneys, heart, nerves, eyes, and blood vessels. In addition, circulation is affected, which places a person at risk of infection, especially in the legs and feet. In the United States 25.8 million children and adults, or 8.3 percent of the population, have diabetes. Among those over age 65, 10.9

million, or 26.9 percent of all people in that age group, have diabetes (American Diabetes Association 2011).

There are two categories of diabetes. Type 1 diabetes mellitus, or insulin-dependent diabetes mellitus, is identified as an absolute deficiency of insulin and can be diagnosed at any age. This type is thought to be an autoimmune disorder.

Type 2 diabetes mellitus, or non-insulin-dependent diabetes mellitus (NIDDM), is the most prevalent and affects mostly older people, especially those who are obese. People with type 2 diabetes have a cellular resistance to insulin and may have reduced, normal, or elevated insulin levels. Of interest to the fitness leader is the fact that exercise and weight reduction, along with diet and medication if recommended, can improve blood glucose control in type 2 diabetes. Exercise has an insulin-like effect on the system in addition to reducing body fat. Most people with diabetes are at higher risk of heart disease and stroke than those without diabetes. Exercise can combat the buildup of LDL cholesterol (the artery-clogging agent), which increases with insulin resistance in the blood lipids.

The fitness leader should minimize the potential for hypoglycemic events among diabetic participants. Hypoglycemia (low blood sugar) occurs when too little glucose is in the blood. The participant may have taken too much insulin, not eaten enough, or exercised too strenuously. The participant may feel hungry, weak, and dizzy and may tremble and perspire. This situation can become a serious medical event if not addressed immediately. A hypoglycemic person needs simple carbohydrates, such as orange juice or any sugary substance. Your observation makes all the difference in keeping people with diabetes exercising safely. See the section "Emergencies" in chapter 2 for a review of procedures if a medical emergency occurs during your exercise class.

Refer to "Physical Activity and Type 2 Diabetes" (Hawley and Zierath 2008) in "Suggested Resources" to further your understanding of and effectiveness for participants with this disease. Also, see table 1.8, Diabetes: Teaching Tips, at the end of this chapter.

Hip Fracture or Replacement and Knee Replacement

Some participants in your exercise program may be receiving physical therapy for a hip fracture, a total or partial hip replacement, or a knee replacement. The most important things to find out about a participant with hip and knee problems is how long it has been since the surgery, the precautions recommended by the physician, and how you can assist the person in achieving therapy goals. The physician and therapist will be specific with guidelines for exercise postsurgery.

A participant who has dementia may not remember the surgery or therapy, so be sure to check with staff or family to be current with any fractures or replacements.

As with all orthopedic issues and injuries, the fitness leader needs to identify who will assist with participant transfers from a wheelchair to a chair, bed, or toilet. The new fitness leader should ask for specific protocols according to the site where she or he is teaching. Transfers should only be done by qualified therapists or aides and caregivers with appropriate training. Fitness instructors should not attempt to transfer participants unless specifically trained and approved by the staff on site. Refer to table 1.9, Hip Fracture or Replacement or Knee Replacement: Teaching Tips, at the end of this chapter.

Hypertension

Hypertension (high blood pressure) is considered a silent killer because no symptoms occur in its early stages, although routine blood pressure readings offer early detection. Any adult blood pressure above 140 over 90 is considered high. The 140 represents the systolic blood pressure (highest pressure in the arteries at any time), and the 90 is the diastolic blood pressure (lowest pressure in the arteries at any time). An estimated 37 percent of U.S. adults have prehypertension of 120 to 139 over 80 to 89,

and nearly one in three adults has hypertension according to ACSM (2009a).

When blood pressure is higher than average, the heart needs to work harder, stressing it and putting greater demand on the arteries. Possible consequences include enlargement of the heart and arteriosclerosis (hardening of the arteries). Hypertension also increases the risk of stroke.

Some of the causes of hypertension are related to lifestyle and diet. In addition, some medications, such as birth control pills, steroids, decongestants, and anti-inflammatories, increase the risk of high blood pressure (Kaiser Permanente 2010).

The origin of some cases of hypertension is unknown. In such cases, physicians often advise that patients cut back on sodium and fat in their diets and add moderate exercise to their weekly schedules. These lifestyle modifications help physicians evaluate the origin of the hypertension and decide on the necessary treatment.

One known risk factor for hypertension is inactivity. Exercise is a positive intervention for hypertension. A moderate-intensity aerobic exercise program supplemented by resistance training (also of moderate intensity) is recommended to decrease both systolic and diastolic blood pressure (ACSM 2010, 249). "Exercise remains a cornerstone therapy for the primary prevention, treatment, and control of HTN" (ACSM 2004a, 546). Refer to table 1.10, Hypertension: Teaching Tips, at the end of this chapter.

Multiple Sclerosis

Multiple sclerosis (MS) is a progressive and degenerative neurologic disorder that affects the central nervous system. An insulating fatty sheath, called myelin, protects the nerve fibers in a healthy person. With MS, this protecting layer is damaged, which consequently impairs the function of the affected nerves in the brain and spinal cord.

Like most diseases, MS differs in different people. Symptoms can range from mild to severe; there can be remissions for years or no remissions. This disease afflicts young to middle-aged adults. More women than men are affected. The origin of the disorder is unknown.

A person with MS may need a wheelchair for mobility. As the disease progresses, people with MS may need assistance with all activities of daily living. A young person with MS may live in a long-term care facility because of the complexity of his or her needs. Along with physical limitations, emotional difficulties related to the loss of independence and function affect many people with MS, especially because the loss occurs at a much younger age than in people without MS. The joints need to move through their range of motion to keep the person as functional as possible. Range-of-motion exercises are always recommended. Stretching is also important to add to an exercise program. A common symptom of MS is weakness. Sometimes the weakness is exacerbated by lack of movement and exercise. This can be a teachable moment to help clients become more aware of when they begin to feel fatigued. At this point, they should stop all activity and rest so that they can conserve the energy that they have. Exercise programs are good for those living with MS because of the social connectedness in addition to any of the movements they are able to perform. The MS Society (www.nationalmssociety.org) has many excellent resources for clients at all levels of this disease. Refer to table 1.11, Multiple Sclerosis (MS): Teaching Tips, at the end of this chapter.

Osteoporosis

Osteoporosis is a disease characterized by low bone density. This density loss leads to brittle and porous bones. Osteoporosis is a major health threat to an estimated 10 million Americans, 80 percent of whom are women (Williamson 2011, 265). Osteoporosis is considered a silent epidemic because the disease is often not detected in the early stages (although a bone-density test can offer early detection) until there are visible signs, such as loss of height; a forward-curved upper back; or broken bones in the hip, wrist, or spine. In gen-

eral, the more visible the signs are, the more advanced the disease is. An estimated 34 million Americans have lower-than-normal bone mass (osteopenia) (Williamson 2011), which is considered the precursor to osteoporosis. As the body ages, some natural declines occur in bone mass. In addition, loss of bone mass can result from use of steroid medications, vitamin and mineral deficiencies (particularly D and calcium), heavy drinking, smoking, a thin and small-framed body, insufficient weight-bearing exercise, and low estrogen levels in women (ACSM 2009a).

Osteoporosis primarily affects postmenopausal women. Osteoporosis among menopausal women results from a decrease in estrogen levels. As estrogen levels decrease, bone thinning and bone loss occur. Most of the bone loss occurs in the early stages of menopause. Postmenopausal women have less bone loss, but they may still be losing more bone than their systems replace.

Regardless of the cause of bone loss, as osteoporosis advances, the risk of bone fractures increases. When the bones are weakened, the potential for bone fracture during exercise increases. Most fractures take place in the vertebrae, hips, and wrists. In part II, we provide specific safety precautions for those with osteoporosis for helping prevent bone fractures during exercise.

A participant may have severe spinal deformity that impedes his or her ability to stand up straight (kyphosis). This condition can be the result of osteoporosis. Because kyphosis alters a person's center of gravity and impairs balance, the risk of falling increases. In addition, the forward movement of the shoulders and head can confine the chest enough to impair breathing

The statistics for falls and hip fractures related to osteoporosis are staggering. Twenty-four percent of people with hip fractures over the age of 50 will die within the first year after the fracture, and others may lose functional ambulatory ability and require nursing home care. Knowing whether a fall occurred because of an osteoporotic fracture (organic fracture) or whether a fracture was a result of the fall is important. The need for safe and effective exercise programs to improve balance and strength along with flexibility are a primary intervention for this condition.

Many older adult participants in your class will have some level of osteoporosis or osteopenia. An estimated 90 percent of residents of long-term care facilities have osteoporosis. The California Department of Health Services, Institute for Health and Aging states that this high percentage causes 1.5 million fractures yearly. Exercise is an important intervention in this disorder. Although osteoporosis is not reversible, exercise can at least slow down the age- and inactivity-related decline in bone mass (ACSM 2009a). Bone mass can be increased with consistent relatively high-intensity resistance training and weight-bearing endurance exercise (ACSM 2004b, p. 1985), but such exercise is contraindicated for those with advanced osteoporosis. Refer to table 1.12, Osteoporosis: Teaching Tips, at the end of this chapter.

Parkinson's Disease

Parkinson's disease is a degenerative and progressive neurologic disorder that affects both movement and posture. Neurotransmitters within the brain help relay signals from the peripheral nervous system to the brain. The neurotransmitter dopamine is significantly reduced or destroyed in this disease process. The symptoms related to this reduction are resting tremors, slow movements (bradykinesia), postural instability, uncontrolled movements (dyskinesia), involuntary cessation of a movement (freezing), gait disorders, and shuffling. Changes also occur in the volume of the voice. In some cases dementia is related to this disorder.

Exercise can help participants with Parkinson's improve motor performance, trunk rotation, eye–hand coordination, and stability and balance during walking. Exercise can improve muscle volume and strength (ACSM 2009a). In addition, exercise can help with some of the nonmotor symptoms such as depression,

constipation, pain, genitourinary problems, and sleep disorders.

Remember to speak slowly and directly to this participant so that he or she can process and then respond to you. Avoid adding movements together. One movement at a time is much more successful. Being a part of an exercise group is also beneficial to this participant, who may be avoiding social settings because of embarrassment related to his or her symptoms.

Note *Health Professionals' Guide to Physical Management of Parkinson's Disease* (Boelen 2009) in "Suggested Resources" to further your understanding of participants with this disease. Refer to table 1.13, Parkinson's Disease: Teaching Tips, at the end of this chapter.

Sensory Losses

Many older adults are living with one or more sensory losses, such as loss of vision, hearing, or sensation. Singularly or in any combination, these losses challenge a person who is attempting to master the environment and stay functionally independent.

You need to be aware of any sensory limitations a participant has to ensure that the participant can exercise safely to his or her full potential. For example, using clear verbal descriptions and reducing distracting background noises can help participants with vision and hearing losses. Being aware of body position at all times is important for participants with sensory loss. Additional strategies for teaching participants with sensory losses are reviewed in chapter 3, and you can find teaching tips in table 1.14 at the end of this chapter.

Traumatic Head Injury

Traumatic head injury occurs when the head collides with another surface. This collision causes the brain to impact on the inside of the skull. Besides causing the direct brain injury, a head trauma may create secondary issues and injuries such as edema (an excessive amount of tissue fluid) and ischemia (a local and temporary deficiency of blood supply because of obstruction of the circulation to a body part).

Table 1.7   Depression: Teaching Tips

Characteristic	Exercise and safety tips
Fatigue	Start slowly and establish easily achievable and realistic goals.
Anger and frustration	Encourage participants to use exercise as a way to vent some of these feelings. A brisk walk or aerobic exercise of any type can help to alleviate these emotions. Group support is also beneficial in reducing some of these symptoms. Try to listen without giving advice or making judgments.
Negative outlook	Keep a positive attitude and encourage depressed individuals to participate. Remember to offer positive feedback and compliments. Try to keep your interaction with the participant lighthearted.
Difficulty with decision making	Be encouraging and involve participants in making decisions. Do not offer too many choices.
Insomnia	Ask participants how they slept the night before exercising. If they appear fatigued, suggest a lighter workout than usual. Be observant for signs of overexertion. Encourage participants to spend time outside during the day, because sunshine helps improve the quality of sleep.
Decreased interest or pleasure in daily activities	Remind the participant in private that decreased interest in activities is a symptom of depression and that exercise can help. Also, encourage socializing with other members of the class.
Lack of sunlight stimulation	Many depressed people spend most of their day inside, away from sunlight. Sunlight not only improves the quality of sleep but also can decrease symptoms of depression. If possible, arrange for your exercise session to be in a location with ample daylight as long as it does not present a glare to the group and participants' ability to watch the leader.
Lack of physical activity	Regular exercise (both aerobic and resistance training) is associated with increases in the brain chemicals endorphins and serotonin. Both of these can reduce the symptoms of depression.
Anxiety	Deep breathing (see chapter 4) and relaxation (see chapter 7) help decrease anxiety.

From E. Best-Martini and K.A. Jones-DiGenova, 2014, *Exercise for frail elders*, 2nd ed. (Champaign, IL: Human Kinetics).

Table 1.8 Diabetes: Teaching Tips

Characteristic	Exercise and safety tips
Low tolerance to heat and cold	Avoid exercising in hot environments, because such settings increase the risk of heat injury for those with neuropathy (disease of the nerves). Avoid exercising in cold environments, which can impair circulation.
Poor circulation in legs and feet	Remind participants to wear comfortable and properly fitting shoes. Participants should be aware of positioning of feet and legs. Participants should avoid crossing the legs and feet.
Vision problems	Avoid exercises that can increase blood pressure (isometrics or too much exercise with arms overhead), which can harm the retinal blood vessels.
Potential for hypoglycemia (insulin reaction), the symptoms of which include faintness, sweating, dizziness, hunger, loss of motor coordination, rapid pulse, or confusion	See the section "Emergencies" in chapter 2 and be sure to check the policies for medical emergencies specific to the setting that you teach in. Recommend that participants carry a medical ID.
Limited endurance	Remind participants to take breaks and not to overexert themselves.
Possible low blood sugar (type 1 diabetes)	Remind the participant to check his or her blood sugar level before class. If it is low (under 70 milligrams per deciliter), the participant should eat a snack before any physical activity. The greater the physical activity is, the more complex carbohydrates should be eaten. During exercise, blood glucose levels should be in the range of 100 to 250 milligrams per deciliter.
Taking beta blockers for heart problems	Be especially observant of participants who take these drugs, because they mask the symptoms of an insulin reaction.
Potential for dehydration	Remind participants to stop for water breaks.

Table 1.9 Hip Fracture or Replacement or Knee Replacement: Teaching Tips

Characteristic	Exercise and safety tips
Decreased functional mobility	Remind participants to move slowly and deliberately. Remind participants to be aware of balance.
At risk of falls	Focus on safety in ambulation and transfers to and from a chair. Promote balance and strengthening exercises.
Pain	Participants should move only through a strain-free and pain-free range of motion while exercising. Teach deep-breathing exercises along with relaxation techniques for pain management and reduction (see chapters 4 and 7).
For total and partial hip replacements	To prevent hip dislocation, the participant should follow these recommendations unless his or her physician or physical therapist recommends otherwise: • Do not bend at the hip more than 90 degrees. • Avoid sitting in low-seated chairs. Keep knees lower than the hips. • Do not cross the legs. • Avoid internal rotation (pointing the toes inward).
For total knee replacement	Pain can be a problem with knee replacements. Follow the pain tips given earlier. There are no limitations on upper-body exercising. The participant may be able to bear full weight with no limitations on exercise.

From E. Best-Martini and K.A. Jones-DiGenova, 2014, *Exercise for frail elders*, 2nd ed. (Champaign, IL: Human Kinetics).

Table 1.10 Hypertension: Teaching Tips

Characteristic	Exercise and safety tips
Shortness of breath	Offer frequent rest periods; participants should not overexert themselves.
Limited endurance	Aerobic exercises are encouraged, because they reduce systolic blood pressure and help to increase endurance. High-intensity exercise, however, should be discouraged.
Increased blood pressure with exercise	Avoid continuous over-the-head work with or without weights, because this activity increases blood pressure.
General recommendations	People with blood pressure above 180 over 110 should be encouraged to add endurance training only after initiating drug therapy (ACSM 2009a). Stress reduction and relaxation exercises (see chapter 7) decrease blood pressure and should be encouraged. Remind participants to breathe while exercising so that blood pressure does not become elevated. Isometric exercises should be avoided, because they can elevate blood pressure.

From E. Best-Martini and K.A. Jones-DiGenova, 2014, *Exercise for frail elders*, 2nd ed. (Champaign, IL: Human Kinetics).

Table 1.11   Multiple Sclerosis (MS): Teaching Tips

Characteristic	Exercise and safety tips
Inability to tolerate heat	Locate the participant close to ventilation. Avoid exercising in hot environments.
Limited energy reserve	Remind participants to take breaks. Teach energy-conservation techniques. Participants with limited energy need to prioritize physical activities.
Decreased coordination (increased risk of falls)	Keep the environment safe and clear of obstacles. Provide space between seats. Do not hurry from one movement to another. Allow extra time to move from one exercise position to another. Keep exercise movements simple.
Possible vision deficits	Locate the participant close to the leader. Use contrasting colors for instructional materials, because the participant may have problems with color discrimination. Keep the environment free from clutter.
Loss of feeling in limbs, numbness, tingling (paresthesia)	Be aware of the participant's body positioning in a chair, because the participant may not detect sitting incorrectly. Observe the placement of feet and hands to avoid injury.
Spasticity (including foot drag, stiffness, or lack of control of one or both legs), muscle weakness, potentially limited range of motion	Begin exercises slowly because the participant may be deconditioned and weakened in addition to experiencing spastic weakness. All movements should be slow. Avoid having any one muscle group do too much work. Eliminate neck exercises if the participant has any weakness or loss of control of neck muscles.
Possible impairment of respiratory function	Be aware of any breathing difficulties. If they are observed, have the participant stop exercising.
Decreased range of motion	Never force any stretch or movement. Remind the participant always to move within a pain-free range of motion.
Loss of muscular coordination trunk or limbs (ataxia)	Encourage participants to keep their arms close to their sides, which can alleviate tremors.

From E. Best-Martini and K.A. Jones-DiGenova, 2014, *Exercise for frail elders*, 2nd ed. (Champaign, IL: Human Kinetics).

Table 1.12 Osteoporosis: Teaching Tips

Characteristic	Exercise and safety tips
Kyphosis, need for sensory input, increased risk of falling	Avoid exercises that increase spinal flexion (bending forward at the waist). This position can increase risk of vertebral fractures. Avoid overload of the back. Be aware of safety hazards in the environment, because participants may not have a clear view of surroundings because of their posture. Provide exercises that bring the shoulders back, expand the chest, and enhance the participant's ability to stand straighter, stronger, and with better balance. This posture can be encouraging for people with kyphosis.
Bone fractures	Fractures can occur spontaneously with decalcified (brittle) bones (osteoporotic fractures). Avoid exercises that involve leaning forward over the knees, particularly in combination with stooping over. Fast, jerky movements should be avoided at all times. Remind participants always to sit slowly and stay in control of their movements.
Anxiety	Because of the risk of fractures, many people are anxious about becoming physically active. They need emotional support and a safe environment in which to exercise.
Chronic back pain	Seated resistance exercises are encouraged, because they help build muscle strength and prevent falls while exercising. If approved, standing resistance and weight-bearing exercises can help increase both bone density and back strength.
Risk of falling	Avoid any exercises that impair balance. Encourage a good seated posture. Remind participants always to wear shoes that have a nonskid bottom. Exercises should focus on building up the larger muscle groups to cushion a fall if it occurs.
Stiffness	Always have participants start exercising slowly to warm up the joints and muscles.
Fatigue	A stooped position can impair the participant's pulmonary function and thus limit endurance. Watch for signs of fatigue, and encourage participants to rest between exercises as needed. Self-monitoring is important. Participants need to stop when they feel fatigued.

From E. Best-Martini and K.A. Jones-DiGenova, 2014, *Exercise for frail elders*, 2nd ed. (Champaign, IL: Human Kinetics).

Table 1.13 Parkinson's Disease: Teaching Tips

Characteristic	Exercise and safety tips
Resting tremors	Holding light weights and performing relaxation techniques (see chapter 7) help decrease tremors.
Rigidity	Reciprocal (moving backward and forward) and rotational (turning on an axis) physical exercises help decrease rigidity.
Stooped posture	Remind participants often to be aware of their posture. Encourage exercises such as backward shoulder rotation.
Slow movements (bradykinesia)	Take extra time to complete each movement. Have the participant warm up muscles slowly and change positions slowly. Break exercises into steps.
Postural instability	Frequently remind participants to be aware of their posture. Encourage the participant to walk with larger steps and try to lift the foot off the floor with each step. A good posture exercise is standing with the back against a wall and having the back of the head (if possible, while keeping the chin level), shoulders, buttocks, calves, and heels touching the wall, while envisioning good posture.
Acceleration or abbreviation of walking movements (festination)	When festination occurs, have the participant stop, breathe, and reposture before beginning to walk again. Remind the participant to allow a good space between the feet for balance before walking.
Uncontrolled movements (dyskinesia) and shaking movement of limbs (ataxia)	Physical activity can help reduce dyskinesia and ataxia. While seated, have the participant follow your movements: Stretch the arms out in front of the chest, clench the fists, and release. Slowly bring the arms to the sides and shake them out. Breathe deeply.
Freezing of movements	If freezing occurs during ambulation, have the participant stop moving, ensure good distance between the feet, slowly sway from side to side, and then proceed with walking. Sometimes the side-to-side movements of dancing can help to break the freeze. Because of the great risk of falling, these tips should be performed on a one-to-one basis. Walking is a recommended physical activity. Marching in place is a good variation. Chair exercises and slow stretching exercises are also advised.
Motor problems, motor memory problems	Repeat directions and follow up with visual demonstrations. Participants should exercise slowly without any jerky movements.
Difficulty with oral or facial control	Speech can become faint and facial expressions may lessen. To combat both of these, include breathing exercises (e.g., pronouncing "AEIOU," smiling, singing, and whistling).
Dementia	Use visual cues to teach exercises. Break exercises into easy steps. Keep it simple.
Depression	Focus on the abilities and functions that the participant still has. Exercise, social connectedness, and having fun help to decrease symptoms of depression.

From E. Best-Martini and K.A. Jones-DiGenova, 2014, *Exercise for frail elders*, 2nd ed. (Champaign, IL: Human Kinetics).

Table 1.14   Sensory Losses: Teaching Tips

Characteristic	Exercise and safety tips
Vision loss	Use large print for written materials. Remember always to use dark-colored print on a white background for ideal contrast. Remember that your verbal description and verbal pacing dictate how participants learn the exercises. Participants with vision loss have greater sensitivity to light and may take longer to adjust to changes in light levels. Avoid clutter in the environment. When sitting down, participants should feel the chair with their hands for proper positioning.
Glaucoma	Avoid any position that increases blood flow to or fluid in the eyes, such as bending over and letting the head hang below the heart.
Hearing loss (often a hidden, or undetected, disability)	Remember to speak at a normal volume. Do not shout. Keep the pitch of your voice normal, and make direct eye contact with the listener. Music playing in the background can be both an annoyance and a distraction from exercising safely. Be visually demonstrative so that participants can use your body language as a cue. Use gestures. Rephrase your directions if they are not clearly understood. Remind participants who wear hearing aids to bring the arms close to the ears but not touch them when such movements are required in an exercise.
Communication losses, including expressive aphasia (inability to express oneself), receptive aphasia (inability to receive information clearly), or global aphasia (both)	Make directions simple and demonstrate them visually. Give participants positive feedback on their performance.
Loss of sensation	Participants may not feel heat, cold, or pain in their hands or feet, so keep them in a safe position.

From E. Best-Martini and K.A. Jones-DiGenova, 2014, *Exercise for frail elders*, 2nd ed. (Champaign, IL: Human Kinetics).

Table 1.15   Traumatic Head Injury (THI): Teaching Tips

Characteristic	Exercise and safety tips
Poor judgment	Keep the environment structured and keep directions simple to follow.
Disinhibition	Maintain a low-stimulus environment. Set limits for appropriate and inappropriate behavior in a social setting. You may need to remove the participant from the group and work with him or her one on one.
Possible hemiparesis	Encourage the participant to work with the affected side by having the strong arm help move the affected arm or leg in exercises. Be aware of participants' positioning in the chair during seated exercises, because they may not be able to feel whether they are sitting safely. Remind the participant to keep the affected arm on the lap for protection and to avoid letting it hang over the side of the chair.
Poor balance and coordination	Encourage participants to focus on their posture while sitting in a chair. They should sit all the way back in the chair. If they fall to one side or their affected arm hangs over the side of the chair, verbally remind them to reposition. Have them use the strong hand to pick up the affected arm and place it in their lap. Use exercises that involve both sides of the body to enhance balance and coordination. Exercise movements that take the participant off the midline or center of balance help build balance control. Some exercise ideas are ball toss or kicking. Trying to catch a ball on the affected side enhances both balance and body awareness.
Difficulty planning and carrying out movements	Keep movements simple. All movements and follow-through deserve positive feedback. Hand-over-hand assistance may be necessary. Ask permission to help and approach the participant slowly while making eye contact.
Perceptual problems	Help participants more easily differentiate between the foreground and background of signs and written materials by using strong color contrast, such as black and white.
Speech and language problems	Speak clearly and give simple directions. Look directly at the participant. Give him or her extra time to respond.
Overstimulation	Balance active and passive behaviors in the exercise class. The participant needs frequent breaks to stay relaxed.
Frustration, with potential for aggression and catastrophic reactions	Because frustration is a common emotional response after head injury, do not overchallenge participants. They need to feel successful in performing simple steps.

From E. Best-Martini and K.A. Jones-DiGenova, 2014, *Exercise for frail elders*, 2nd ed. (Champaign, IL: Human Kinetics).

REVIEW QUESTIONS

1. Gerokinesiology is a new term that was coined to define specific curriculum necessary to standardize exercise programs for older adults and frail elders. List four of the nine areas identified as training modules in this curriculum.

2. The following are recommended for your interactions with people with Alzheimer's disease and related dementias:

   a. Focus on their strengths rather than their limitations, to enhance their self-esteem.

   b. Look beyond the behaviors and limitations and more at the person.

   c. Communicate clearly, patiently, and compassionately.

   d. Regardless of the level of dementia, show respect and care.

   e. Encourage physical activity for well-being and prolonged physical functioning.

   f. All of the above.

   g. *a, c,* and *d* only.

3. List four characteristics of dementia.

4. Participants with _____ typically experience pain in the hips, knees, or other weight-bearing joints, resulting from the progressive breakdown of articular cartilage (tissue that covers and protects the end of the bones).

5. Chronic obstructive pulmonary disease (COPD) is an umbrella term that includes these three pulmonary disorders:

6. Some of the causes of hypertension are related to

   a. lifestyle (poor diet, lack of exercise, and so on)

   b. some medications (such as steroids, birth control pills, anti-inflammatories, decongestants)

   c. unknown origin in some cases

   d. all of the above

   e. *a* and *b* only

7. Define the following symptoms of Parkinson's disease:

   a. bradykinesia

   b. festination

   c. dyskinesia

   d. ataxia

8. A participant with hypoglycemia may have all of the following symptoms except (*circle one*)

   a. hunger

   b. weakness, dizziness, or trembling

   c. shortness of breath

   d. perspiration

   e. all of the above

   f. *a, b,* and *d* only

CHAPTER

2

The Exercise Program:
Make It Motivating, Safe, and Effective

Research shows that for many aging individuals,
participation in whole-person health programs
slows the aging process and promotes independence.

—Jan Montague

LEARNING OBJECTIVES

After completing this chapter, you will have the tools to

- understand how the wellness model fits into the design of a physical fitness program,
- assist participants in designing individual and realistic fitness goals,
- develop a functional fitness class that includes all components of a safe and comprehensive program,
- manage safety issues and emergency situations with how-to checklists, and
- identify how many levels of physical function will be included in the design of your program.

Physical exercise is important for all people regardless of their limitations or existing health conditions. This message was one of the key points in a report by the U.S. Surgeon General (1996). From this report and the growing interest in physical activity in older persons, the U.S. Department of Health and Human Services (2008a) designed the *Healthy People 2010* objectives and the National Institute on Aging created *National Blueprint: Increasing Physical Activity Among Adults Age 50 and Older* (AARP et al. 2001). In 2010 the Centers for Disease Control and Prevention published

State Indicators Report on Physical Activity (CDC 2010). This report provides information on each state's progress in improving health and physical activity for all ages. In addition, it measures each state's progress toward achieving specific recommendations defined in the 2008 guidelines and from *Healthy People 2020* objectives (www.cdc.gov/physicalactivity/).

Healthy People 2020 has established new guidelines and goals for the years ahead. Older adults are identified as a population needing more light, moderate, or vigorous leisure time physical activity. This new report has a secondary goal of reducing moderate to severe functional limitations in older adults. Specifically, these reports state the need for all communities, agencies, and businesses to promote physical activity among their members and for all people to become more physically active both to increase quality of life and to decrease the health care needs of our aging population. In support of this need for more physical activity, the American College of Sports Medicine (ACSM) along with the American Medical Association (AMA) created a joint initiative titled "Exercise is Medicine." The primary goal of this collaboration is to "encourage all physicians to assess and review every patient's physical activity program every visit" (ACSM and AMA 2009). This initiative is an incredible support system for every fitness program, leader, and participant.

Whether you are a seasoned fitness instructor or are new to the field, this chapter walks you through a few of the most important areas in developing a safe and effective exercise program.

The exercise program provided in part II is designed to be customized for each participant. When working with the frail elderly and adults with special needs, you must observe and assess their abilities and limitations and consistently evaluate their need for exercise modifications. Additionally, you need to hone your motivational skills so that participants are encouraged to keep coming back to your classes. In so doing, they can see and experience the results of their involvement in physical activity.

WELLNESS AND THE WELLNESS MODEL AS A TREE

Wellness is the totality of body, mind, and spirit—everything that you think, feel, and believe has some effect on your state of health (Montague 2011). We use this approach for a healthy lifestyle that will support our health and quality of life. Wellness is the root and philosophy associated with programs that

look at each of us with many dimensions that work in perfect collaboration. These branches are physical, emotional, creative expressive, cultural, vocational, cognitive, social, spiritual, and environmental wellness.

The wellness tree (figure 2.1) is a visual description of how each element or dimension of our lives affects the other. All of these branches help us focus on lifestyle choices and our own role in living our best life one day at a time. Well-being is an active process that is integral to all health management and prevention approaches. Regardless of disease and health issues, wellness is attainable by each of us. Physical health and wellness really set the stage for all of us in our pursuit of a life worth living. Many participants will join your fitness program because of a recommendation by a doctor or therapist. After they join your program, they become part of a group and begin to make new friends, have fun, and find other new interests. Along with all of that, they become more physically fit. Many things can blossom from the mere act of getting started! This chapter looks at how to motivate participants, adhere to safety guidelines and industry fitness standards, and incorporate your experience as a leader into your exercise program.

Physical activity is one dimension of wellness. Each dimension is interconnected and important in the pursuit of well-being and quality of life. The wellness tree in figure 2.1 illustrates how these dimensions tie into every aspect of our lives. The physical dimension is a core element because it helps strengthen all the other branches of the tree. The newest dimension of the wellness model is environment, added by the International Council on Active Aging (ICAA 2010a). Colin Milner, the president of ICAA, believes that environment influences the way that we exercise, engage our minds and spirits, and socialize and can enhance participation levels.

In reading this chapter's description of how to design a motivating, safe, and effective exercise program, keep in mind that the fitness program, while focusing primarily on

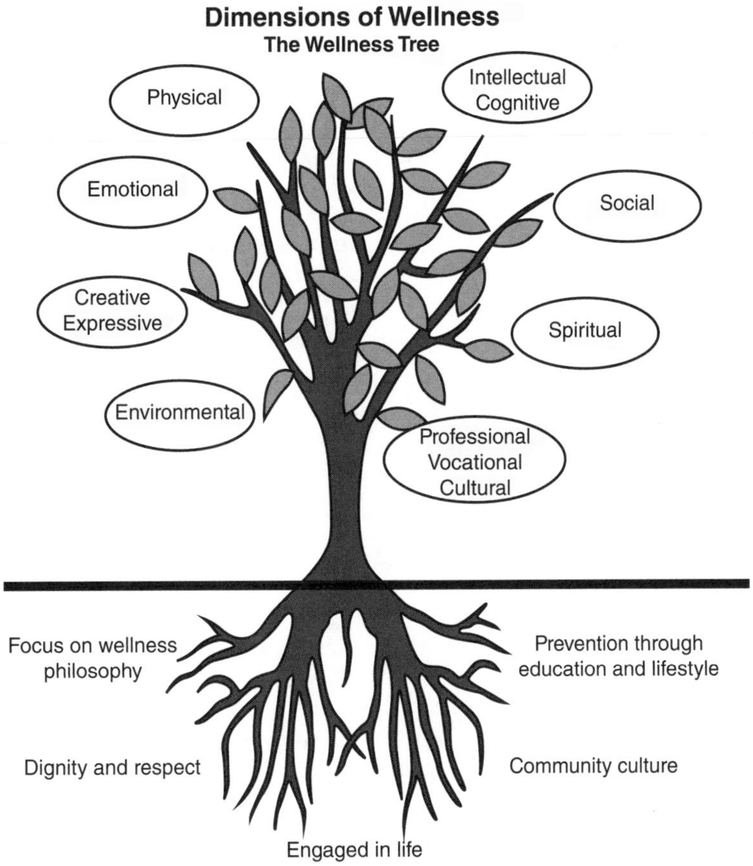

Dimensions of Wellness
The Wellness Tree

- Physical
- Intellectual Cognitive
- Emotional
- Social
- Creative Expressive
- Spiritual
- Environmental
- Professional Vocational Cultural

Focus on wellness philosophy

Prevention through education and lifestyle

Dignity and respect

Community culture

Engaged in life

Figure 2.1 The wellness tree illustrates that all aspects of our lives contribute to the various dimensions of wellness and our overall well-being. The environmental dimension was added by the ICAA in 2010.

From Best-Martini, E., Weeks, M.A., and Wirth, P. *Long Term Care for Activity Professionals, Social Services Professionals, and Recreational Therapists, Sixth Edition.* Enumclaw, WA: Idyll Arbor. Used with permission.

the dimension of physical activity, can interact with and affect other aspects of a participant's overall well-being.

MAKE IT MOTIVATING

Do you ever wonder what draws people to an exercise class and what makes it a success? Participants attend for various reasons. Some are encouraged by family, therapists, or facility staff to attend exercise programs. Others come because they seek social interaction. And some attend because they have always been physically active and are continuing to pursue their interest. Most people come looking for experiences other than strictly exercise.

Importance of Motivation

Motivation is the force that initially brings participants to your class and brings them back. Personal motivation is a powerful tool. Do your best to be aware of each participant's motivation and goals. This awareness gives fitness leaders better insight into who the participant is, what he or she needs from them, and how to personalize the exercise program.

Participants may be motivated to achieve intrinsic or extrinsic goals. Intrinsic goals come from within the individual. For example, I may want to join an exercise class because I want to lose weight or try something new. These are self-directed motivators—intrinsic goals.

Extrinsic goals are external motivators. For example, I may pursue training to achieve a certificate or award.

Generally, extrinsic motivators vary over the stages of our lives, but the intrinsic motivators give us the staying power to continue. Both the intrinsic and the extrinsic motivators are important. At times, people may need more external motivators to keep them going until they feel the internal benefits from the experience.

As the leader of the fitness class, you should find ways to help motivate each participant intrinsically or extrinsically. You first need to persuade participants to come and participate in the exercise class. Continuity and frequency of exercise can help your participants see and feel the personal benefits of physical activity—a powerful intrinsic motivator. Seeing and feeling these benefits can increase participants' motivation if their individual goals are being met. When participants experience success and notice how their exercising has affected their day-to-day life, be sure to have them share their story with the class, which can be a powerful extrinsic motivator. Hearing about the success of others is uplifting and motivating.

Creating realistic goals for each participant is crucial for motivation. The next section presents important points to remember in creating goals with and for your participants.

Goal Setting

You can instill confidence in your participants by assisting them in identifying and achieving their goals. Many older adults have not established goals for fitness. You can help them determine their goals. People who set specific health- and exercise-related goals are more likely to adhere to their programs, and people who identify realistic fitness goals have more success in achieving them. We recommend that you have participants identify and write down their first fitness goal. This goal is first created with collaboration from the leader and the individual participant and is written on the "Medical History and Risk Factor Question-

naire" (appendix A4). A copy of this is kept by the fitness leader and by the participant on request. In addition, the goal is added to the "Fitness Leader's Log" form found in appendix A6.

Good fitness goals have these qualities:

- Realistic (i.e., achievable) for the individual.
- Specific and measurable. (The more concrete the goal is, the easier it is to measure success.)
- Time-based, to provide some schedule in which to work. (Goals may be short or long term.)
- Easily modified when circumstances change.

Let's look more closely at these four areas of fitness goal setting

- **Setting realistic goals**. Some participants want to achieve goals that are not realistic for them at the time. The fitness leader should encourage them to be realistic in setting goals and expectations. Help them set goals that can be achieved and then built upon. For example, one of your participants, Mr. Judd, tells you that he wants to start walking again without a walker. Remember that the goal needs to be realistic, and encourage him to discuss the goal of walking without a walker with his physician or physical therapist. The physician or therapist may then send a note to you requesting a focus on specific exercises that reinforce their treatment or therapy goals. From this information and your assessment and observations, you can better define and clarify realistic functional fitness goals. The "Medical History and Risk Factor Questionnaire" (appendix A4) and "Statement of Medical Clearance for Exercise" (appendix A2), especially any special recommendations or specific comments from the physician, will help you gather and document helpful information for goal setting. The following is an example of a realistic goal: "Mr. Judd will participate in a seated exercise program two to three times a week to increase his activity level and learn the chair stand."

• **Setting specific and measurable goals**. Goals help the participant see his or her progress step by step. Break the larger goal into obtainable steps. Mr. Judd may not currently be able to walk without a walker, but that may be a long-term goal if it is approved by his physician. For that reason, we start by obtaining the physician's approval. If a goal is not realistic, we help the participant identify goals that are more realistic to work toward. The fitness leader must realize that settings will have varying protocols for obtaining the physician's approval, establishing goals, and working with the individual participant. By breaking the goal of walking unaided into the short-term goals of strengthening specific muscles, for example, a participant can look for small changes and experience success. Remember that the more specific the goal is, the easier it is to measure success and progress. The following is an example of a specific and measurable goal: "Mr. Judd will participate in a seated resistance-training program three times a week with a special focus on building strength in his quadriceps, hamstrings, and triceps so that he can complete a chair stand."

• **Setting time-based goals**. Change takes time. Participants should begin exercising slowly. Never rush fitness goals. Determine how much time is needed to see the benefits of the exercises. Keep breaking down goals into obtainable steps and keep participants working on short-term goals first. This approach allows them to have small successes along the way to obtaining long-term fitness goals. You do not need to establish a specific date, but you should project how long you expect them to be working on a specific goal. With this timeline, the participant and you can evaluate progress and, if necessary, reassess the goal. Use your attendance records to reinforce how long a participant has been involved in exercising. The following is an example of a goal that encompasses realistic, specific, measurable, and time-based qualities: "Mr. Judd will participate in a seated resistance-training program three times a week with a special focus on building strength in his quadriceps, hamstrings, and triceps so that he can complete a chair stand with chair-arm assistance in 3 months."

• **Modifying the goals**. The frail elderly and adults with special needs can experience fatigue, lack of sleep, changes in vision and hearing, new medical conditions, emotional or memory difficulties, and other changes that negatively affect their exercise participation and abilities. These changes can be discouraging to the participant and can alter fitness goals. By redefining goals together, you can help the participant succeed at his or her level of ability. One fitness goal may be simply to maintain the current frequency, intensity, and duration of exercises. Goal setting is a cyclic process. When change occurs, you reevaluate the goal, make sure that it is realistic for the participant's new level or need, make it specific and measurable, and then set a new schedule. The following is an example of a modified goal: "Because of a new diagnosis of Parkinson's disease and associated tremors, Mr. Judd will maintain his current goal of an arm-assisted chair stand for the next 3 to 6 months rather than progressing to an independent chair stand."

Maintaining current functional levels rather than progressing them is a realistic goal for many frail elderly participants. Discuss these issues with them individually. You will find that most older adult participants are realistic and will appreciate your recommendations.

You can keep track of these changes on the "Fitness Leader's Log" form (appendix A6). Significant changes can also be noted on the "Medical History and Risk Factor Questionnaire." After fitness goals are established, remind participants of all the benefits of their hard work in exercising. These reminders are both motivational and educational to the participant.

Benefits of Exercise

Some participants in your class may be physically active, but others may continue to live sedentary lives. In addition, many of your participants may be dealing with multiple medical disorders along with physical frailties. The benefits of exercise may not be easy for them to see in the beginning. Part of your role as fitness leader is to educate your participants about the benefits of exercise. You need to help them see how these are relevant to their own lives and health. One of the best ways to make exercise relevant is to correlate an exercise with an everyday function. See table 5.3 in chapter 5 for examples of functional benefits of seated and standing resistance exercises and table 7.3 in chapter 7 for examples of functional benefits of seated and standing stretching exercises. You may copy these tables for your participants as a motivational tool.

One example of a functional benefit of a resistance exercise is walking up the stairs. When the correlation is clear, the participant can see why strengthening specific lower-extremity muscles such as the quadriceps will benefit them. Another example is looking behind you, as if to see who is calling you from behind. From a seated position, this movement takes flexibility to twist and rotate the head toward the shoulder. Flexibility and stretching exercises enhance the participant's ability to look over the shoulder. Lifting objects and reaching for objects are other useful examples. When participants are able to recognize these exercise benefits for themselves, the benefits become intrinsic motivators. The exercise program thus becomes relevant to the participant.

Promoting independence and maintaining or improving function are two of the greatest benefits and goals of an exercise program for frail elders and adults with special needs. By seeing an improvement in physical endurance and strength, a participant can begin to see himself or herself as a more active and vital person. This perception can transform a previously sedentary person into an active and more independent person. This person achieves functional fitness—the ability to perform activities of daily living (ADL) such as pushing, pulling, lifting, squatting, balancing, and sitting and standing erect that enhance well-being and quality of life. By providing exercises and movements that mimic the movements and activities of daily living, the participant

will be able to complete everyday activities with greater ease, strength, flexibility, and confidence. Many times the participant cannot see or feel the difference from exercising. Ask him or her to think about a task or ADL that used to be difficult. Ask the person how it feels now. This task may be getting in or out of a wheelchair or chair, walking up a set of stairs, carrying groceries, getting in and out of a car, leaning down to pick up something, and so forth. By correlating the function to an activity of daily living, the participant can experience positive changes in his or her functional fitness.

You will find a list of physiological and psychological benefits from the World Health Organization (1997) in appendix B1. You can make copies of this and hand them out to your participants. You can refer to them often and post enlarged copies in the exercise room for reference. These educational handouts can be extremely motivating.

MAKE IT SAFE

In addition to being motivating and effective, your exercise class needs to be safe. At any age, physical exercise carries risks. As an instructor working with frail elders and adults with special needs, you need to know your participants' limitations, their established goals, and any exercises that are contraindicated for them. Concern for safety not only helps you be a better teacher but also instills confidence in your participants. Frail elderly people typically have fears of failing, falling, and looking foolish. Being assured of safety builds confidence, security, and competence along with overcoming these initial anxieties related to physical activity.

Hierarchy of Physical Function

The following hierarchy of physical function (figure 2.2) will help the fitness leader determine which level of exercise a specific participant should be best suited to at a specific time. The levels will change according to levels of participation, changes in health issues, and any chronic disorders. You are probably already aiming your exercise program at a general level

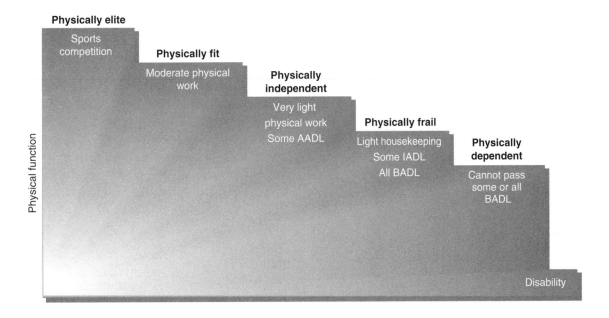

Figure 2.2 Hierarchy of physical function of the old (75–85 years) and oldest-old (86–120 years). AADL = advanced activities of daily living; IADL = instrumental activities of daily living; BADL = basic activities of daily living.

Reprinted, by permission, from W. Spirduso, 2005, *Physical dimensions of aging*, 2nd ed. (Champaign, IL: Human Kinetics), 264.

in this hierarchy. With an understanding of frailty and special needs from chapter 1, you can incorporate the following information into the final design of your exercise class. This design will aim your fitness instruction to the right level. Participants will be challenged and will maintain or improve in functioning, but they will not be posed with unrealistic expectations that could lead to injury.

The levels of the hierarchy of physical function are the following:

1. **Physically elite**—elderly at the highest level of the hierarchy who train on a daily basis and compete in competitions with their age group.

2. **Physically fit**—elderly who exercise two to seven times a week for health, enjoyment, and well-being.

3. **Physically independent**—elderly who do not exercise but have retained the capacity to function, although they may be in delicate health with meager reserves. Most old to oldest old are in this category.

4. **Physically frail**—elderly who are frail (see chapter 1 for definition) and are at high risk for instability and potential loss of function leading to a possible disability.

5. **Physically dependent**—elderly who are at the lowest level of the hierarchy and depend on others to assist in some or many daily functions.

New Standards for Accessibility

Fitness leaders need to know about environmental safety issues pertaining to special needs and disabilities. The American Disability Act of 1990 (ADA) gave specific guidelines for space, signage, and accessibility issues. The new 2010 standards for accessible design include play areas, gyms, recreational facilities, and more. To find these, go to www.ada.gov.

Some of the new additions include accessible paths of travel with handrails along walking surfaces; stable, firm, and slip-resistant floors; clear floor or ground space between two pieces of exercise equipment; provision of written materials, amplifiers, and large print materials for those with sensory deficits; and permission for service animals to be on the property. The new guidelines differentiate between already existing buildings and structures, historic structures, and newly constructed structures.

Safety starts with knowing your participants. The first step is obtaining medical clearance from their physicians.

Medical Clearance

The responsibility of the fitness leader is to know and understand each participant's abilities and limitations. The first source of information about these issues is the physician. Every participant should have a physician who oversees his or her health. The initial step in making exercise safe is to request information regarding health issues and limitations from the physician.

The "Statement of Medical Clearance for Exercise" in appendix A2 is a sample form for the physician to complete to give the participant clearance to take part in the exercise program. Review this form and feel free to adapt it to suit your setting and program. This form can be faxed or mailed to the physician's office. If the physician thinks that a patient has too many medical issues to address in a classroom setting, the physician may not give his or her approval. The form also includes a comments section where the physician can write in any limitations or cautionary notes for the fitness leader. Appendix A3 is a sample cover letter that you can fax or mail to the physician with the medical clearance form. Note any details about contraindicated exercises or limitations on the completed form and then file it.

Assessment

As mentioned in the earlier section on motivation, your participants come to exercise class for varying personal reasons. Regardless of their motivations for attending, you need to understand their current limitations, medical conditions, and ability. Without this information, you cannot ensure that their fitness goals are safe and appropriate. Many types of forms can be used to assess a person's fitness level and needs. We suggest using some or all of the following forms that suit your population and work setting:

- The "Medical History and Risk Factor Questionnaire" (appendix A4) allows the fitness leader to gather information about the current physical status of a participant. This questionnaire is a tool to use in the evaluation for establishing fitness goals. It records both past and current health issues and identifies any current functional limitations and fitness goals. If you do not currently have a form to use, feel free to adapt this form to your program needs.
- We also recommend that you have each participant complete the "Exercise Program Informed Consent" form (appendix A5). By signing this form, participants state that they consent to participate and understand the risks of the program. This form is completed along with requesting the physician's approval.
- The "PAR-Q & You" fitness questionnaire (appendix A1) is another widely used form designed to assess an individual's readiness to begin exercising. If a respondent answers yes to one or more of the questions, be sure to have that person check with her or his doctor before starting the exercise program. We recommend always obtaining a physician's approval as a safety guideline.

If you are not using a standard form provided in our appendixes or by your facility, be sure that you gather the information shown in "Assessment Checklist" during the assessment.

The assessment process begins with your initial interview and conversation with a participant. In this interview, you will begin to gather the information needed to assess the participant's strengths, limitations, and goals for joining.

The "Medical History and Risk Factor Questionnaire" form records an informational baseline—the participant's starting point, previous medical history, and initial fitness goals. All other observations and records are compared with this initial baseline. If you create a progress or attendance board, record the results

ASSESSMENT CHECKLIST

- ☐ Initial interview
- ☐ Previous lifestyle and exercise information
- ☐ Review of medical and social history
- ☐ Identification of existing conditions
- ☐ Identification of previous injuries and conditions
- ☐ Physician's approval and recommendations or precautions
- ☐ Therapeutic recommendations and precautions
- ☐ Results and information from any previous fitness testing

From E. Best-Martini and K.A. Jones-DiGenova, 2014, *Exercise for frail elders,* 2nd ed. (Champaign, IL: Human Kinetics).

of testing by date. Such a board, which is an extrinsic motivator, visually conveys a participant's progress.

Recognize that the assessment process varies from setting to setting according to participants' functional abilities and ability to live independently. Some fitness leaders teach and assess participants in more than one setting. You may gather some or all of this information listed earlier, depending on the protocols and procedures of the setting of your program.

Assessment in Retirement Communities and Senior Centers

In a life-care or other retirement community or community senior center, you may lead exercises for physically active and independent elderly participants. For instance, participants may live in their own houses or apartments and may receive assistance with some areas of daily living. Their level of assistance is important for you to know. For example, a participant may live at home but receive physical therapy for injuries from a recent fall or recent fracture. The participant may have someone helping with food preparation, temporarily helping him or her transfer from a chair to bed, and so on. Participants in an exercise class at a senior center also may have special needs that are not visible to you. During the initial assessment, be sure to ask about areas of personal care with which they need assistance. Their answers

will help you understand their current level of physical functioning.

Assessment in Assisted-Living or Residential Care Facilities, Adult Day Health Centers, or Skilled Nursing Settings

Specific federal and state regulations require that exercise programs be offered in assisted-living or residential care settings (the residents of which need some level of assistance with activities of daily living), adult day health centers (a day program that provides nursing supervision, therapists, and social workers), and skilled nursing settings (convalescent care). Residents live in or regularly visit these settings for some medical reason. They may have limitations in activities of daily living or memory loss that prevents them from living alone. Adult day health programs have physical, occupational, speech, and recreation therapists on staff along with social workers and activity directors to provide a medical model—a medical team approach. These settings provide you with much support for exercise assessment.

Those in skilled nursing settings need 24-hour nursing supervision. Participants are often in frail physical condition and depend on staff for one or more of their activities of daily living. The staff in these settings may already have a form for assessing functional fitness (a person's ability to perform daily activities) and for requesting the physician's approval. Because the approach to care in skilled nursing facilities is interdisciplinary, staff also provide you with support in the assessment process.

Safety Guidelines

Let's look at safety issues in the exercise class. Both the leader and the participants have many safety issues to consider. The "Safety Guidelines

SAFETY GUIDELINES CHECKLIST

Safety guidelines for the leader

☐ Be sure that each participant has medical clearance from his or her physician.

☐ Be sure that all participants breathe continuously during the exercises. Holding their breath can increase their blood pressure.

☐ Watch for signs of overfatigue or other indications that the activity level is too demanding.

☐ Avoid too many exercises that involve overhead movements. Continuously raising or holding the arms overhead (especially while holding weight) can raise blood pressure.

☐ Be vigilant while teaching. Always monitor how participants respond to the exercise.

☐ Exercise should never cause pain. Have a participant stop exercising if he or she experiences any pain. (Refer to figures 2.3 and 2.4.)

☐ Avoid combining any resistance exercises with exercises that involve turning or bending the spine.

☐ Avoid teaching full neck rotations. Each head and neck movement should be completed separately and slowly.

☐ Be aware of the environment and any potential safety hazards (including a room that is too hot or too cold).

☐ Ask your participants how they felt after the last workout the next time you see them so that you can give them appropriate guidance for the next class.

Safety guidelines for the participant

☐ Be aware of your posture in a chair or a wheelchair.

☐ Do not try to compete with other participants. Everyone needs to exercise at his or her own pace and within his or her own ability.

☐ Avoid jerking or thrusting movements while exercising.

☐ During standing exercises, be sure to hold on to a steady chair, a handrail, or the wall for safety.

☐ During seated exercises, do not raise both feet off the ground at the same time. This can add undue stress to your back.

☐ When you are leaning or bending forward during a seated exercise, be sure to support yourself by placing your hands on your knees.

☐ Prevent dehydration; take water breaks during the exercise class.

☐ Don't overdo it. Mild muscle soreness lasting up to a few days and slight fatigue are normal. What are not normal are exhaustion, sore joints, and unpleasant muscle soreness.

From E. Best-Martini and K.A. Jones-DiGenova, 2014, *Exercise for frail elders*, 2nd ed. (Champaign, IL: Human Kinetics).

Checklist" can serve as a quick reminder and adds to your safety awareness. It is broken into two parts—one for the leader and the other for the participants. These lists emphasize that the responsibility for exercise safety lies with both the leader and the participant. Additionally, chapters 4 through 7 have sections that cover safety precautions for each exercise component (warm-up, resistance training, aerobics, and stretching). Each chapter offers general safety precautions and specific ones for those with special needs.

Emergencies

One of the fitness leader's most important safety responsibilities is dealing with medical and other emergencies. As the fitness instructor, you need to have an emergency plan in case something unexpected happens. Request a copy of the emergency policy and procedures from the staff at the facility where you teach. The policy and procedures both for medical emergencies and for natural disasters are important for you to know. The policy should outline the command structure in an emergency. You should know exactly who to call on site if an emergency occurs in your class. If no such policy is in place, design a simple plan of action to follow in case of any emergency in the classroom. If your teaching setting does not provide a first-aid kit, we recommend that you carry your own to your fitness classes.

We recommend that you have both a completed "Medical History and Risk Factor Questionnaire" (appendix A4) and a signed "Statement of Medical Clearance for Exercise" (appendix A2) for each of your participants. Keep a log on each participant that includes the information gathered from those forms. Know their diagnoses, previous medical histories, and the medications that they are taking. Many medications have side effects that can alter mood, balance, and coordination. Knowing this information can make all the difference in an emergency. On the log, be sure to note a contact person and phone number for each participant. Many of the settings for exercise classes, including retirement communities, day centers, and hospitals, have these records available. If not, use the form in appendix A6—"Fitness Leader's Log"—to keep all this information together.

Along with having information about individual participants, familiarize yourself with the environment in which you teach. Look around for the items listed in "Emergency Checklist."

EMERGENCY CHECKLIST

Make sure that you know where each of these items is before you need them in an emergency.

- ☐ Closest staff desk or station
- ☐ Telephone
- ☐ Microphone
- ☐ Door alarms
- ☐ First-aid kit
- ☐ Water faucet
- ☐ Fire extinguisher
- ☐ Fire sprinkler placement
- ☐ Closest available wheelchair
- ☐ Emergency exit

From E. Best-Martini and K.A. Jones-DiGenova, 2014, *Exercise for frail elders,* 2nd ed. (Champaign, IL: Human Kinetics).

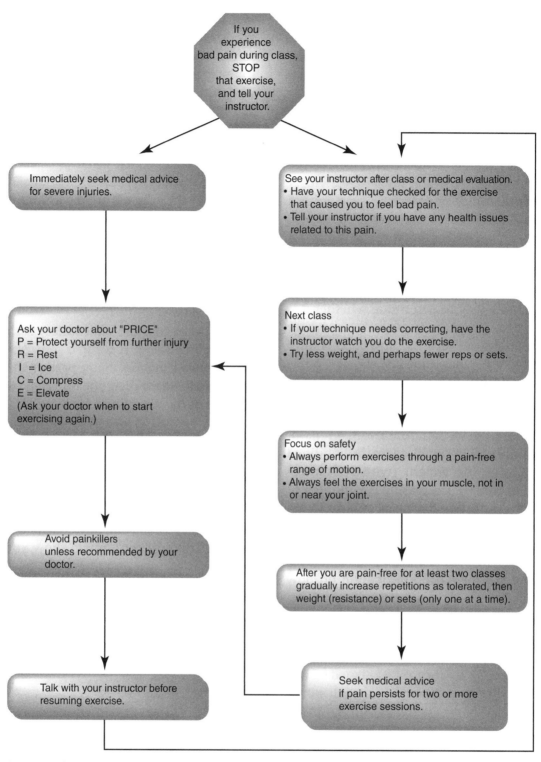

Figure 2.4 Tips for responding to bad sensation, or pain.

From E. Best-Martini and K.A. Jones-DiGenova, 2014, *Exercise for frail elders,* 2nd ed. (Champaign, IL: Human Kinetics).

LARGE-GROUP SAFETY CHECKLIST

☐ With a large group, your need for good observation and communication skills increases. Safety becomes more challenging when you are unable to be fully attentive to all participants.

☐ Be prepared for new participants to join before you know their limitations and needs. Consider seating them next to you for the first few sessions.

☐ Keep all equipment and supplies within safe reach and in a safe location.

☐ Do not keep weights, if used, at each participant's place. Instead, keep them close to you on a cart, and distribute them when needed.

☐ You may limit the exercise class to just the warm-up session to make a larger group more manageable. Refer to "Duration of Warm-Up" in chapter 8 for how to extend warm-up exercises (chapter 4) into an entire class.

☐ When possible, create two smaller exercise groups instead of one large one.

☐ Find a qualified coleader to make two pairs of eyes available. You both may lead, or one can lead while the other spots participants.

☐ Review the room setup charts in chapter 3 (figures 3.1 and 3.2) for guidance about the physical setup of the room and the arrangement of participants and supplies. The seating arrangement depends on the number of participants in the class. When you plan the room layout, remember to take into account the space needed for wheelchairs, leg-extending foot pedals on the wheelchairs, and walkers (when using them as an exercise prop for standing exercises).

From E. Best-Martini and K.A. Jones-DiGenova, 2014, *Exercise for frail elders,* 2nd ed. (Champaign, IL: Human Kinetics).

MAKE IT EFFECTIVE

An exercise program is effective when it focuses on function, fitness, and fun and meets the needs and goals of individual participants. Effectiveness includes consideration of motivation (without motivation people will not come to class), safety (if a person becomes injured, he or she will not be able to exercise), and the following points:

- In collaboration, the participant and the leader need to set realistic goals.

- The leader needs to observe and remain informed about each participant's current functional status.

- The exercise program should be based on current evidence-based fitness standards.

- The exercise class needs to adhere to safety guidelines.

- The exercise components (described in the next section) need to follow a structured sequence as reviewed in part II of this book.

Let's look more closely at the exercise components.

Effective Use of the Exercise Program Components

The components of the exercise programs that are offered in this book are

- warm-up (chapter 4),
- resistance training (chapter 5),
- aerobic training and dynamic balance (chapter 6), and
- cool-down (chapter 7).

Each of these components is important and has specific goals and benefits.

1. Warm-up exercises ensure a smooth transition between the resting and exercising states. Warm-up includes posture, breathing, range-of-motion exercises, and stretching exercises.

2. Resistance exercises enhance the strength and endurance of participants' major muscle groups.

3. Aerobic exercises enhance cardiovascular endurance, usually by means of sustained large-muscle activity (e.g., walking, swimming, cycling, and so on). Dynamic balance exercises have been added to this second edition with aerobics (i.e., exercises 6.1–6.12) for improving participants' balance while moving and for decreasing risk of falls.

4. Cool-down exercises ensure a smooth transition between the exercising and resting states. Cool-down includes stretching exercises to increase flexibility in the major joints, particularly in injury-prone hip, trunk, and shoulder areas. Relaxation, stress reduction, and breathing techniques can be included in this component or taught to participants to use outside class.

Table 2.1 helps you understand the effective use of each component. Chapter 8 provides many options for combining the exercise components into an effective exercise program. For example, for beginners or as a buildup to resistance training, you may start by teaching only the warm-up component—gentle exercises that are easy to learn and appropriate for all participants. With the information in chapter 8, you will be able to customize comprehensive exercise programs.

Balance, Core, and Agility Training

Notice that table 2.1 includes benefits related to balance, core, and agility. Training to achieve these benefits is important to the older adult and frail elder population, especially because of their role in preventing falls. Although balance, core strength and stability, and agility are natural outcomes of the comprehensive exercise program presented in this book, they can also be trained for specifically. You can add separate sessions to train these skills, or you can build an extra few minutes of training in these areas into your regular exercise sessions.

Balance

Balance is a person's ability to control the body's center of mass (COM) from either a static or moving position to offer a base of support to the body. Static balance refers to maintaining balance in a stationary position, and dynamic balance is maintaining balance while in motion. You will find balance training exercises and tips in this chapter as well as in chapters 4, 5, 6, and 7 so that as the fitness instructor, you can either add in balance exercises or create a class specifically designed to focus on balance training.

The fitness leader must understand the multidimensional aspects of balance when working with this population. Balance strategies will give you the tools to determine which exercises will work best with your participants. You may have a participant who is strong and flexible but is experiencing balance issues that are directly affecting daily life and challenging his or her independence. Although a participant may visually appear to be at a high level of functional fitness, he or she may have limitations because of balance issues that limit all other aspects of fitness and activities of daily living. This is true for participants performing both seated and standing exercises.

To understand what affects balance, we first need to understand how this intricate system works. Balance is a fine symmetry between three systems: the sensory system, the motor system, and the cognitive system.

• The sensory component includes our vision, somatosensory system (sensations to the body through the skin and environment such as touch, pain, pressure, joint and muscle positions [proprioception]), and the vestibular system (the inner-ear function of balance that

Table 2.1 Components of an Exercise Program

Component	Includes these exercises	Repetitions per exercise[a]	Duration of a single exercise or repetition	Duration per 45- to 60- minute class	Major benefits
Warm-up	• Range-of-motion (ROM) • Low-intensity aerobics	3–8	1–2 seconds per repetition	10 minutes minimum	• Increases internal body temperature • Injury prevention • Static balance
Resistance training	• Body-weight exercise[c] • Resistance exercises	8–15	6 seconds per repetition	15–30 minutes	• Muscular strength and endurance • Core strength and stability • Static balance
Aerobic training	• Aerobic exercises	Varies	Varies[b]	15–30 minutes	• Cardiorespiratory endurance • Dynamic balance • Agility
Balance training	• Dynamic and static balance activities • Postural and core strengthening	Varies	Varies	15–30	• Balance • Fall prevention
Cool-down	• Stretching exercises[d]	1–4	10–30 seconds per stretch	5–30 minutes	• Improved flexibility
	• Relaxation techniques • Stress reduction techniques	Varies	Varies	5–30 minutes	• Relaxation, stress reduction

[a]Several factors determine the number of repetitions, such as the component of exercise, the level of fitness of the participant, the level of progress for that exercise, day-to-day variations in the participant's physical state, and the total amount of time available for the exercise class.

[b]Varies according to the type and beat of the music.

[c]Body-weight exercises are exercises in which body weight, such as the weight of the arms or legs, serves as the resistance.

[d]The cool-down from aerobics also includes range-of-motion and low-intensity aerobic exercises.

responds to movements of the head). (Vertigo occurs when there is an imbalance in this system.) The vestibular system is the organ of adaptability that helps us detect motion and determine whether that motion is our body moving or the environment around us moving (Best-Martini 2011). For example, if you are sitting in your car when it goes through a car wash, you may feel as if the car is moving when it is the environment outside your car that is moving.

• The motor system is the central nervous system. The motor system responds to the sensory input.

• The cognitive system creates the motor movement response necessary to negotiate the environment.

A physiological change to any of these three systems can affect balance. The fitness leader needs to watch the participant closely to help identify potential causes of balance problems, which may be a combination of a few of these areas.

Possible reasons for balance problems:

• History of falling
• Poor posture and weak postural control
• Weak core
• Weak joints
• Weak muscles
• Tight muscles
• Limited range of motion
• Osteoporosis
• Loss of sensation in extremities
• Unsteady gait
• Poor response or reaction time to movement
• Inner ear problems and vertigo
• Postural hypotension
• Cognitive changes or impairment
• Vision problems
• Lack of body awareness
• Distractibility

• Medications
• Alcohol use
• Nutritional deficits
• Dehydration
• Using assisted devices improperly
• Poor shoes
• Unsafe living environment, such as uneven flooring or tripping hazards (ACSM 2004b, p. 1991)

As you can see from this list, balance issues can result from many causes, and all of these can lead to a fall. Some of these reasons can be resolved or improved by exercising, such as strengthening muscles and joint stability, improving posture, building core strength, increasing response time to movement, working on body awareness, and gait and agility skills. We can make some recommendations for the other reasons that cannot be addressed in an exercise program. These recommendations should be discussed on a one-to-one basis after the class.

The balance exercises in table 2.2 enhance balance, weight shift, good posture and looking ahead instead of down at the feet, and power and speed (agility) training. Look for the balance symbol throughout the book to identify exercises that enhance balance. The beauty of balance training is that it can develop the skill so that balance can be restored or enhanced. Like any skill, balance needs to be practiced often, both in and out of class. Balance is like dancing, the more you practice, the better you will become.

Core and Core Stability

The core is the central part of the body that includes the spine, pelvic girdle, and hip joints. Twenty-nine muscles attach to these locations. All movement begins from this core region. The deeper inner core stabilizer muscles cannot be seen, but they help stabilize the spine before the more superficial outer core muscles move the spine. The inner core muscles are the transverse abdominis (hidden under the six-pack abs), the multifidus (muscles that lie along

Table 2.2 Exercises to Improve Balance

Balance exercises	Seated	Standing	Reference and instructions
EXERCISES FOUND IN THIS BOOK, *EXERCISE FOR FRAIL ELDERS, 2ND EDITION*; SEE THE SECTIONS "ILLUSTRATED INSTRUCTION"			
Hip Rotation	X	X	Exercise 4.3, Hip Rotation
Standing Crane Pose		X	Exercise 4.5, Toe Point and Flex Hold a ball in the hands in front of the chest and overhead for extra challenge.
Alphabet Toes	X	X	Exercise 4.6, Ankle Rotations Lift one foot and write the letters A through C; switch feet and write the same letters. Add more letters when participants are ready.
Center of Gravity Awareness	X	X	Exercise 4.23, Torso Rotation Hold a ball in the hands to the front, side, or overhead for extra challenge.
Alternate Heel Lifts	X	X	Exercise 6.2, Alternate Heel Lifts
Alternate Kicks	X	X	Exercise 6.10, Alternate Kicks Hold a ball in the hands to the front, side, or overhead for extra challenge.
Alternate Toe Touches to Front	X	X	Exercise 6.5, Alternate Toe Touches to Front For an extra challenge, hold a ball or rod in the hands to the front after stepping forward is comfortable.
Alternate Toe Touches to Sides	X	X	Exercise 6.7, Alternate Toe Touches to Side Hold a ball or rod to the front for extra challenge.
Chair Stands	X	X	Exercise 5.12, Modified Chair Stands Various progressions are used in this strengthening and balance exercise.
OTHER EXERCISES			
Colored Spot Walk	X	X	See *FallProof, 2nd ed.*, p. 141 (Rose 2010) for exercises using colored spots. Dynamic weight transfer exercise improves anticipatory control to improve balance.
Four-Corner Marching	X	X	*FallProof, 2nd ed.*, p. 140 (Rose 2010) Dynamic weight transfer exercise improves anticipatory control to improve balance.
Round the Clock	X	X	Move one foot toward each hour of a clock—clockwise and then counterclockwise. This exercise emphasizes both weight shifting and power and speed (agility) movements.
Toe Raise	X	X	*FallProof, 2nd ed.*, p. 232 (Rose 2010) Raise the toes off the floor until weight is on heels only.

(continued)

movements using ankle strategies and a faster response time to get back to their center of gravity.

Agility training helps to compensate for some of the age-associated changes in balance and speed. For example, a client may be experiencing vision problems, spinal changes because of osteoporosis, and a hesitancy to increase the speed of movements and gait because of fear of falling again. This combination slows speed and response time and increases the likelihood of another fall. So adding speed and power (agility) to simple seated and standing exercises helps build a participant's skill level. By using agility along with ankle and hip strategies (Rose 2010), the participant will be building strength, balance, and the ability to recover quickly from a loss of balance experience. Agility training helps identify the importance of rapid limb movement to balance recovery (Signorile 2011). After successfully recovering from a potential loss of balance, a participant begins to build success in movement and skill. At this point the skill translates into an activity of daily living.

Some of these translational skills and drills can be found in *Bending the Aging Curve* (Signorile 2011) and are listed in table 2.4. In addition, the aerobic exercises in chapter 6 will help develop agility in frail elders.

Falls and Fall Prevention

Falls occur for many reasons, some of which can be found in the list of factors influencing balance earlier in this chapter. One of the goals of our exercise programs for frail elders and adults with special needs is to prevent falls by becoming stronger and more flexible, becoming more aware of the physical environment, and building balance and agility skills. The strength, flexibility, and awareness of our bodies in the surrounding environment are the framework for fall prevention.

Some statistics from the Centers for Disease Control and Prevention show the necessity for incorporating fall prevention into a functional fitness class:

- The chances of falling and of being seriously injured in a fall increase with age.
- In 2009, the rate of fall injuries for adults 85 and older was four times that for adults 65 to 74.3 years of age.
- Over 90 percent of hip fractures are caused by falls, and of those hospitalized because of a fracture, four out of five will be admitted to a long-term care facility for a year or longer.
- In 2008, 82 percent of fall deaths were among people 65 and older.

Table 2.4 Training and Translational Matching Exercises

Power, balance, and speed	Both	Strength, balance, and control
Functional reach drill	Heel stand	Skating drill
Pillow stands	Heel walk	Lateral advances
Triple-line drill	Lateral throw	Back-to-back handoff
Lateral shuffle drill	Forward and backward passes	Chest pass
Forward and backward cone drill	Truckin' drill	Overhead and lateral throw
Zigzag drill	Dual tasking	Soccer kicks
Cone-touch drill	8-foot (2.4 m) up-and-go drill	Broom hockey
Speed and stride drill	Ladder drills	Step drill
Hexagon drill	Chair drills	Scarf drill
Star excursion drill	Coin pickup drill	Book drills
	Gallon jug drill	Ball-and-pylon drills
	Dot drills	Floor coin pickup drill

Reprinted, by permission, from J.F. Signorile, 2011, *Bending the aging curve: The complete exercise guide for older adults* (Champaign, IL: Human Kinetics), 262.

These statistics from the Centers for Disease Control and Prevention (CDC 2011) are shocking to read but important for fitness leaders to be aware of. Our comprehensive exercise routine will help you develop a program that can prevent your participants from contributing to these statistics. One of our greatest rewards is watching an older adult get stronger, build balance and agility skills, increase flexibility, prevent falls, and have greater quality of life.

Effective Exercise Program Design

To be effective, an exercise program must meet individual participants' needs and adhere to current standards of fitness programming for older adults. The American College of Sports Medicine and the American Heart Association recommend that older adults engage in endurance exercise with moderate intensity 30 to 60 minutes per day in at least 10-minute bouts, accumulating at least 150 to 300 minutes of moderate-intensity endurance exercise per week (ACSM 2009b). The exercises presented in part II of this book adhere to the standards set by the American College of Sports Medicine, the American Council on Exercise, the American Heart Association, the American Senior Fitness Association, the National Strength and Conditioning Association, the U.S. Surgeon General, and the U.S. Department of Health and Human Services. See chapters 4 through 7 for specific guidelines for warm-ups, resistance training, aerobics and dynamic balance, and stretching exercises. Chapter 8 will help you put these exercise components together into an effective exercise program design. Table 2.5 summarizes the FIT (F for frequency, I for intensity, and T for time) guidelines for resistance training, aerobics, and stretching.

We highly recommend that you know your participants' abilities and limitations and introduce exercise slowly. Start with 1 or 2 days a week if that is all they can physically or mentally tolerate. If participants cannot attend two exercise classes a week, suggest types of exercises that they can try on their own (with their physician's approval). The ACSM (2009b) recommends that you use a gradual approach, perhaps doing just one type of exercise, with

Table 2.5   Exercise Program Design for Older Adult Fitness

Exercise component	Frequency	Intensity	Time
Resistance training	2 to 3 days per week on nonconsecutive days when doing a full-body workout	Initially, perform 8 to 15 repetitions of a resistance exercise at an exertion level perceived as very slight to slight (an RPE of 1 to 2). Progress to "somewhat hard" (an RPE of 4) when appropriate, after learning excellent technique.	Not applicable
Aerobics	3 to 5 days per week	3 to 4 on the RPE[a] scale ("moderate" to "somewhat hard")	20 to 30 continuous minutes of low to moderate work
Stretching	2 to 3 days per week	Stretches should be taken only to the point of tightness or mild intensity, not pain.	10 to 30 seconds per stretch, except 5 seconds or less for neck stretches

[a] An RPE (rating of perceived exertion) scale is a useful tool for monitoring exercise intensity; see table 6.3.

the long-term goal of adding other forms of exercise. As participants' strength and endurance increase, you can help them increase the frequency, intensity, time, and type of exercises. In addition, make the program one that people will want to be members of. If the experience is positive and people are enjoying each other as much as the exercises, you have added the secret element of fun. The fun of physical activity is what brings people back to re-create the experience and encourages them to include physical activity in their lives on a regular basis.

SUMMARY

The frail elderly and adults with special needs benefit greatly from physical activity. They can show a greater response to exercise than older adults who are more active. This audience needs fitness leaders who are aware of motivational, safety, and professional standards for making their exercise successful and effective.

The first key to creating a successful exercise program is motivation. Motivation may come from intrinsic motivators such as losing weight or trying something new. It also may stem from extrinsic goals such as pursuing advanced training or achieving an award. Fitness leaders need to understand participants' intrinsic and extrinsic goals because these motivators keep participants coming back to an exercise class. The wellness model can be used to help participants identify realistic goals. Motivational strategies such as realistic goal setting can keep participants motivated both intrinsically and extrinsically over time because participants see and feel improvement in their functional fitness, mood, strength, and flexibility as they progress.

The second key to creating a successful exercise program is safety. As noted in this chapter, physical exercise carries risks at any age. Make your exercise class safe for each participant by obtaining a physician's medical clearance, conducting an assessment to establish appropriate

fitness goals, and being prepared for emergencies and pain issues during class. A safe exercise program is designed with both the individual's and group's strengths and limitations in mind. Your vigilant observations during class can ensure that participants are exercising at a level that is appropriate for them. The hierarchy of physical function in older adults will help identify the correct levels for your participants. Following established and recommended safety guidelines including the new ADA guidelines are the base of the program. Reviewing educational handouts and planning regular group discussions on safety topics will keep safety at the forefront of your exercise class.

The third key to creating a successful exercise class is effectiveness. An exercise program is effective when it meets the motivational and safety needs of participants, as mentioned earlier, but also meets certain professional standards. These professional standards include effective use of the exercise program components. The four main exercise components offered in this book are warm-up, resistance training, aerobic training and dynamic balance, and cool-down. We have also added a section on balance, core, and agility in this chapter. Each of these components is important and has specific goals and benefits that contribute to a well-rounded exercise program. The components follow guidelines from the U.S. Surgeon General, U.S. Department of Health and Human Services, and other leading organizations in the field of health and fitness such as the American College of Sports Medicine, the American Council on Exercise, the American Heart Association, the American Senior Fitness Association, and the National Strength and Conditioning Association.

The combination of motivation, safety, and effective program components helps you create an exercise class that meets individual as well as group goals. A well-designed program promotes functional independence at all levels and offers a rewarding and enjoyable experience to participants.

REVIEW QUESTIONS

1. Define and give an example of (*a*) intrinsic motivation and (*b*) extrinsic motivation.

2. Write a fitness goal for an older adult that is (*a*) realistic, (*b*) specific and measurable, and (*c*) time based.

3. The client in question 2 has been newly diagnosed with rheumatoid arthritis. What would be an example of modifying the fitness goal?

4. Define functional fitness.

5. The *Red Cross First Aid Manual* describes nine symptoms that require immediate professional medical attention. List four of these.

6. If a participant is experiencing pain during an exercise class, he or she should (*circle one*)

   a. push through the pain

   b. increase the intensity or timing

   c. stop exercising immediately

7. An effective exercise program includes four components. List one benefit for each of the following:

   a. warm-ups

   b. resistance training

   c. aerobics

   d. cool-down (stretching)

8. List the five levels of the physical function in older adults hierarchy scale.

9. List nine dimensions of the wellness model.

The Leader:
Tips and Strategies for Success

People must believe that leaders understand their needs
and have their interests at heart. . . . Leaders breathe life into
the hopes and dreams of others and enable them
to see exciting possibilities that the future holds.

—Kouzes and Posner

LEARNING OBJECTIVES

After completing this chapter you will have the tools to

- identify specific leadership skills needed to lead a class for people with special needs;
- incorporate the three-step instructional process into your teaching methods;
- implement tips and strategies for participants dealing with sensory, cognitive, and communication issues; and
- define balance, core, and agility and integrate them into the exercise program.

Frail elders and adults with special needs who participate in your exercise class look to you as the leader to exhibit the qualities expressed in the quotation that opens this chapter. You need to determine and monitor what your participants need from you as their fitness leader.

This chapter discusses how to develop leadership skills and how to incorporate leadership strategies in your exercise class. We share with you our own tips for positive leadership.

CREATING A SENSE OF FUN AND COMMUNITY

What activities do you look forward to attending? Most likely they are activities that are interactive, educational, and fun. You may look forward to going because of the instructor or the other participants. An interactive, educational, and fun atmosphere is what you want to instill in your class. The following sections present some strategies for creating a warm and welcoming environment, promoting common goals for the group, and encouraging friendships and social support.

Creating a Warm and Welcoming Environment

As mentioned in chapter 2, participants join your group for various reasons. As you become more familiar with individual participants, you can begin to facilitate social interaction among them. As participants get to know one another, a sense of community begins to develop. Here are some ways to encourage a warm environment.

- Be organized and ready for your participants to arrive. They receive the message that you are eagerly awaiting their arrival.

- Have everyone wear name tags during class so that they can learn each other's names.

- Be sure that participants feel welcome. Know each person's name and welcome participants by name. Ask what they prefer to be called. Never assume that elderly people prefer to be called by their first name.

- Avoid using terms such as "sweetie," "honey," or "guys." These terms can make participants feel uncomfortable and insulted.

- As a group, choose a name for your exercise class.

- Create a display board that describes the exercise class. The board can include photos of participants, group goals, and reminders.

- Have the class create new names for the exercises in part II. Names that your class originates can be easier for participants to remember. The naming process helps them feel that the class belongs to them, which is a good motivator.

- Put the group's name on exercise supply items. The name can be painted on exercise towels, vests, T-shirts, or hats to reinforce a sense of teamwork.

- Keep an attendance chart on a large board to show the attendance and progress of participants. This board can be a visual motivator for participants.

- Acknowledge individual successes. You can show physical progress through a photo timeline.

- Help participants feel the fun of physical activity. Be sure to laugh and encourage a sense of playfulness. Be sure that no participant misinterprets your laughter as ridicule.

Promoting Group Goals

First, help each participant in your class identify his or her individual goals (see the section "Goal Setting" in chapter 2). Having group goals helps to create a sense of fun and community. The goals are group goals because all members and leaders create them together. The focus on establishing realistic and obtainable individual goals also applies to group goals.

Here are some ideas for group goals:

- To feel welcome

- To know the names of other participants

- To see personal progress through attendance records and photos

- To be aware of posture and positioning

- To be able to identify the muscles targeted by specific exercises

- To describe the muscles involved in the exercises

- To build endurance and muscular strength

- To have fun and feel part of something special

- To present the exercises to other groups

- To understand the physiological and psychological benefits of physical activity (see appendix B1)

Encouraging Friendships and Social Support

Many of your participants may live in settings other than their own private homes. Previous relationships with family and friends may have been altered by this relocation. Recreation and wellness programs can promote a sense of culture and community that help people again feel part of a social network. Social activity and friendships help people stay well as much as physical activity through exercise does. The importance of adult friendship was researched by Rosemary Blieszner and Rebecca G. Adams. One of their findings was that "good friends are critically important to successful aging. . . . Friends can be more important to the psychological well-being of older adults than even family members are" (Blieszner and Adams 1992, 112). You can help create feelings of ease, warmth, and friendship within the exercise group. Be sure that your room is set up before the class so that participants come into a welcoming environment. Advance preparation helps create a friendly setting where people feel safe and comfortable.

New friends are one of the most important elements that you can offer to participants. The wellness tree reminds us that all branches and dimensions of the wellness model are intertwined. All of them carry the same importance in working toward whole-person wellness. We need all these dimensions to be as strong and involved as the others. You can encourage friendships and nurture a sense of community within the group in subtle ways. Here are some ideas:

- After you are familiar with the group, seat people next to one another for specific reasons. For example, a gregarious person can be encouraging to one who is less confident. A new participant can be seated next to the leader to be introduced to the group.
- Use exercises and activities that encourage participants to look at one another, such as having them say an initial "hello" to the person seated next to them or tossing a balloon while calling out the name of the intended catcher.
- Promote socialization and friendship within your group. Participants are interested in each other's lives and experiences. For participants who have communication losses and cannot share their stories with others, if you know about their lives, ask whether they would like you to share their stories.
- Acknowledge the absence of any member. Other participants may wonder and worry about why someone is missing, even if they do not verbalize their concern. Remember that confidentiality is important. Check with the staff and the participant in question before sharing personal information about him or her.
- Always be honest so that participants learn to trust you.
- Be compassionate. If a participant is in the hospital, you could bring a get-well card to class for others to sign. Your concern gives participants the message that they are part of a community of caring people.
- Depending on the size of your group, you may want to celebrate birthdays. You can also celebrate other occasions, such as holidays and exercise accomplishments.

HOW TO SET UP A GROUP EXERCISE CLASS

Your responsibilities as a fitness leader begin before the first class meeting takes place. The following sections offer some tips for preparing for your class and some important issues to consider before teaching frail elderly participants and adults with special needs. After reviewing the setup, you should consider the organization and use of supplies and equipment. The final section can help you decide whether to use music in your class.

TIPS AND STRATEGIES FOR PREPARING THE CLASS

☐ Identify good candidates for participation in the class.

☐ Request physician's approval or physician's orders for each participant. A sample form for this purpose appears in appendix A2. The staff, the participant, or family members can assist you in filling out the cover letter and form to submit for the physician's approval and signature. Review the physician's recommendations with the participant. See chapter 2 for more details.

☐ Send an approval notice to the participant's family or responsible party if the participant is not living at home.

☐ Establish individual goals with each participant. See chapter 2 for more details.

☐ Keep a binder containing the medical clearance forms and "Fitness Leader's Log" (appendix A6) for all participants.

☐ Be familiar with specific recommendations and issues identified by the physician on the medical clearance form.

☐ Depending on the setting of your class, let the appropriate staff members know who will attend and what time the class starts. Some of your participants may need assistance with personal care or transportation before class.

☐ Remind participants (and any staff members who help them dress) to dress casually and wear athletic shoes or walking shoes.

☐ Have your attendance displays and informational materials ready for use.

From E. Best-Martini and K.A. Jones-DiGenova, 2014, *Exercise for frail elders*, 2nd ed. (Champaign, IL: Human Kinetics).

Handling Challenging Behaviors

The fitness leader's goal is to understand each participant's needs. In addition, the leader needs to step back and look closely at the group in its totality. This group is composed of many personalities, emotional needs and issues, physical needs, cognitive limitations, and mental health issues such as depression, apathy, and more. When leading a group, the leader has the group as the priority rather than the individual. The needs of the group versus the individual create the group dynamics. The group dynamics and group process help create a cohesiveness and culture in the group. Best-Martini, Weeks, and Wirth (2011) list some common challenges that require understanding, skill, and sensitivity from the leader:

Passivity

Anxiety

Lack of response

Loneliness

Feelings of uselessness

Cognitive losses

Apathy

Depression

Wandering

Hyperactivity

Confusion

Embarrassment

Low self-esteem

Dependency

Short attention span

Sensory losses

Anger

You may need to address in your class one or more of these issues, depending on the setting and the number of participants. Each of these challenges requires a response in either your attitude or your action as the leader. Your sensitivity will help you to determine the best response. Suppose that you are beginning a new exercise in your class. Five participants are not moving or responding to your verbal and physical cues. Before you jump to the conclusion that your teaching style is weak, look more closely at these individuals. They may not be responding because they are embarrassed, are passive by nature, are depressed, have low self-esteem, or have visual and auditory losses. Lack of participation may occur for many reasons. By getting to know your individual participants, you will be able to help them become more active and feel better about themselves.

The fitness leader needs to know as much as she or he can about each participant and then be responsible for creating the group experience. Participants look to the leader to take control, address behaviors or issues that arise, motivate, and always keep the group goals and procedures moving smoothly throughout the session. These management and teaching techniques are skills that take time to learn and master. Here are some tips:

- Create a positive environment. Consider the diversity of individuals' needs—to feel connected, get fit, learn, grow, share the experience, and have fun—as you create your fitness program.
- Be proactive. Intervene immediately when one person's behavior is distracting the focus from the group process.
- Be a clear communicator. Listen well and repeat verbal cues when necessary.
- Set your group goals and encourage participants to do their best at whatever level they are able. This approach is empowering.
- Remind the group that each person's opinions and input are important and should be respected. This reminder reduces potential personality conflicts within the group and sets the ground rules.

- Promote a buddy system so that social interaction begins to occur quickly.
- Be a good role model. Show respect and expect others to do the same.
- Come up with a personal plan for how you would deal with a variety of scenarios, because they always come up. Trading notes with experienced coworkers and colleagues can be helpful.
- Dealing directly with a behavior is always better than hoping that it will go away. Other participants will get worried and begin to lose confidence in the leader if problems are not addressed.
- If one participant always seems to take over with conversation or a behavior, talk to him or her after the class and see whether you can better understand the person and his or her needs. Sometimes this type of participant needs a leadership role to stay focused (taking attendance, greeting people as they enter, counting aloud with the leader).
- Interpret challenging behavior compassionately. Every behavior is a means of communication for people who are unable to communicate their needs or understand their environment.
- Create a safe and cohesive group. Some elderly participants have unresolved emotional issues. These issues turn into challenging behaviors with regressed elders. Find ways to help them feel safe and part of the group. This approach will help prevent challenging behaviors from arising.

Setting Up the Room and Supplies

The physical environment of your class needs to be looked at closely. A good room arrangement can enhance interaction between the participants and the fitness leader. Remember that environment is one of the components of a wellness program, because it has an effect on participants' overall well-being. We recommend that you create a chart of your room layout. Room setup varies with the size of the group. Figures 3.1 and 3.2 show various room setups. Figure 3.1 shows two schemes—the semicircle and open box—for setting up for a group of 15 or fewer participants; the chart in figure 3.2 is for more than 15 participants. We highly recommend an assistant or coinstructor for larger groups. See "Checklist for Setting Up the Furniture, Equipment, and Supplies" for further help in preparing your class site.

The list of equipment in appendix B4 offers ideas about the supplies and equipment that can work well for your group. As you add to your collection of exercise equipment and supplies, we recommend the purchase of a cart with wheels to store and transport them.

Resistance bands and tubes are inexpensive and safe resistance-training tools, but exercises that use these devices can be more challenging for the instructor to explain and demonstrate and for the participants to perform than exercises that use free weights. Resistance bands and tubes can be tied to wheelchair arms or bed rails for push-and-pull exercises. Bands and tubes come in at least three different resistances—light, medium, and heavy—and can be doubled up to increase the workload. Sponges of various sizes and shapes can be used to squeeze and grip for improving hand strength.

Vinyl-coated weights can be less intimidating than traditional metal dumbbells, especially for beginners, and their color coding allows easy weight identification. You can use these

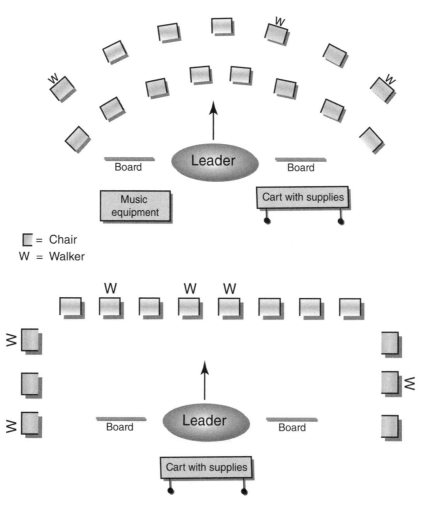

Figure 3.1 Room setup for 15 or fewer participants: (*a*) semicircle and (*b*) open box.

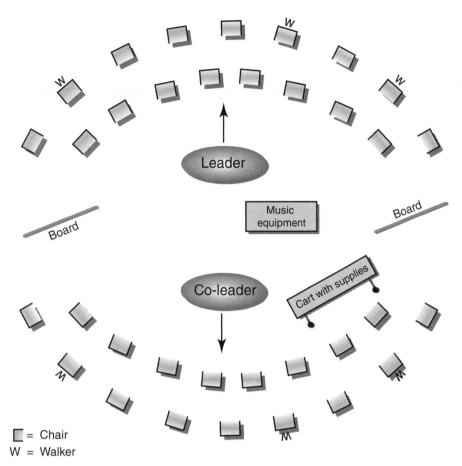

= Chair
W = Walker

Figure 3.2 Room setup for more than 15 participants.

colors to encourage participants' progress. For example, one possibility is to award a red ribbon for mastering a red weight. Be creative.

When your budget does not allow for conventional resistance-training equipment, you can make your own weights, such as a sock or glove filled with rice or sand. A long tube sock works best (knot the open end or tie the two ends together). Refer to appendix B4 for additional creative ideas.

If your work setting has a physical therapy department or medical supply office, the associated staff may be able to recommend additional resistance-training products and distributors. A medical supply office might be able to order soft surgical tubing, which can be cut into 5- or 6-foot lengths to be used as resistance tubes for push-and-pull exercises. The facility or instructor may purchase the equipment in some cases, or participants may pay for their own.

Deciding Whether to Use Music

Another important issue to consider is whether to use music during the exercise class. Music is optional. The decision to use music or not will be up to you as the fitness leader. Remember that safety and participant success should always come first in making this decision. Ask your participants whether they would like music during the class. If you decide to use music, ask the participants for their favorite types of music to help create a sense of community within your group.

Using music (appropriate for the group and component of exercise) offers several advantages:

- Music creates a welcoming environment.
- Music can set the mood.
- Music can motivate and bring a smile to the face of participants.

CHECKLIST FOR SETTING UP THE FURNITURE, EQUIPMENT, AND SUPPLIES

Furniture

☐ Have the room set up before participants arrive.

☐ Determine whether the chairs should have arms or no arms. This consideration is important for proper exercise technique and individual safety needs. Doing exercises in chairs without arms is easier, but participants with balance problems who are at high risk of falls may feel more secure in chairs with arms. Most fitness leaders need to be flexible and make do with the chairs available at the class site. Keep in mind that some of your participants will probably be seated in wheelchairs.

☐ Arrange chairs and remember to allow space for wheelchairs within the circle.

☐ Arrange the furniture so that participants are not looking into the sun or glare. Their backs should be to the window or light whenever possible.

☐ Arrange the furniture so that all participants can focus on the leader. You can sit in the middle of a circle, a semicircle, an open box group setup diagram (as illustrated in figures 3.1 and 3.2), or double circles, depending on the size of the group.

Equipment and Supplies

☐ Find a corner or other out-of-the-way location to store any walkers that will not be used. Many participants feel more secure knowing that their walkers are directly behind their chairs. A walker with brakes can make a good prop for some of the exercises; for example, it can facilitate the transition from sitting to standing.

☐ If you decide to use music, have the media close by so that you can change the music or lower the sound when needed. A sound system may already be set up at the site so that you do not need to bring your own equipment.

☐ Eliminate competing sights and sounds. If a television is in the room, be sure that both the sound and the picture are turned off.

☐ Set up all your visual props, such as a poster of muscles, attendance records, name of the group, inspirational pictures, or the exercise routine in large print. Display them in an uncluttered way. You can vary the visual props according to seasonal themes or the type of exercises that will be done.

☐ Focusing on an object at about eye level is a good technique for promoting balance. You can put a mark or line on the wall at a height of about 5 feet 2 inches to 5 feet 7 inches (160 to 170 cm) for those who stand while exercising. You can display a beautiful poster or picture for participants to focus on instead of a bare wall. These visual aids can also be used in the relaxation and visualization exercises found in chapter 7.

☐ Make a copy of the exercises in part II. You can place them on a clipboard for your reference while teaching.

☐ Keep exercise supplies and equipment in a convenient location so that you can pass them out safely and quickly when needed. Appendix B4 describes various types of equipment that can enhance your class.

☐ Place exercise equipment in a safe place not readily accessible to participants who could injure themselves by misusing it. You need to control the use of weights to ensure safety.

From E. Best-Martini and K.A. Jones-DiGenova, 2014, *Exercise for frail elders,* 2nd ed. (Champaign, IL: Human Kinetics).

- Music can awaken the spirit and energize participants with extreme limitations of movement. Even if they can move only their toes or fingers, they can tap along with the music.
- Music might be used during certain parts of the program but not others.
- Music adds variety to the exercise class.
- Music of a specific type fosters camaraderie among the people who helped select it.

Using music has some disadvantages as well:

- Music can be a distraction and can decrease attention span.
- Music can drown out your instructions to participants.
- Participants with hearing losses may find the music irritating when it is too loud or the pitch is too high.
- Some music can overstimulate participants who are trying to follow directions.
- Participants have different individual and cultural tastes in music. The music that one person may love to exercise to may be disliked by another.

If you decide to use music, we offer the following tips:

- You can play soft music or sounds of nature to welcome participants and begin the warm-up.
- Be sure that whatever type of music you use is in sync with the specific exercises. For example, music played during the welcome should be soft and inviting. The warm-up should have music with sustained, flowing sounds that encourage participants to take their time in their movements and to be aware of their breathing and posture. The aerobic component can use lively, faster-paced music. You might not play any music during the resistance-training component so that everyone can focus on counting and form. The cool-down should have relax-

ing music that again promotes slower movements.

- Many older adults favor music that was popular when they were in their teens and 20s for long-term reminiscing. People who have grown up with music, however, continue to appreciate and listen to new sounds. Do not limit yourself or your participants. If you decide to use music, take the opportunity to introduce new types of music so that participants feel more a part of today's world.
- Listen carefully to participant feedback and consider what the majority of participants want and enjoy.

Because of the variety of individual tastes, we do not recommend specific music. In the section "Media Resources, Music" in "Suggested Resources," we list some companies that you can contact for exercise music resources. In addition, you can create your own playlists from iTunes or listen to Pandora Playlists, which is an app for smart phones, iPods, and iPads.

OPENING YOUR EXERCISE CLASS

Begin each session with a welcome and a description of the upcoming exercise routine to give structure to the class. After the welcome, tell the participants what is to be covered in the class. This review can help alleviate participants' anxiety regarding exercising. Remind the group about the importance of safety. Safety comes first in all aspects of the exercise program. You can also use this time to educate participants about exercise, health, healthy lifestyles, prevention, and wellness. The following sections look at the welcome, safety, mobility, and education in more detail.

The Welcome

The welcome establishes the tone for your class and sets the stage for all group work. In addition to establishing rapport with your group, you can also use this time to observe each member and to detect individual needs.

Tips for the Welcome

- Always start the class with a welcome. You can greet each person individually by name and shake his or her hand. While welcoming each person, you can ask how he or she is feeling that day.

- While you are greeting participants, observe each person closely. Are they responsive to your greeting? Do they have their hearing aids on?

- Are there any new participants whom you have not met yet? Do they have medical clearance to participate? If not, you can encourage the participant to move through the range-of-motion component only and observe the rest of the class. Then, after class you both can talk about the medical clearance process and any special needs this person may have. Work with the person after class on the details of seeking medical clearance.

- Be observant. Does anyone appear to be sleepier than usual? Does anyone exhibit a change in mood or attitude? These are possible signs of emotional stress, new medications, or overmedication. They also are possible indicators of a change in medical status.

- Open the class with a friendly greeting, such as, "Welcome to our exercise class. I am happy to see each of you here today."

- You can begin the class by announcing the day's inspirational or fitness theme or simply the date.

Physiological and emotional changes frequently go unnoticed by those who work with frail elders and adults with special needs. Your observations can make all the difference in avoiding an emergency. This point brings us to the importance of safety.

Focus on Safety

Safety is the cornerstone of any good exercise program. Every aspect of your fitness class or program is based on a clear understanding of safety issues. A major role of the leader is to instill this focus on safety in the participants. While you have everyone's attention during the welcoming phase of the class, use this opportunity to remind them about safety during the class.

Safety Reminders

- Remind participants about the importance of good posture.

- Remind participants to follow you closely to ensure that they are using proper exercise techniques.

- Remind participants to breathe continuously during all exercises.

- Remind participants to cease exercise immediately if they experience any pain.

- Remind participants who need assistance with getting in and out of a chair to ask for help before getting up.

- Remind participants to go at their own pace and not to feel that they need to compete with others.

- Remind participants to be aware of one another while exercising in a crowded space.

- Remind participants to put exercise equipment and supplies in a safe location so that no one will trip over them.

Safety is important both within and outside the class. Your goal is to emphasize the importance of everyday safety to participants. Outside class, safety concerns are related to walking, transferring from a chair to a walker, navigating steps and stairs, and eliminating fall risks in the home environment. Refer to chapter 2 for a review of general exercise safety guidelines and the "Safety Guidelines Checklist."

Mobility and Transfer Issues

Your involvement in mobility and transfer issues will vary according to the site that you are working in. In most licensed settings you will be walking only with participants cleared by staff as being safe to ambulate. Never assume that a participant has good mobility skills. Check with staff. In addition, in a licensed setting you will not transfer participants from a wheelchair to a chair unless given approval or training by staff. Check with staff for specific protocols.

Wheelchairs

Some or many participants joining your exercise class will be using wheelchairs, walkers, or canes. Depending on the setting, you may want a participant to transfer or be assisted with a transfer from his or her wheelchair to a chair during the class. You should never attempt to transfer a participant from a wheelchair to a chair unless you have been trained in transfer techniques and have received approval to do so.

If the participant states that she or he is able to transfer independently, be sure to clarify with a staff member that the participant has both the ability and approval to do so. This practice will lessen the potential for accidents or falls.

If the participant stays in the wheelchair during class, be aware of the following:

1. Allow more space between chairs in the circle.
2. Be sure that the wheelchair brakes are locked before the participant starts exercising.
3. Remove leg rests (if any).
4. Be aware that some upper-body movements and exercises may be limited from a full range of motion because of the wheelchair arms and wheels.
5. When possible and safe, have the participant in a regular chair because the goal is to maintain or improve functional fitness.

Walkers

You will often have to walk by the side of someone with a walker and stand by to assist in terms of assuring that the chair is well situated and that the participant can navigate the surrounding space. Here are a few safety reminders for walkers in the classroom:

1. Keep the walker close to the participant or within view so that he or she can see where it is. Walkers are the key to independence for those who need them. Be sensitive to this issue.
2. Be sure to observe how the participant uses the walker. Ideally, you should have a refresher class on proper positioning and use of a walker. If physical therapists or restorative aides are present at your setting, ask for a short in-service on this topic.
3. If many of the walkers look alike, consider adding a name tag or some visual tag like a license with the participant's name to differentiate walkers.
4. The walker can be used as an exercise prop or aide to help a participant get up and out of a chair, and a walker is particularly useful with standing exercises. Place the walker in a convenient location in front of the participant's chair and provide standby assist (one-on-one assistance) when possible. The Modified Chair Stand (exercise 5.12), a key functional resistance exercise, can be a good starting point for introducing standing exercises using a walker for assistance.

Canes

Canes come in many styles according to need and adaptability. Canes should be placed in the corner of the room or against a sidewall. Canes can cause significant accidents if they are improperly placed or leaned against furniture. If not properly placed during class, they are easy to trip on and can cause injury.

Prevent accidents and falls in your classroom. Focus on safety with equipment at all times. Next, we will focus on another valuable aspect for your fitness class—educating your participants.

Focus on Education

Schedule time in your exercise class outline for an educational component. The welcome, opening section, or closing section of the class are good opportunities for a focus on education. Take time to help participants fully understand the role that they play in improving their functional fitness and independence. This understanding is created through education.

Education affects individual behaviors and builds the motivation that is needed to change a sedentary lifestyle. By seeing improvements in physical endurance and strength, participants can begin to see themselves as active and vital people. Their lifestyles and attitudes can improve dramatically. This personal perspective is extremely important for you to take into account.

We recommend that you provide your class with information about fitness, wellness (the constant, deliberate effort to stay healthy physically and emotionally to achieve the highest potential for well-being), and healthy lifestyle issues. You might want to cover a specific topic over several classes, such as improving balance and fall prevention. Remember to cover only topics that are within your scope of practice and expertise. In addition, be sure that your educational references, recommended readings, and handouts are current and appropriate

for your client base. "Suggested Resources" at the end of this book can be used to identify for reputable references.

Table 3.1 offers some topics for your focus on education. We have included useful and informative material throughout the book that can be used as handouts, including the following:

- Figure 1.1, Frailty
- Table 1.1, Common Medical Disorders
- Figure 2.1, The wellness tree
- Figure 2.3, Good sensation versus bad sensation, or pain
- Figure 2.4, Tips for responding to bad sensation, or pain
- Table 5.1, Common Myths and Facts About Resistance Training
- Table 5.2, General Resistance-Training Guidelines for Older Adults
- Table 6.2, General Aerobic-Training Guidelines for Older Adults
- Table 7.2, General Stretching Guidelines
- Appendix B2, "Muscles of the Human Body"

Table 3.1 Educational Topics for Fitness and Wellness

Topic	Activity
Diet and nutrition	During the class, take a break to drink water. During the break, discuss the importance of diet and hydration.
Stress	While leading the stretching portion of the exercise program, discuss why relaxation is beneficial and how it helps decrease stress and anxiety. Refer to chapter 4 (the sections on deep three-part breathing) and chapter 7 for more information. Remind participants to breathe deeply for stress reduction. Bring an inspirational quote to each class.
Physiological and psychological benefits of exercise	Use appendix B1 to reinforce instruction about the benefits of exercise.
Healthy lifestyles	Have a theme for each class, such as staying active mentally and physically, sleeping well, or making the home environment safer.
Wellness model	See figure 2.1 for this model. This is a good time to talk about all of the things in our lives and lifestyle that work together to keep us well. The wellness tree is a good visual reminder that we want to focus on all aspects of our health.
Muscle anatomy	Have participants get to know all the muscle groups that the exercises work. Appendix B2 offers a visual aid for you and your participants.

Many participants will take educational handouts with them and review them further. These handouts reinforce the information that you discuss during the exercise class.

LEADING YOUR EXERCISE CLASS

We want to present some tips and strategies that can help you successfully lead a class for frail elders and adults with special needs. The three-step instructional process (table 3.2) gives you a structure in which to teach exercises safely and effectively. This technique is a foundation; later in this chapter we present specific tips and strategies for teaching participants with communication, cognitive, and sensory losses. In addition, you will find tips and strategies for adding balance, core stability, and agility exercises to the routine in chapter 2.

Three-Step Instructional Process

The three-step instructional process helps you lead exercise for frail elders and adults with special needs safely and effectively.

In step 1 you demonstrate and describe each exercise. In step 2 you observe and evaluate your participants as they follow your lead. In step 3 you give your participants constructive, positive feedback (verbal or nonverbal instruction, assistance, and recommendations) as they continue to follow your lead. Feedback (step 3) can also be given between exercises. Steps

1 through 3 flow naturally together. While applying these steps, pay attention to how your participants learn best.

Step 1: Demonstrate and Describe

Describe how to do the exercise as you demonstrate it. Choose words that enable your participants to feel successful. For example, say, "Move your elbows toward each other," instead of saying, "Move your elbows together." Questions that are sensitive to your audience can be an effective way to describe how to do the exercise. For example, say, "How close can you comfortably move your elbows toward each other?" Keep your instruction positive and encouraging: "The farther apart your elbows are from touching, the more potential you have for improvement." "Notice how your elbows get closer over time."

Demonstrate every exercise with proper technique and speed. Avoid the temptation to do a speedy demonstration. Remember, you are modeling the exercise (showing how to perform it). If any of your participants has trouble following you, demonstrate the exercise without words, not even counting. Always keep those participants dealing with visual impairments as close to you, the leader, as possible.

In beginning classes and for new participants or people with poor carryover skills (those unable to apply or carry over techniques previously learned), such as those with memory

Table 3.2 Three-Step Instructional Process

Step 1. Demonstrate and describe the ABCs of each exercise.
Action
Breathing and other safety tips
Counting

Step 2. Observe and evaluate (SEE each participant).
Safety precautions
Exercise technique
Each individual's needs

Step 3. Give group and individual feedback.
Verbal
Visual nonverbal
Physical nonverbal

loss, follow these *ABCs* to demonstrate and describe exercises:

• **Action**. Briefly describe and demonstrate the exercise technique: the start position, highlights of the movement phase, and the finish position, which is always the same as the start position. Chapters 4 through 7 provide insight regarding exercise. The arrows in the photographs of these chapters indicate the direction of movement for each exercise.

• **Breathing and other safety tips**. Briefly describe safety tips as you continue demonstrating (which are highlighted for each exercise in the "Exercise and Safety Tips" of the "Illustrated Instruction" sections in chapters 4 through 7). Also, we encourage you to review the general safety guidelines in chapter 2. Two important safety criteria are correct posture and breathing. Teach your participants good posture and proper breathing, particularly not holding their breath. Your participants cannot hold their breath if they are counting aloud. Therefore, have them count aloud, especially in beginning classes and large groups where it

is not possible for you to check each participant's breathing.

• **Counting**. Demonstrate the exercise about two more times as you count aloud. Counting varies with different types of exercise. Table 3.3 summarizes how and why to count with warm-ups, resistance training, aerobics, and stretching exercises. Participants need to count aloud during resistance exercises because breath holding during those exercises presents a higher risk of increasing a participant's blood pressure. If participants are counting aloud, you know that they cannot be holding their breath. Counting keeps participants engaged and can create a lively atmosphere. Count in the dominant language of the group or have the participants take turns counting in their primary language.

After participants become familiar with the pace of the exercises by counting, instruct them to focus on their breathing instead of counting. If participants get off rhythm, recommend that they resume counting aloud. Remind your participants to count if you regularly have new

Table 3.3 How Counting Varies Among the Different Components of Exercise

Components	Repetitions	How to count[a]	Why count
Warm-up	3–8	"1, and, 2, and, 3, and . . ." "1, and" = 1 repetition = 2 seconds.	For slow and smooth pacing
Resistance training	8–15	"1, 1, 1, up, 1, 1, 1, down, 2, 2, 2, up, . . ." (or out and in instead of up and down). "1, 1, 1, up" = 1 repetition = about 6–8 seconds.	For slow and smooth pacing To ensure that participants are not holding their breath
Aerobics	1 or more	Varies according to the type and beat of the music.	To get and keep the pace
Stretching	1	Count silently or visually with the second hand of a clock. Stretches are held for 10 to 30 seconds (the same count on each side), except neck stretches, which are held only 5 seconds per side.	To start and stop the stretch

[a]First, announce the number of repetitions of each exercise. Then count the repetitions of each exercise aloud, except for stretching.

participants or lead a large group without an assistant.

You will develop your own style of counting for each exercise component. For instance, you can look at the second hand of a clock to time a stretching exercise rather than counting aloud for a quieter, more relaxing atmosphere. Do what works best for you and your participants.

During step 2, observing and evaluating, counting can be a distraction for the instructor. You should initially count aloud, however, to get the participants started. If the participants' counting fades during the exercise or if you notice anyone not counting, resume counting aloud with the participants.

If you do not have new participants in your class, you might use less demonstration and description of the exercises as your participants become more experienced. When they know the exercises, try skipping step 1. At that time, you can use just steps 2 and 3. Individuals with poor carryover skills need at least a short demonstration and description of the exercises at every class.

Step 2: Observe and Evaluate

After a demonstration and description of the exercise (step 1), have participants follow you in performing the exercise. Observe and evaluate each participant. When observing and evaluating, pay attention to these areas, which you can remember by the acronym *SEE:*

*S*afety precautions: Observe to ensure that participants are following general and specific safety guidelines for each exercise.

*E*xercise technique: Observe the technique.

*E*ach individual's needs: Observe how this exercise addresses each participant's health needs and fitness goals (when possible).

The performance of your class determines the need for further cueing. No two classes are the same. You may have time to evaluate only the first two areas, especially if you are a new instructor or your participants are beginner exercisers. As you become more comfortable teaching the exercises and as your participants become more experienced, you can begin to consider each person's needs in your evaluation. Do your best to make time at the beginning of class to find out how your participants are feeling, and find out how they responded to the exercises at the end of class. If possible, let them know other times when you are available to discuss questions or concerns.

Step 3: Provide Feedback

After your observation and evaluation of the class, as participants continue the exercise to its completion, give them feedback based on your observation and evaluation. The three types of feedback are verbal, visual nonverbal, and physical nonverbal.

Verbal Feedback

Keep your verbal feedback clear, concise, and positive. Be specific. Here are some examples of verbal feedback:

- Remind participants to count and not to hold their breath: "Mr. Judd, remember to count with us so that we all keep the same pace."
- Ask pertinent questions to inspire active participation: "Does anyone know what leg muscle helps us get up out of a chair? The quadriceps helps us get up, and that is why the leg march exercise is so important."
- Acknowledge what they are doing well (individually or as a group): "Look at how much farther Mr. Judd can move through this exercise. What an improvement! Good work!" "Remember when we had a hard time completing 15 minutes of exercise? Now we are exercising for more than an hour. This is great progress!"
- Adjust the pace or rhythm: "Let's slow down our pace as we get ready to start our stretches."

• Motivate your participants to perform their best: "Let's look at this attendance board. It shows us how long we have been exercising together. It also shows us that each of you has progressed from 1-pound weights to 3- and 5-pound weights. Fantastic!"

Visual Nonverbal Feedback

When giving visual nonverbal cues, make sure that all your participants can see you. Here are some examples of visual nonverbal feedback:

• Demonstrate further from a different position or location.
• Show illustrations, such as a muscle anatomy chart (such as appendix B2).
• Speed up or slow down your performance to adjust the pace or rhythm.
• Motivate your participants to perform their best by gestures such as clapping or a thumbs-up.

Physical Nonverbal Feedback

When giving physical nonverbal cues, remember to touch a participant only after he or she has given you permission. Here are some examples of physical nonverbal feedback:

• Gently assist a participant through the exercise. (Try using verbal or visual nonverbal cues first.)
• Adjust equipment.
• Motivate your participants to perform their best by physical acknowledgments such as a pat on the back. Although physical touch can be nurturing for older adults, especially those living alone, be cognizant that not everyone feels comfortable with physical touch.

You can also give feedback between exercises. Beginning classes need more feedback between exercises as participants learn safety precautions and proper exercise technique. The pace of the class is slower, which helps prevent overexertion. As your participants become more experienced, minimize feedback

between exercises to maximize exercise time. Ultimately, you can flow gracefully from one exercise to the next.

You should only interrupt your leading of the exercise to give participants feedback when the benefits of assisting individual participants outweigh the benefits of remaining in front of the class. Use your best judgment. As your participants learn exercises, they benefit greatly from one-on-one attention. If you have an assistant or coleader, you have more opportunity to help your participants individually.

Leadership can be seen as a dialogue. For this dialogue to take place, people must be able to understand and respond to each other, which requires listening well and the ability to understand and interpret the words spoken. This dialogue becomes a challenge if any of the participants are dealing with communication losses, cognitive losses, or sensory losses. For participants with these losses, nonverbal descriptions and dialogue can be as important as or more important than verbal descriptions and dialogue. But if someone has had a stroke with paralysis on the left side, rely more on verbal instructions, using fewer gestures (American Senior Fitness Association 2012c). Both your verbal and nonverbal communication skills need to be direct and clear to the participant. Let's look at strategies for teaching participants with communication, cognitive, and sensory losses.

Teaching Participants With Communication Losses

Participants who have communication losses, such as aphasia, require both verbal and nonverbal cues from the leader. They may understand but not be able to express their thoughts (expressive aphasia), or they may not be able to understand or interpret information (receptive aphasia). Some participants may experience both receptive and expressive aphasia (global aphasia). Such participants comprehend best with a multisensory approach. For a multisensory approach, you need to use visual and tactile aides to clarify directions and to provide physical, visual, and verbal cuing. Nonverbal and multisensory approaches help participants understand and learn better. Here are some communication strategies to incorporate into your leadership style.

- Keep good eye contact with the participants. They need to see your demonstration and hear your directions.
- Repeat directions and information.
- Add nonverbal cues.
- Use your facial expressions and positive nods of your head to reinforce a job well done.
- Treat each participant as an intelligent person.
- Participants dealing with communication losses may look closely for visual cues and reinforcers. Be sure that you are a good model for them. Look professional and always wear athletic shoes and appropriate attire. Avoid too many contrasting colors in your outfits. It may be difficult to see you and your cues if your outfit looks too busy.
- Give participants time to respond to you. It may take them a little longer.
- Try to eliminate distractions in the surrounding environment while you are trying to communicate. Extraneous noises and activity can decrease participants' comprehension.
- Avoid using any language or form of communication that may seem demeaning to participants, such as referring to them with endearments.
- Speak to participants as you would to a friend in conversation but maintain a professional demeanor.

Teaching Participants With Cognitive Losses

Most settings that have frail elders and adults with special needs include someone who has some cognitive loss (an inability to perform normal cognitive functions, such as judgment,

problem solving, communication, interpretation of environmental stimuli, memory, abstract thought, and paying attention). People with cognitive losses respond well to multisensory instruction because the sensory memory is the most intact.

Here are some leadership strategies for teaching participants with cognitive losses:

- Treat each participant as an intelligent person. Cognition is only a small part of who we are. People with cognitive losses still have many skills and talents.
- Smile and help all participants feel welcome.
- Keep your directions simple.
- Slow down your conversation, maintaining a respectful tone of voice and a suitable tempo for the exercises.
- Make good eye contact and remember that nonverbal cues work well.
- Use many colorful visual props. They add the element of fun, which helps participants reduce their anxiety regarding their ability to understand directions in addition to encouraging attention.
- Repetition reinforces learning and is a successful strategy when working with people with any level of memory loss.
- Provide structure and routine in each session. This continuity helps participants retain information.
- Allow extra time for participants with cognitive losses to respond to questions or directions. They may need longer. Practice patience.
- Keep the environment as uncluttered and quiet as possible to keep it from being overstimulating.
- Give participants a lot of positive feedback.
- Provide cueing when needed.
- Break down instructions and exercises into smaller steps to make them easier to understand and follow. This strategy is called task segmentation. The steps are

then added together to perform the complete task. Task segmentation can be used to teach new skills or forgotten skills.

- Be aware that many participants can no longer retain a learned skill from class to class. You may need to teach the same skills and exercises repeatedly, because they may seem new to some people with cognitive losses.

- Remember that participants with cognitive losses want to communicate normally and that they feel frustrated when they struggle with words.

The cueing strategies in table 3.4 have proved successful in teaching participants with cognitive losses. Table 3.4 also provides some examples of implementing these strategies.

Teaching Participants With Sensory Losses

Some of your participants may have sensory losses. Besides undergoing the normal physiologic changes of aging, many elderly people experience a loss of one or more of the five senses (sight, hearing, taste, touch, and smell). The most noticeable sensory losses affect sight and hearing, but less obvious sensory losses are still significant. A participant may have a loss of sensation in the hands and feet, and you need to know this. A person with a sensory loss may feel removed from the experience enjoyed by other participants. Participants with sensory losses need clear directions and visual or auditory reinforcements. Here are some leadership strategies for teaching participants with sensory losses:

- Use gestures and physical examples of what you verbally describe. The gestures need to be dramatic to emphasize the directions. The gestures can include facial expressions.

- Always check to be sure that participants are wearing their glasses or hearing aids.

- Seat participants with visual or hearing losses near you.

Table 3.4   Cueing Strategies for Teaching Participants With Cognitive Losses

Cueing technique	Example
Visual demonstration	Demonstrate the exercise for the participant. Look directly at the participant and speak clearly and simply. Be sure that you make eye contact and encourage the participant to mirror, or copy, your movements. Perform the visual demonstration slowly.
Verbal prompts	Clearly state to the participant how to do the exercise: "Mr. Williams, move your fingers as if you are playing the piano."
Physical prompts	Physically initiate the movement for the participant. Always ask permission before physically touching a participant: "Mr. Williams, may I help lift your arms to get you started?"
Physical assistance	Physically assist the participant with the exercise. This type of cueing helps move the participant through the exercise even if he or she is unable to perform it alone. This step is a hand-over-hand movement in which the leader assists the participant with her or his hands. "Mr. Williams, look how we are playing the piano together hand in hand." Always ask permission before physically touching a participant.
Feedback	Give immediate feedback and reinforcement for the exercise and interaction. "Well done, Mr. Williams. Thank you for participating with me."

Adapted from R.P. Katsinas, 1995, *Excess disability*. Presented at American Therapeutic Recreation Society Conference, Louisville, KY.

- Show large illustrations of specific exercises as a visual aid. The illustrations of specific exercises found in chapters 4 through 7 can be enlarged for this purpose.
- Provide exercise props that help reinforce the movements and techniques. Scarves and resistance bands help reinforce movements. Scarves are also colorful sensory enhancers. Pinwheels can be used during breathing exercises to help participants see their breath at work.
- Write the names of the muscles and the exercise on a large board. Have participants read and repeat them to reinforce the information.
- The loss of sensation (touch) can leave participants unaware of a region of their bodies, so always be sure to focus on the area that is moving, such as a leg, an arm, or the fingers. Encourage participants to touch this part to enhance body awareness and circulation.

CLOSING YOUR EXERCISE CLASS

The closure of the class is as important as the opening and welcome. Just as you began the class with a warm welcome and acknowledgment of individual participants, you address some closing remarks to the group and some to each participant individually. After the participants have said good-bye and the class is formally over, you still have some additional items to complete.

The Closing

The closing of the group should be integrated naturally into the framework of the exercise class. The final component of an exercise class, the cool-down, is intended to slow down the pace, stretch the muscles, and encourage participants to relax. While cooling down and encouraging relaxation, your voice should soften but still be audible to those hard of hearing. Some participants may be looking forward to the end of the class, whereas others may wish that the group could stay together longer. Remember that some of your participants attend for the social and emotional connections rather than physical exercise. You should establish a clear signal that the class is about to end. This signal is important to provide structure, especially for participants with sensory or cognitive losses. Here are some tips for closing the group.

- After the relaxation segment, look around the group and acknowledge the efforts of each participant.
- Thank everyone for coming and participating.
- Review safety and educational tips. Ask the participants if they have any questions or areas that need further review.
- Be sure to address progress and accomplishments. Positive feedback is important.
- Remind participants of the next session date and time. Remind participants about any specific exercises that you recommend they do before the next session.
- After you officially close the group, begin to assist individual participants. Some participants may need you to get their walkers, which may have been placed behind the chairs or to the side of the room. Always check the name to be sure that participants are walking away with the correct walkers, canes, and personal belongings.
- Complete the attendance board chart while the group is still together (if you are using one).
- Be sure that you have collected all supplies, weights, water bottles, and towels.
- Look around to ensure that no one has forgotten any personal adaptive devices or equipment.
- If you are playing music, keep it on low until all participants have left.

- You want all participants to leave feeling positive about the experience, themselves, and you. The success that they feel will motivate them to return. As a fitness leader, you can help participants feel successful by giving positive and clear feedback.

Feedback

One of your most important roles as the fitness leader is to give feedback to your participants. The frail elderly and those with special needs are often unaware of their progress, especially if they are insecure about or lack confidence in their physical abilities. They need someone else's verbal reinforcement to help them see how well they are doing.

Feedback can be both general and individual. General feedback is for the entire class; for example, you might say, "In the past 2 months, each of you has gained flexibility. We can see this when we compare your arm flexibility with the initial pretest." Individual feedback pertains to one participant; for example, you might say, "Ms. Jones, I wanted to comment on how much improvement I see in your ability to complete the balance exercises without holding onto the chair." The feedback that you give needs to be specific and concrete, and you should give it when you observe a change or improvement. By doing so, you can correct improper form before it becomes a habit. Individual feedback can also be given one on one after class. Use this approach for participants who are easily embarrassed in the group setting.

The progress of some of your participants may seem slow and, at times, doubtful. If a participant feels discouraged, he or she should look first at the length of his or her involvement in the class. You can keep count on a board or form how many sessions he or she has attended and mention the progress reflected on the board. Your feedback thus moves from general to the individual's own progress. Even having a new board is a positive statement for the individual participants

and the group as a whole. These boards also reflect changes in fitness. Sometimes just reviewing and reminding participants about their improvements helps them see that they are meeting fitness goals. Newer participants can feel encouraged with the results that they see in other members.

Another way of providing feedback and tracking progress is to take photographs at different times. One of our participants, Anita, had a right-side cerebrovascular accident (stroke) that affected her entire left side. When Anita started the exercise class, she had no movement in her left arm. We encouraged her to keep a soft ball in her left hand and try to squeeze it. She also moved her left arm with her right hand during exercises. After 6 months, she was feeling discouraged and saw no improvement. We were able to show her before and after photos that told the story better than any words could have. Her left arm was moving through almost 90 percent range of motion, compared with no range of motion at the beginning.

All feedback needs to be honest and genuine. Be aware that some people do not take suggestions well. Always focus on the positive and acknowledge improvement. Then mention any recommendations and finish with a compliment. This format balances progress made in the past with goals to work toward in the future.

Finishing Touches: Organizing Supplies and Taking Attendance

Your class is over for the day. After helping participants gather their belongings and saying good-bye, you are now ready for the finishing touches: reorganizing the supplies, cleaning them with an antibacterial spray or cloth, and taking attendance for the day. The ideal approach is to take attendance while participants are present, which can be an extrinsic reward and motivator. But you might complete more detailed attendance logs after the official ending of the class or after organizing the supplies and equipment. Attendance records may include dates, attendance, and exercise details, such as length of aerobic component, sets, repetitions, and weights used (see appendix B5, "Fitness Training Log").

You have many things to remember that you may want to jot down. But first, take care of the physical environment and supplies. See "Finishing Touches Checklist" for things to do after class. Some participants will be willing and able to assist with finishing touches.

SUMMARY

This chapter is for and about you, the fitness leader. Success as a fitness leader begins with creating a sense of fun and community within your group. Participants join an exercise class for a variety of reasons. Some come to exercise, whereas others are looking for new friends. You, as the leader, create an environment that can nurture friendships and social support. Never forget the importance of fun. Fun brings back the enjoyment of new experiences and the rapture of being human.

Another important responsibility is setting up the group exercise class, from setting up the room and organizing the supplies and equipment to deciding whether or not to use music. This point may seem simplistic to the new leader, but the experienced leader knows that good organization is one of the bases for a successful class experience. Your participants will feel more secure and confident in you when they can see that you are well prepared.

Next, we discussed helpful tips and strategies for opening your class. We all know that first impressions are important. Many of your participants will feel nervous or anxious about starting to exercise. You need to make them feel welcome and begin to build their confidence. Your participants look to you as a role model and for guidance, support, and consistency. Your safety and educational reminders during the class reinforce the exercise and its relationship to functional skills needed in their everyday lives.

Successfully leading an exercise class starts with a safe and effective instructional plan. The three-step instructional process works hand in hand with the more specific tips and strategies for teaching participants with communication, cognitive, and sensory losses. In addition, we offered tips and strategies for balance, core stability, agility, and fall prevention. These techniques have been successful in our work with frail elderly participants and adults with special needs for many years.

Finally, we presented helpful tips and strategies for closing your exercise class. You can use this time to give feedback both to the group and to individual participants. The "Finishing Touches Checklist" that you read provides tips

---

FINISHING TOUCHES CHECKLIST

☐ After the participants have departed, organize the supplies and equipment. You should have an inventory sheet that itemizes everything you brought to class. Ensure that each item is accounted for.

☐ Supplies and weights used in the class should be sprayed down with a mixture of equal parts water and alcohol (exception: resistance bands and tubes). Place them on a towel and leave them to dry while you organize the other supplies. All supplies should be clean, properly stored, and ready for the next class.

☐ Depending on the setting of your exercise class, time between activity groups may be limited. Be sure to give your participants ample time to depart and yourself ample time to get organized before the next event.

From E. Best-Martini and K.A. Jones-DiGenova, 2014, *Exercise for frail elders*, 2nd ed. (Champaign, IL: Human Kinetics).

and strategies for organizing after your class and preparing for the next class.

You have come to the end of part I, which has given you essential information about the participant, the exercise program, and the leader for planning a successful exercise program for frail elders and adults with special needs. In Part II you will learn the fine points for implementing a safe and effective exercise program, including warm-up (posture, breathing, range-of-motion, and stretching exercises), resistance training, aerobic training and dynamic balance, and cool-down stretching and relaxation. Answer the following review questions. We encourage you to redo the ones from chapters 1 and 2 to discover what you remember and to identify areas to review. Focus on fun!

REVIEW QUESTIONS

1. List four tips for setting up a group exercise class.

2. Identify one reason that music might not be a good addition to the class.

3. List the steps of the three-step instructional process.

4. T or F. It is only appropriate for you to interrupt your leading of the exercise to give an individual feedback when the benefits of assisting an individual outweigh the benefits of remaining in front of the class.

5. Participants with _____ aphasia may understand but not be able to express their thoughts. Participants with _____ aphasia may not be able to receive or understand information clearly. Participants with _____ aphasia may experience deficits in both receiving and expressing themselves.

6. _____ loss is defined as an inability to perform normal thought processes, such as judgment, problem solving, communication, interpretation of environmental stimuli, memory, abstract thought, and paying attention.

7. List three leadership techniques that will help you communicate with a participant dealing with visual losses.

Part II

Implementing an Exercise Program for Frail Elders and Adults With Special Needs

In chapters 4 through 7 you will learn how to teach warm-up (posture, breathing, range-of-motion, and light stretching), resistance, aerobic and dynamic balance, and cool-down (comprehensive stretching and relaxation) exercises for frail elders and adults with special needs. Along with the exercises are specific teaching instructions to get you started and variations and progression options (VPOs) to keep your exercise classes interesting and progressive for repeat participants. Each exercise has a seated position and a standing variation. Many adults with special needs are able to stand but not get up off the floor; therefore, floor exercises are not included. In chapter 8 you will learn how to put warm-up, resistance, aerobic and dynamic balance, and cool-down exercises together into a safe and effective fitness program. A primary goal of this exercise program is to promote functional fitness. Remember that functional fitness is the ability to perform activities of daily living such as pushing, pulling, lifting, squatting, balancing, and sitting and standing erect that enhance well-being and quality of life. Although part II of the book is geared toward class or group instruction, the information is also useful when working one on one with this population. Thus, the terms *student*, *client*, *resident*, and *patient* can be used interchangeably with *participant*, and *session* and *appointment* can be used interchangeably with *class*, the term used throughout part II.

Chapters 4 through 7 cover the following topics:

- **Safety precautions**—general and specific for individuals with special needs
- **Exercise guidelines**—evidence based, with additional recommendations for target population
- **Basic seated exercises**—24 ROM, 12 resistance, 12 aerobic and dynamic balance, and 12 stretching
- **Basic standing exercises**—a significant step for progressing and varying a functional fitness program

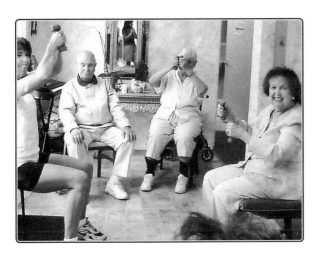

- **Variations and progression options**—for each of the basic seated exercises
- **Illustrated instruction**—a step by step instructional guide to the exercises

Chapter 8 shows you how to take all the tools you've gained from chapters 4 through 7 and create fun, varied, and progressive exercise routines for one person to a class full of challenging individuals.

BASIC SEATED EXERCISES

The basic seated exercises are ideal for people just beginning an exercise program, particularly those in wheelchairs or who are at risk of falling when they stand. You will find an even easier variation of some of the basic seated exercises in "Variations and Progression Options." All 60 exercises can be performed in wheelchairs or chairs with or without arms. Chairs without arms, however, are preferable if they are safe for a participant, because they allow greater range of motion of the limbs. Also, a chair with a vertical, straight back can aid the participant in achieving proper posture. These exercises are also ideal for instructors, both beginning and experienced, who are getting to know their participants' strengths and limitations. Seated exercises minimize concerns over participants' falling. As participants improve their functional fitness with the seated exercises, they also improve their ability and stamina for standing exercises.

BASIC STANDING EXERCISES

Each basic seated exercise has a standing alternative that can replace the seated one, be alternated with it, or be taught at the same time to accommodate a class of participants with diverse needs. In chapter 8 you will find out when to implement standing exercises, benefits of standing exercises, when seated exercise are preferred over standing exercises, and advantages of teaching the seated and standing exercises simultaneously. Despite participants' level of fitness, it is easier to initiate an exercise class or program with everyone seated and then progress toward standing exercises at a comfortable pace as you learn about their strengths and current limitations. Of the countless options, you may choose to lead one exercise component, such as the warm-up, in the seated position and then lead the rest in the standing position.

When a participant is ready to do standing exercises, he or she can start with one or two and gradually progress to as many as comfortable. Even participants who are generally capable of performing all standing exercises have the option of doing some or all seated instead, especially if they feel unusually fatigued or unsteady on their feet. Participants can sit down anytime, even in the middle of an exercise, and rejoin the others who are doing the seated exercises and stand again when they are ready.

You will find the standing exercises in the illustrated instruction sections for each basic seated exercise at the end of chapters 4 through 7 in the variation and progression options sections.

VARIATIONS AND PROGRESSION

Chapters 4 through 7 provide several variations and progression options (VPOs) in the illustrated instruction sections for each of the basic seated 24 range-of-motion, 12 resistance, 12 aerobic and dynamic balance, and 12 stretching exercises. We recommend that you introduce these exercises after your participants have learned the basic seated exercises, with the exception of the easier variations. Some classes—for example, a large class without an assistant in a long-term care facility—may offer limited opportunity for extensive progression (progressively more challenging exercise), but varying the basic seated exercises can add pizzazz to your class. Other classes may outgrow seated exercises and progress to the standing VPOs that offer participants the greatest benefits for functional mobility and increased independence. The variations and progression options enable you to be creative and flexible with a functional fitness program over the years and to meet participants' special needs. Additionally, in chapter 8 you will find many other ideas for varying and progressing the exercises.

ILLUSTRATED INSTRUCTION GUIDE

The instruction guides at the end of chapters 4 through 7 have a consistent, reader-friendly format for illustrating and describing each basic seated exercise:

- A concise description and photographs of the exercise
- Exercise and safety tips
- Variations and progression options

A photograph and description is provided for standing exercises and other VPOs that need further explanation. Also, you will find this new balance symbol in this second edition in the VPOs of chapters 4 through 7 to help you quickly identify the exercises that enhance balance.

PUTTING THE EXERCISES TOGETHER

In the final chapter, you will discover how to put it all together into a safe and effective exercise program (or just a session or class) to promote functional fitness that incorporates one or more exercise component—warm-up, resistance training, aerobic training and dynamic balance activities, and cool-down (stretching and relaxation)—from chapters 4 through 7. You will also learn how to design, schedule, modify, progress or maintain, and monitor a smart functional fitness program for people with diverse special needs and levels of fitness.

Chapter 8 gives other practical information for orchestrating a functional fitness class, such as

- how to extend a single warm-up, resistance-training, aerobics, balance, stretching, or relaxation component into an entire class;
- how to determine when a participant is ready for standing exercises;
- when seated exercises are preferred over standing ones;
- how to teach the seated and standing exercise at the same time;
- when to introduce intermediate-level (challenger) exercises or the VPOs; and
- how to integrate warm-up, resistance, aerobic and dynamic balance, and cool-down exercises into a comprehensive fitness program.

With the exception of the aerobic exercises, we recommend that all exercises be done in the order given. But you may instead alternate upper- and lower-body exercises, which helps to prevent fatigue and adds variety to your fitness class. You can do one or more upper-body exercises and then alternate with one or more lower-body exercises. Find a pattern that is easy to remember. The exercises are numbered to help you keep track of where you are.

Part II will give you the tools to teach seated and standing warm-up, resistance, aerobic, and cool-down exercises confidently and competently. You will also learn how to put together a dynamic fitness program and to vary and progress your classes so that they are fun and functional. "Suggested Resources" in the back of the book will help you build a strong knowledge base for becoming an outstanding exercise leader of frail elders and adults with special needs.

Warm-Up:
Posture, Breathing, Range-of-Motion, and Stretching Exercises

One advantage in growing older is
that you can stand for more and fall for less.

—*Monta Crane*

LEARNING OBJECTIVES

After completing this chapter, you will have the tools to

- teach a safe and effective warm-up component of an exercise session for frail elders and adults with special needs;

- design a creative and progressive warm-up using 24 range-of-motion exercises, numerous variations and progression options, and other warm-up exercises;

- apply important safety precautions and guidelines for leading a warm-up session;

- focus on fall prevention by personalizing your instruction of seated or standing warm-up exercises for a class of people with varying fitness levels and one or more special needs.

This chapter provides practical safety precautions, guidelines, and specific teaching instructions for leading a safe and effective warm-up—the first component of an exercise or functional fitness session—in an individual or group setting. The warm-up exercises focus on joint range-of-motion (ROM) exercises (photographed and described near the end of the chapter) and include good posture, deep-breathing, and light stretching exercises appropriate for frail elders and adults with special needs. *Light* is defined as fewer stretches held for a shorter time than the comprehensive stretching routine of the cool-down phase (see chapter 7). Low-intensity aerobic exercises (see chapter 6) may be used instead of or in conjunction with ROM exercises for the movement part of the warm-up. Always have your participants warm up to prepare them for exercise and to help prevent muscle and joint injury.

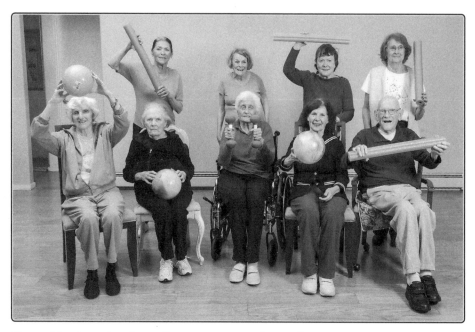

Figure 4.1   Seated and standing exercises can be taught at the same time.

Start with the basic seated warm-up exercises, which all your participants can learn. Participants who are able to stand safely can carefully progress to the basic standing warm-up exercises. The seated and standing exercises are designed to be taught at the same time to accommodate people with varying levels of fitness and diverse special needs. Figure 4.1 illustrates how manageable it is to lead the seated and standing exercises simultaneously.

In this chapter, we first discuss general safety precautions for warm-ups and then specific safety precautions that should be taken for participants with a variety of special needs. Next we present general guidelines that apply to the four parts of the warm-up:

1. Posture awareness
2. Deep breathing
3. Joint range-of-motion exercises
4. Stretching

We then provide specific instructions for leading a seated warm-up and a standing warm-up, each of which incorporate the four parts of a warm-up. The chapter ends with photos and instructions for 24 joint ROM exercises.

SAFETY PRECAUTIONS

Warm-up exercises are safe for frail elders and adults with special needs when appropriate guidelines and precautions are observed. The following general safety precautions and specific safety precautions for those with special needs can help you lead safe warm-ups and keep your participants injury free. Now could be a good time to review the general exercise "Safety Guidelines Checklist" in chapter 2. To assist your learning process, you may photocopy the following "General Safety Precautions Checklist for Warm-Ups" and the general exercise "Safety Guidelines Checklist" in chapter 2.

These general warm-up safety precautions for older adults also apply to those with special needs. The next section, "Specific Safety Precautions for Those With Special Needs," will further the safety and effectiveness of your exercise program for those with special needs.

Specific Safety Precautions for Those With Special Needs

Your class can focus on one or more special needs. For example, you might lead a class for individuals with arthritis, multiple sclerosis, or any condition likely to decrease normal range of motion (the degree of movement that occurs at a joint). Such a group could greatly benefit from a mild ROM program that gently moves every joint through its full, strain-free or pain-free range of motion daily. Teaching participants with similar special needs as opposed to

GENERAL SAFETY PRECAUTIONS CHECKLIST FOR WARM-UPS

☐ Follow the physician's special recommendations and comments for each participant on the "Statement of Medical Clearance for Exercise" (appendix A2).

☐ Remind participants to observe recommendations from their physicians. Remember that you, your participant, or his or her representative may follow up with the physician who has not made any recommendations or has made a recommendation that seems inappropriate, such as "No exercise." Another good time to follow up is when a participant's condition has improved or progressed.

☐ Never skip the warm-up period. If a participant is late for class and misses the warm-up, he or she may do whatever activity the class is doing at a lower intensity for 10 minutes. For example, the participant can do resistance exercises without weights or aerobics at low intensity for 10 minutes. If the participant is capable of an independent warm-up, walking or aerobics equipment (if available) may be a preferred alternative.

☐ Always spend at least 10 minutes on warm-up exercises to reduce the incidence of cardiovascular complications (ACSM 2010; American Senior Fitness Association 2012a, b, c) and help prevent muscle and joint injury.

☐ Focus on fall prevention. During standing exercise have a chair centered closely behind all participants—who can have day-to-day variation with their balance ability—so that they can sit down easily if needed. When they are seated, make sure that participants are safely positioned in their chairs.

☐ Warm up the back in a vertical position (as in exercise 4.21, Pelvic Tilt and Back Arch [Challenger]; 4.12 Rowing; 4.13 Close the Window) before twisting (4.24) or bending (4.22) the trunk sideways (American Senior Fitness Association 2012a, b, c).

☐ During upper- and lower-body ROM exercises, instruct participants to lift arms and legs only as high as comfortable while maintaining erect posture. Remind participants with hip replacements to raise their feet one at a time and only an inch (2.5 cm) or less off the floor to prevent hip flexion of more than 90 degrees.

☐ Instruct participants to avoid hyperextending—locking or extending a limb or part beyond the normal joint ROM—particularly the elbow and knee. In a straight or standing position, instruct participants to keep them soft, not bent.

☐ Do not exercise both legs at one time. Always keep one foot planted firmly on the floor while exercising the other leg to help prevent lower-back strain.

☐ Continually encourage your participants to maintain good posture and breathe fully while exercising and throughout the day. Avoid shallow breathing and especially holding the breath, which can increase blood pressure and decrease enjoyment of physical activities.

☐ Continually encourage participants to stop when they are fatigued, rest, and rejoin the class when they are ready.

☐ Focus on fun and safety, number one!

a class with a variety of special needs can be an easier way to start a class, though doing so is not always possible.

Following are some specific safety precautions for leading warm-up exercises for people with special needs, generally with conditions beyond an early or mild stage. For example, a person with mild symptoms of multiple sclerosis may have no limitations on ROM exercises, whereas one with severe symptoms may have difficulty with all ROM exercises. Additionally, a safety precaution for a chronic special need may be applicable only during an acute phase of a participant's condition. Therefore, these safety precautions may not apply all of the time to every person with a special need addressed in this section. Remember that anyone's performance ability may vary from day to day.

As you are getting to know your participants, also bear in mind that they may have one or more invisible, or silent, special needs, such as osteoporosis (that may be undiagnosed) or a previous hip or knee replacement, that the physician did not indicate on the medical clearance form or the participant is unable to communicate to you. Therefore, focus on the side of safety in your classroom as you apply the following information on specific safety precautions. For example, for those at risk of osteoporosis who are not able to communicate their special needs or have not been recently tested, apply the precautions for osteoporosis.

Keep in mind that this section will have some specific safety precautions that apply to other components of exercise but will be found only in this section because the warm-up component is included first in all exercise program designs.

Alzheimer's Disease and Related Dementias

- Some warm-up exercises require the instructor to be extra observant with participants who may not remember directions or pose a risk of copying others who are doing an exercise that is contraindicated for their condition. Have these participants sit near you in clear sight. If participants have other special needs,

make sure that they follow the specific safety precautions for that special need.

- When leading range-of-motion exercises that are performed on one side and then the other, slowly move uninterruptedly from one side to the other. For example, give a visual and verbal cue such as "change sides." Then, after you see them change sides, continue relevant cueing. This approach helps those with memory issues to remember what side they just exercised.

Arthritis

- A thorough warm-up is especially important for participants with arthritis whose joints may need extra time to reduce stiffness and prepare for exercise.

- To maintain joint ROM and mobility, encourage those with arthritis to perform ROM and stretching exercises carefully every day (one to two sessions per day), even when inflammation (redness, heat, swelling and pain) is present.

- Flexibility (ROM and stretching) exercises performed with low-intensity and controlled movements do not increase symptoms or pain (Rahl 2010, 184).

- When a joint is significantly inflamed, suggest that participants perform one to three (Arthritis Foundation 2009, 258) slow and gentle ROM exercises, moving through a comfortable or functional ROM. For instance, although about 90 degrees is normal wrist flexion range, a range of only about 45 degrees is needed for daily activities. In a class setting when others are doing more repetitions, during the in-between time suggest an exercise that the participant can enjoy and benefit from, such as three-part deep breathing.

- If mild ROM exercises exacerbate inflamed joints, rest may be needed.

Cerebrovascular Accident (CVA, Stroke)

- See also the safety precautions for those with coronary artery disease (heart disease).

- Providing clear warm-up instruction is extremely important to participants who have experienced stroke. If a participant has paralysis on the right side, focus on leading exercises mainly by demonstration, using few verbal instructions. If there is paralysis on the left side, rely more on verbal instructions, using fewer gestures (American Senior Fitness Association 2012c).

- Always have participants keep the head above the heart when bending forward, because of the danger of increased vascular pressure within the brain and the risk of stroke. We have excluded such exercises from this book. Teach stroke survivors, those at risk for stroke, those with uncontrolled proliferative retinopathy (see the section "Diabetes"), and glaucoma to pay particular attention to this precaution when bending forward to tie shoes, pick up items from the floor, and so on.

Chronic Obstructive Pulmonary Disease (COPD)

- A thorough warm-up period is critical for participants with COPD for gradual increases in ventilation, heart rate, blood pressure, and blood flow to exercising muscles (AACVPR 2006, 43).

- Caution participants to avoid holding the breath with all exercises including warm-up, ROM, and stretching exercises to prevent straining the respiratory and cardiovascular systems.

- Arm ROM exercises can cause shortness of breath sooner than leg ROM exercises. If you combine arm and leg exercises, give participants permission to do just the leg exercises because they provide a better warm-up than arm exercises alone.

- Remind participants with COPD to practice diaphragmatic breathing (see "Seated Three-Part Deep-Breathing Exercise" emphasizing the abdominal movement with "Instructions for Three-Part Deep Breathing, Part 1" later in this chapter) with pursed-lip breathing while exercising. If a participant is experiencing *dyspnea* (difficulty breathing, with rapid shallow respirations) or *hyperventilation* (increased rate and depth of breathing) have him or her stop exercise and practice just the breathing.

Coronary Artery Disease (CAD, Heart Disease)

- A thorough warm-up is critical for participants with cardiovascular problems. As CAD progresses the heart's oxygen supply is reduced, and a thorough warm-up can decrease the likelihood of inducing cardiac ischemia (deficiency of blood and oxygen to the heart), which can occur with sudden, intense physical activity (ACSM and AHA 2007).

Depression

- Teaching with an upbeat style and promoting positive peer interaction can have an uplifting effect, in addition to the potential mood-elevating benefit of exercise per se. Throughout class notice

---

Instructions for Pursed-Lip-Breathing[a]

1. Breathe in slowly through your nose. Keep your mouth closed.
2. Pucker (purse) your lips as if you were going to whistle.
3. Breathe out slowly through your pursed lips.[b]
4. Repeat several times or until breathing calms.

Encourage participants with COPD to practice this technique throughout the day.

[a]Have participants first practice pursed-lip breathing alone and then combine it with diaphragmatic breathing.

[b]The exhalation should take two to three times as long as the inhalation. Start with a 2-second inhalation and a 4-second exhalation.

participants' facial expressions and what makes them smile.

- During class inspire participants to practice good seated posture and good standing posture when they are able to stand. Better posture can lead to better self-image and attitude. Capitalize on opportunities to acknowledge or compliment a participant's improved posture, even if the improvement is slight.

- Sitting erect will enable a participant to use more lung capacity with the three-part deep-breathing exercise, which can be energizing and uplifting.

- Good posture, deep breathing, and inspiring imagery can be a powerful combination for alleviating depression. Refer to the visualizations that accompany instructions for good seated and standing posture later in this chapter.

- After establishing rapport, encourage participants to practice good posture, deep breathing, and positive imagery throughout the day.

- Depression may affect a person's motivation and adherence to exercise. Therefore, encourage regular exercise for its vast benefits including mood elevation.

Diabetes

- Ensure that participants on insulin or insulin secretagogues are monitoring their blood sugar before and after class. When preexercise glucose levels are below 100 milligrams per deciliter, carbohydrate needs to be ingested to prevent hypoglycemia (ACSM and ADA 2010, 2285; Rahl 2010, 210; ADA 2008, S22). If appropriate, recommend that the participant carry a high-carbohydrate snack with him or her (Rahl 2010, 218), recommended by the health care provider.

- A snack or change of insulin dosage may be needed 30 to 60 minutes before exercise (Rahl 2010, 214; ACSM 2009a).

- Ensure that participants with peripheral neuropathy (a long-term complication of diabetes that may include sensory loss in the feet) are wearing proper footwear to prevent sores or ulcers (ACSM and ADA 2010, 2286; Venes 2009).

- Instruct participants with uncontrolled *proliferative diabetic retinopathy* (advanced microvascular retinal damage) to avoid activities that increase intraocular pressure and hemorrhage risk, such as hanging their head below the heart (ACSM and ADA 2010, 2286). Refer to the last point of the section "Cerebrovascular Accident (CVA, Stroke)."

Frailty

- Regular, safe movement, such as joint ROM exercises, is essential for the goal of restoring function, as best as possible, for frail individuals. Encourage regular class attendance and a home ROM program (if appropriate), starting with one or two key ROM exercises, such as exercise 4.5, Seated Toe Point and Flex, or exercise 4.6, Seated Ankle Rotations, that loosen up the ankles and may aid gait and balance.

- Address other possible special needs that frail participants present.

Hip Fracture or Replacement

- When the participant receives medical clearance for a maintenance exercise program, strive to maintain the degree of muscle control and ROM that the participant achieved in physical therapy and progress from there.

- Avoid ROM exercises that involve internal rotation (turning the leg inward), hip adduction that crosses the midline of the body (crossing the legs), and hip flexion (decreasing hip joint angle, such as by bending forward at the hip or lifting the thigh toward the upright torso) of more than 90 degrees to reduce the risk of hip dislocation, unless the participant has written clearance from a physician indicating that those specific movements are not contraindicated. Otherwise, if a participant is sitting in a chair that allows the knees to be lower than the hips, he or she may raise the foot 1 inch (2.5 cm) off the floor during exercises that involve lifting the foot off the floor.

Hypertension

- If a person's resting systolic blood pressure is greater than 200 mm Hg or diastolic blood pressure is greater than 110 mm Hg, he or she should not exercise (ACSM 2010, 249).
- Teach participants to avoid holding their breath, including with controlled breathing, to prevent unnecessary elevation of blood pressure.

Multiple Sclerosis and Parkinson's Disease

- Range of motion can be significantly reduced for those with these chronic neurologic conditions. Encourage participants to do the version of each ROM exercise that best serves them.
- Instruct anyone with any trouble controlling neck movement to avoid neck ROM exercises because of the increased risk of injury.
- Avoid standing when performing upper-body ROM and combined upper- and lower-body ROM or any exercises requiring the use of both hands (unavailable for holding on for safety) when balance is an issue.

Osteoporosis

- When osteoporosis is advanced, standing exercise may not be safe because of the risk of falling and because body weight alone can fracture spinal vertebrae. Stay with the seated exercises to eliminate the risk of falling, particularly in a class setting.
- Avoid spinal flexion. Avoid ROM exercises that involve spinal forward flexion (shortening the front of the torso), par-

ticularly in combination with stooping, which increases the risk of vertebral fractures (American Senior Fitness Association 2012a, b, c; Williamson 2011, 283; ACSM 2009a, 275; Minne and Pfeifer 2005).

- For exercise 4.21 (Seated Pelvic Tilt and Back Arch [Challenger]), instruct the participant to keep the spine erect, by not collapsing the torso forward (spinal flexion), when the pelvis is tilted backward while performing the pelvic tilt. This precaution is appropriate for an entire class (with or without osteoporosis); no one benefits from slumping.
- For exercises 4.22 (Side Reach), 4.23 (Torso Rotation), and 4.24 (Twist), participants should avoid twisting movements (Minne and Pfeifer 2005), particularly in combination with stooping (ACSM 2009a, 275). If the participant has milder osteoporosis and medical clearance for spinal movements, he or she should perform these ROM exercises slowly within a small, narrow ROM with good posture.
- Promote good posture. Encourage participants to sit and stand with their best posture throughout the class and day. They should always avoiding slumping or torso flexion, which can cause collapse of the anterior vertebrae.
- Instruct participants to scoot their buttocks back as far possible when sitting in chairs, ideally chairs with a vertical, straight back for the best support. Refer to "Instructions for Good Seated Posture" and surrounding text later in this chapter about how to use a hand towel for lumbar (lower-back) support.

Sensory Losses

- Give a clear demonstration of the warm-up exercises to participants with hearing loss.
- Describe warm-up exercises precisely and directly to participants with visual impairment.

> **! Safety Tip** For a safe and effective warm-up for older adults, carefully follow the safety precautions and the following evidence-based guidelines.

GUIDELINES

Begin every workout with a warm-up. A 10-minute warm-up is essential for increasing blood flow to the exercising muscles, raising deep muscle temperature, loosening up muscles and joints, increasing joint ROM and function, and helping prevent muscle and joint injury. Table 4.1 shows the duration of various parts of a 10- to 15-minute warm-up. The warm-up exercises are shown in the recommended order, beginning with posture awareness and followed by three-part deep-breathing, joint ROM, and finally stretching. If your class starts late, you can do the 10-minute minimum warm-up.

If you plan to lead both resistance and aerobic exercises in a class, the group needs to warm up only in the beginning if aerobics precede resistance training. If you lead resistance exercises before aerobics, stretch briefly (using the minimal five stretching exercises in table 4.3) immediately after resistance training and follow with several minutes of active rhythmic movement (such as slow walking or low-intensity aerobic leg exercises) before moving on to the aerobic workout.

The following guidelines for each segment of the warm-up apply to leading both seated and standing exercises. Following this discussion of general guidelines, this chapter includes specific instructions for the four parts of a warm-up—posture, deep-breathing, joint ROM, and stretching exercises—for both a seated warm-up and a standing warm-up.

> **! Safety Tip** Give participants frequent, positive verbal cues to tune in to their bodies and to slow down or rest when needed during exercise.

Posture-Awareness Guidelines

Good posture is crucial during exercise and all activities of daily living. Poor posture reduces range of motion and breathing capacity and increases the risk of falling and incidence of pain, particularly in the low back. You can inspire participants' enthusiasm for exercise by taking them from a slumped to an upright posture.

Keep the following guidelines in mind when leading the posture-awareness exercise:

Start Smart

- Teach the posture-awareness exercise first so that your participants can begin exercise with improved posture.
- In the initial stages of teaching the exercises, give frequent reminders about good posture. Before a participant develops the habit of good posture, sometimes a quick positive cue (such as "sit erect" or "sit tall") is necessary before, after,

Table 4.1 Duration of the Segments of a 10- to 15-Minute Warm-Up

Warm-up exercises	Duration
Posture awareness	1/2 to 1 minute
Three-part deep breathing	1/2 to 1 minute
Joint range of motion[a]	8 to 10 minutes
Stretching	1 to 3 minutes

[a]Low-intensity aerobic exercises (see chapter 6) may replace or be combined with joint ROM exercises.

or even during an exercise. Those who are memory challenged may perpetually need reminders.

- When participants have learned the exercises and you flow from exercise to exercise without pausing, give a posture lesson at the beginning of class and offer reminders throughout when needed.

Verbal Instruction and Feedback

- When you observe a participant slumping or overarching the back, try these tips:
  1. Give a general reminder about good posture to the class.
  2. Use positive instructions such as saying "Lift" or "Open your chest," as opposed to "Don't slump." Ask motivating questions, such as, "Are your hips as far back as possible in your chair?" "Is your pelvis in alignment with a natural lumbar (lower-back) curve?"
  3. Give specific encouragement to the participant if he or she still needs it after the general reminder.

- Instruct participants not to hold the body in a rigid or static posture. Promote a relaxed and lifted posture by having participants gently shake their arms after the posture exercise while maintaining the improved posture.

- Look for opportunities to tell the group, "Your posture is looking good."

- Give individuals positive feedback about their posture or other improvements when working one on one or before or after class.

- Encourage your participants to sit erect using postural muscles and not to rest their backs against the backs of their chairs for as long as possible throughout the exercise class (and eventually outside of class) to strengthen core muscles. Instruct them to scoot their buttocks to the back of the chair when they get tired and need support (to minimize slumping).

As Always

- If a participant tends to lift the shoulders while doing the posture-awareness exercise or any other exercise, have him or her stabilize the shoulders by moving them up, back, and down to help keep the shoulders down throughout each exercise.

- Visual imagery can be helpful. For example, to convey the idea of the spine getting longer when sitting or standing erect, say, "Imagine your spine as a piece of elastic thread being pulled out from the top of your head at the same time that it is being pulled at its base" (Diamond 1996, 4).

！ Safety Tip Never physically force anybody into good posture or manually manipulate his or her body.

Three-Part Deep-Breathing Guidelines

The three-part deep-breathing exercise described later in this chapter improves mental focus, which can help your participants concentrate better on your instructions and thus avoid injury. Here are a few simple guidelines for leading the three-part deep-breathing exercise:

- Always teach the seated posture-awareness exercise before deep breathing to inspire those who are slumping to sit erect so that they can use more of their lung capacity.

- Do deep breathing before exercise to relax participants and make them more aware of their bodies.

- Give participants reminders to perform deep breathing at a comfortable pace.

Make sure that they do not strain to keep up with the class or hold back if they have larger lung capacity.

- Teach participants to keep their shoulders relaxed throughout this exercise, particularly when the collarbones rise slightly with the deep breathing in part 3.

- After participants learn this exercise, encourage them to exhale more air from their lungs gradually without straining.

- Try to integrate deep breathing into the exercise session. For example, they can do one three-part deep breath after each stretching exercise to promote deeper relaxation during the cool-down.

- Throughout the class, remind participants to use more of their breathing capacity by sitting or standing with good posture and by breathing less shallowly and more deeply.

! **Safety Tip** If a participant feels light-headed or dizzy during three-part deep breathing, instruct him or her to resume a normal breathing rhythm and to sit down carefully if standing.

Joint Range-of-Motion (ROM) Guidelines

ROM exercises help improve flexibility, musculoskeletal function, balance, and agility in older adults. Continuous, rhythmic ROM exercises are excellent for gently preparing frail elders and people with special needs for exercise. The joint ROM exercises illustrated at the end of this chapter work all the major joints of the body. Follow these guidelines when leading ROM exercises:

Start Smart

- Initially, it may be easier for participants to learn a ROM exercise by doing six to eight repetitions on one side at a time. This way participants can properly learn an exercise on one side at a time before

coordinating both sides simultaneously. There are two exceptions:

1. Seated Up-and-Down Leg March (marching in place).
2. Wrist and ankle ROM exercises: Do both sides together with smaller movements to avoid cooling down.

- After your participants are comfortable with the ROM exercises on one side, you can use one of these movement patterns:

1. Alternate sides—that is, perform the ROM exercise on the right, then left, then right, and so on.
2. Exercise both arms together.

Make It Effective

- Ultimately, for a more effective warm-up, have participants do upper- and lower-body ROM exercises together (e.g., leg march plus butterfly wings).

- Do not rest between repetitions of the same exercise or between different ROM exercises. Keep the movement continuous to increase internal body temperature, a primary goal of warm-ups, but give participants continual reminders to tune in their bodies and slow down and rest when needed.

- Also, include more exercises that use larger muscles, such as marching (exercise 4.1), between or in combination with upper-body exercises, when appropriate.

! **Safety Tip** Avoid doing too many ROM exercises that focus on small muscle groups, such as wrist and finger exercises, which can delay the goal of warming up the body.

Repetitions

- Instruct participants to perform three to eight repetitions (repetitions, or reps, are the number of times an exercise is performed without a break) of each ROM exercise. If the exercise is performed on one side and then the other, it would be three to eight reps on each side. An instruction for an exercise to "repeat in opposite direction" means that the participant should perform three to eight reps in each direction.

- With classes, especially larger ones, begin with more repetitions—six to eight repetitions of each ROM exercise, if well tolerated by participants. Starting with fewer repetitions may not give you enough time to observe and evaluate all participants and give them appropriate feedback with each exercise.

- After the ROM exercises are familiar to the participants, you may lower the number of reps to the lower end of the recommended range of three to eight if you need extra time for the rest of the class, particularly if it is a comprehensive fitness class (described in chapter 8). Remember, however, to have the movement portion of the warm-up be at least 8 minutes in duration.

Timing and Technique

- Perform ROM exercises slowly and smoothly.

- Each repetition of ROM exercises should be about 1 to 2 seconds in each direction, compared with 3 seconds for resistance exercises.

Variations and Progression

- Add some spice to the warm-ups with the variations and progression options described in the illustrated exercises at the end of the chapter. A general way to vary these exercises is to make progressively larger movements but always keep movements within an individual's strain-free and pain-free ROM.

- You may replace the ROM segment of the warm-up with low-impact, low-intensity aerobic activity, such as walking or stationary cycling. Incorporate some upper-body ROM exercises into walking

or cycling, if participants can do them safely. Some of the upper- and lower-body aerobic exercises in chapter 6 can be performed at low intensity as a warm-up.

- Do not use dumbbells or other resistance props for variety with ROM or any other exercises, except with resistance training.

Stretching Guidelines

Warm-up, or preactivity, stretching is intended to prepare the body for exercise, whereas cool-down, or postactivity, stretching promotes flexibility. Here are guidelines for leading the warm-up stretches (for more details on stretching, see chapter 7):

- Do stretching at the end of the warm-up when muscle temperature is elevated (ACSM 2011, 1345), after posture, breathing, and ROM exercises.

- During the warm-up, do a shorter set of stretching exercises (table 4.3 or 4.4) than during the cool-down. Tables 4.3 and 4.4 include critical stretches for body parts that are notoriously tight for most older adults. Tightness can compromise posture, impair balance, and reduce functional mobility.

- Have participants hold warm-up stretches for approximately 10 seconds. (During the cool-down, do more stretches and hold them for 15 to 30 seconds.)

! Safety Tip Remember to have participants stretch after they are warmed-up, to avoid injuring cold muscles and joints.

BASIC SEATED WARM-UP EXERCISES

The basic seated warm-up focuses on a comprehensive set of 24 joint ROM exercises and includes posture, breathing, and stretching exercises (refer to table 4.2). Before teaching these exercises, we recommend that you carefully read this entire chapter and learn the answers to the review questions at the end. Also, if you are a beginner fitness leader or would like to refine your teaching skills, review the three-step instructional process in chapter 3. Then begin by teaching the basic seated warm-up exercises first—as you get to know your participants' strengths and current limitations—before teaching the basic standing warm-up exercises. Seated exercises eliminate the risk for falling while standing. Participants who are able to stand safely can slowly progress to the standing variations of the basic seated warm-up exercises.

Here are instructions for leading the basic seated warm-ups in the recommended order:

(*a*) first posture, (*b*) then breathing, (*c*) then ROM exercises, and (*d*) finally stretching after the body is warmed up.

Seated Posture-Awareness Exercise

Teach good seated posture first to get participants in the habit of exercising with good posture. See "Instructions for Good Seated Posture." A primary objective of this exercise is to teach your participants the natural curves of the spine—a neutral spine (figure 4.2). You know you have achieved a neutral spine when you are sitting as tall as possible with a long

---

Instructions for Good Seated Posture

Verbally explain and physically demonstrate the following exercise. Refer to the surrounding paragraphs for important information for leading this exercise.

1. **Hips**: *Move your hips to the back of your chair.*
2. **Back**: *Sit with your spine erect.*
3. **Knees**: *Put your knees about hip-distance apart over your ankles.*
4. **Feet**: *Place your feet flat on the floor about hip-distance apart and point the toes forward or slightly outward (if that's more comfortable) and symmetrical.*

5. **Hands**: *Place your hands by your sides or on your thighs.*
6. **Chest**: *Take a big breath; feel your belly, ribs, and chest expand; and feel your chest lift upward. Maintain that lifted feeling.*
7. **Shoulders**: *Shrug and then relax your shoulders while maintaining erect posture (see Seated Shoulder Shrugs, exercise 4.11).*
8. **Head and neck**: *Look straight ahead and slightly pull or glide your chin inward and backward.*

Teaching tip: Check each participant for good seated posture. Repeat any step as needed.

Visualization exercises: To help maintain good posture, lead participants in these visualization activities:

1. *"Imagine a golden [or let participants choose their color] string attached to the top of your head, pulling gently upward. Your torso is lengthening with ease into good posture."*
2. *"Imagine something tall, beautiful, and inspiring like a tree or waterfall. Allow the uplifting image to help you sit tall."*

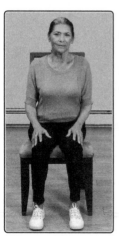 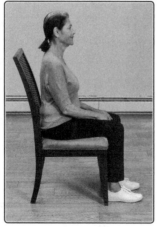

Instructions for good seated posture.

From E. Best-Martini and K.A. Jones-DiGenova, 2014, *Exercise for frail elders*, 2nd ed. (Champaign, IL: Human Kinetics).

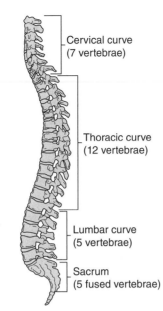

Figure 4.2 The natural curves of the spine.

and lifted spine. Participants will tend to need frequent reminders to maintain this improved posture throughout the class.

To promote good seated posture, or a neutral spine, use a chair with a vertical, straight back, if available. When a participant leans on the back of a chair or wheelchair for support, a pillow or pad may help him or her sit erect, especially if the back of the chair is not straight. To support the natural lumbar (lower-back) curve, a hand towel can be rolled about 3 inches (8 cm) thick (depending on body size) and wrapped with rubber bands.

The position of the pelvis is a key to good posture. Teach your participants the Seated Pelvic Tilt and Back Arch (Challenger) (exercise 4.21), which moves the pelvis forward and backward so that participants can bring the pelvis toward and ultimately into alignment and find the natural lumbar (lower-back) curve. Refer to the variations and progression options of exercise 4.21 for the seated pelvic tilt instructions. Allow extra time for participants to practice the pelvic tilt in class and give them some "homeplay" to practice it at home (if appropriate).

First, make sure participants are able to exercise with good seated posture with back support. Then when they are ready, gradually progress to sitting erect without back support

(for as long as they can while maintaining good posture) to strengthen the postural, or core, muscles. Give participants permission to do what works best for them.

Performing good seated posture effectively with back support on a stable surface is considered an introductory seated balance exercise (Bryant and Green 2009, 534). This exercise is a prerequisite to progressing to a more difficult seated balance challenge, such as sitting erect without back support. For participants not at risk of falling off an unstable surface, cautiously progress to practicing good seated posture on an unstable surface, such as an inflatable disc or stability ball.

Inspire participants to maintain this improved posture throughout the class as well as throughout the day. You may copy "Instructions for Good Seated Posture" for reference during class. You may also enlarge figure 4.2 to use as a visual aid for your class.

If a participant's feet cannot reach the floor, have him or her scoot forward in the chair. If he or she is unable to sustain that position, provide a foot support, such as a phone book or folded towel.

Seated Three-Part Deep-Breathing Exercise

Teach deep breathing in three steps. Verbally explain and physically demonstrate each step to facilitate your participants' learning process. Start with part 1 deep breathing, which concentrates on fully expanding and contracting the abdomen (belly). If possible, check to see whether each participant's abdomen is going out on the inhalation and in on the exhalation. After participants have learned part 1 (this may take one class or several weeks), add part 2, which continues the deep breath from the abdomen into the rib cage. After participants are comfortable with part 2, then present part 3, which continues the deep breath into the chest region.

Step-by-step instructions for teaching three-part deep breathing, which apply in both the seated and standing positions, are shown in the following boxes. Notes to the instructor can be

Part 1 Deep Breathing

To learn effective abdominal breathing, it is helpful for participants to place one or both hands on their abdomen and feel it move in on the exhale and out on the inhale.

1. *Imagine that a small balloon (of a soothing color) is in your abdomen. Place your hands on each side of your abdomen cradling the balloon.*

2. *Exhale fully by contracting your abdomen in toward your spine. Imagine the air is being released from the balloon. Notice your fingers coming closer together. [For participants with shorter exhalation, leave out the last line.]*

3. *Inhale. Imagine your balloon filling with air as your abdomen expands.*

   Repeat steps 2 and 3 as desired. Progress to steps 4 and 5 when participants can perform steps 2 and 3 independently.

4. *Continue for about three (or more) deep breaths at a comfortable pace.*

5. *With each breath, feel more and more relaxed.*

Part 2 Deep Breathing

Continue with the balloon imagery from part 1. Instruct participants, "Place one hand on your abdomen cradling your balloon and move the other hand to the rib cage."

1. *Exhale fully and feel your abdomen pull in toward your spine.*

2. *Inhale and feel your abdomen expand [as in part 1]. Your balloon is expanding past your abdomen into your rib cage.*

3. *Keep inhaling and feel your rib cage expand [for participants with shorter inhalation, leave out the rest of this sentence] as you imagine your balloon softly pressing against the inside of your rib cage.*

4. *Exhale and feel your rib cage contract, slowly letting the air out of your balloon.*

5. *Then pull the abdomen in toward the spine, completely exhaling without strain. Let all of the air out of your imaginary balloon, gently, slowly. [For participants with shorter exhalation, leave out the last line.]*

   Repeat steps 2 through 5 as desired. Progress to steps 6 through 7 when participants are ready.

6. *Continue at a comfortable pace for about three (or more) deep breaths.*

7. *With each breath, feel more and more relaxed.*

Part 3 Deep Breathing

Continue with the balloon imagery from "Part 2 Deep Breathing" or be creative with another image. Participants may find it helpful to place their hands on their collarbones.

1. *Exhale fully, contracting your abdomen in toward your spine.*

2. *Inhale fully by expanding your abdomen [as in part 1].*

3. *Then expand your rib cage [as in part 2].*

4. *Keep inhaling and feel your chest expand and collarbones slightly rise, imagining your balloon filling the inside of your upper chest cavity (softly pressing against the inside of your abdomen, ribs, and upper chest).*

5. *Exhale and feel your collarbones lower slightly and chest contract, rib cage contract, and abdomen contract toward your spine, slowly letting the air out of your balloon.*

   Repeat steps 2 through 5 as desired. Progress to steps 6 through 8 when participants are ready.

6. *Continue for about three (or more) deep breaths at your own pace.*

7. *With each breath, feel more and more relaxed. [Instructor pause.]*

8. *After your last deep breath, take a few moments to enjoy a more relaxed state.*

From E. Best-Martini and K.A. Jones-DiGenova, 2014, *Exercise for frail elders*, 2nd ed. (Champaign, IL: Human Kinetics).

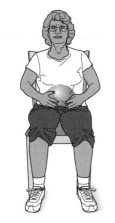

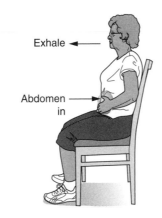

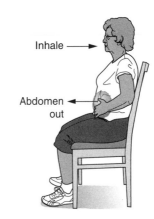

Part 1, step 1: Beginning position.

Part 1, step 2: Exhale.

Part 1, step 3: Inhale.

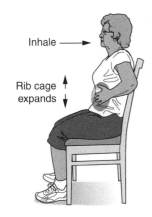

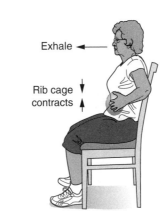

Part 2, step 3: Inhale.

Part 2, step 4: Exhale.

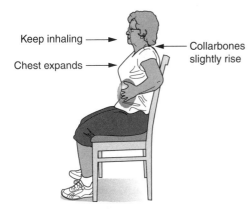

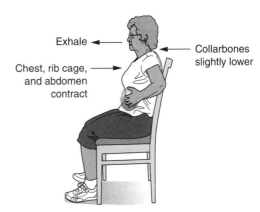

Part 3, step 4: Inhale and chest expands; collarbones rise slightly.

Part 3, step 5: Exhale and collarbones lower; chest contracts.

found in brackets. For variety and to enhance participant learning, experiment with applicable synonyms for the words *contracting* (i.e., tightening, pulling, squeezing), *expanding* (i.e., filling, enlarging, inflating), *exhale* (i.e., breathe out, blow out), *inhale* (i.e., breathe in, inspire), and so on. Observe and ask participants (when appropriate) what words work best for them.

When planning your class, schedule extra time for learning new exercises. Some participants will need more time than others to learn how to coordinate the exhalation with abdominal contraction and the inhalation with abdominal expansion (part 1) and so on. After the initial learning phase, if you schedule the minimum 10-minute warm-up, lead a short posture and breathing segment of about 1 minute. In this case, you do only about three three-part deep breaths before the movement segment (joint ROM or low-intensity aerobics) of the warm-up.

Seated Joint Range-of-Motion (ROM) Exercises

Table 4.2 shows the 24 joint ROM exercises that can be done seated or standing. This comprehensive set of 6 lower-body and 18 upper-body exercises targets the major joints of the body. The ROM exercises are generally organized by lower-body and upper-body groups and more specifically by target joints for a logical flow and to help you and your participants remember these exercises. For variety, you can do the upper-body exercises first and then the lower-body exercises, or you can alternate lower- and upper-body exercises, which can be an easier way to start for frail and deconditioned participants. When alternating upper- and lower-body exercises, it will be easier to keep on track by doing an entire target joint category before moving on to another.

To help you remember and lead the ROM exercises, each target joint category is organized with the same general order of exercises:

1. First, up and down or forward and backward movement: flexion and extension. (Extension is movement that increases the joint angle between adjacent body parts. Flexion is movement that decreases the joint angle between adjacent body parts.)

2. Second, sideward movement: abduction and adduction. (Abduction is sideward movement away from the body. Adduction is sideward movement toward the body.)

3. Third, circular movement: rotation.

4. Fourth, additional movements possible for a specific joint.

The range-of-motion exercises (chapter 4), resistance exercises (chapter 5), and stretching exercises (chapter 7) include intermediate and advanced exercises called challenger exercises. Before introducing these more challenging exercises, give your participants an opportunity to feel comfortable with the other basic exercises. You will also find challenger exercises in the variations and progression options of the illustrated instruction sections of chapters 4, 5, and 7.

Introduce the challenger exercise—4.21, Seated Pelvic Tilt and Back Arch—after your participants are comfortable with the other basic seated ROM exercises. If you choose to do the exercises out of the recommended order, until participants are proficient at 4.21, Pelvic Tilt and Back Arch (Challenger); warm up the back by performing 4.12, Rowing; and 4.13, Close the Window; before the twisting and bending spine ROM exercises (4.22, 4.23, and 4.24). According to the American Senior Fitness Association (2012a, b, c), the risk of injuring the back is minimized by warming it up first with forward and backward movement before twisting and lateral (sideways) spinal movements. Know the specific safety precaution for people with osteoporosis, particularly avoiding spinal flexion.

Begin the warm-up with the posture and breathing exercises before doing ROM exercises and end with light stretching (see tables 4.3 and 4.4). You may make a copy of table 4.2, Basic Warm-Up: Seated or Standing, to refer to during class.

Table 4.2 Basic Warm-Up: Seated or Standing[a]

POSTURE EXERCISE

See "Instructions for Good Seated Posture" and "Instructions for Good Standing Posture" in this chapter.

BREATHING EXERCISE

See "Instructions for Three-Part Deep Breathing" in this chapter.

LOWER-BODY RANGE-OF-MOTION EXERCISES

Target joints	Exercise
Hips	4.1 Up-and-Down Leg March
	4.2 Out-and-In Leg March
	4.3 Hip Rotation
Knees	4.4 Best Foot Forward and Backward
Ankles	4.5 Toe Point and Flex
	4.6 Ankle Rotations

UPPER-BODY RANGE-OF-MOTION EXERCISES

Target joints	Exercise
Shoulders	4.7 Arm Swing
	4.8 Butterfly Wings
	4.9 Shoulder Rotation
	4.10 Stir the Soup
	4.11 Shoulder Shrugs
Shoulders and elbows	4.12 Rowing
	4.13 Close the Window
Wrists	4.14 Wrist Flexion and Extension
	4.15 Wrist Rotations
Fingers	4.16 Hands Open and Closed
	4.17 Sun Rays
	4.18 Piano Playing
Cervical spine (neck)	4.19 Chin to Chest ("Yes")
	4.20 Chin to Shoulder
Spine (back)	4.21 Pelvic Tilt and Back Arch (Challenger)[b]
	4.22 Side Reach
	4.23 Torso Rotation
	4.24 Twists

WARM-UP STRETCHES

See The Minimal Five Stretching Exercises (table 4.3) or The Strategic Eight Stretches (table 4.4) in this chapter.

[a]All seated basic range-of-motion exercises and stretches can be adapted to standing exercises. See the corresponding standing exercise in the variations and progression options of the illustrated exercises at the end of chapter 4 for ROM exercises and chapter 7 for stretches.

[b]Until participants are proficient at 4.21, Pelvic Tilt and Back Arch (Challenger); warm up the back by performing 4.12, Rowing; and 4.13, Close the Window; before the twisting and lateral bending spine ROM exercises (4.22, 4.23, 4.24).

From E. Best-Martini and K.A. Jones-DiGenova, 2014, *Exercise for frail elders*, 2nd ed. (Champaign, IL: Human Kinetics).

Seated Stretching Exercises

Teach seated stretching exercises after the ROM exercises, when your participants are warmed up. Two sets of warm-up stretching exercises for you to choose from appear in table 4.3, The Minimal Five Stretching Exercises, and table 4.4, The Strategic Eight Stretches, both of which are shorter than the comprehensive set of 12 stretching exercises shown in chapter 7. All the stretching exercises are illustrated and described at the end of chapter 7, which also gives safety tips and variations and progression options for each stretch. You may copy tables 4.3 and 4.4 for use during class.

BASIC STANDING WARM-UP EXERCISES

The basic standing warm-up, like the seated one, focuses on a comprehensive set of 24 joint ROM exercises and includes posture, breathing, and stretching exercises. All these exercises were listed previously in table 4.2. These exercises are the standing version of the basic seated warm-up exercises; therefore, the standing exercises can replace the seated ones, can be alternated with them, or can be taught at the same time with the seated ones to accommodate a class of participants with diverse needs. See chapter 8 to learn when a participant is ready to progress

Table 4.3 The Minimal Five Stretching Exercises: Seated or Standing[a]

Basic stretching exercises[a]	Target body parts and muscles stretched	Functional benefits
7.3 Swan	Chest (pectoralis major) Shoulders (deltoids) Front upper arms (biceps)	Posture, balance, using more lung capacity, reaching backward (e.g., personal hygiene, wiping)
7.8 Tib Touches	Back of thighs (hamstrings) Back (spinal erectors)	Posture, walking, grooming (e.g., toenails), dressing, tying shoes, gardening, housekeeping (e.g., making bed, loading and unloading dishwasher and dryer); improved static and dynamic standing balance
7.5 Zipper Stretch	Back of upper arms (triceps) Back (latissimus dorsi)	Reaching upward (e.g., upper shelf), scratching back, bathing, hair washing and brushing, dressing, hooking bra, cleaning
7.12 Calf Stretch	Calves (gastrocnemius, soleus)	Balance, walking (prevents shuffling)
7.7 Spinal Twist	Torso (abdominals, spinal erectors)	Looking behind (e.g., driving), getting in and out of car, passing an item (i.e., a plate), cleaning, loading and unloading dishwasher and dryer

[a]Stretches are in a recommended but optional order, alternating upper- and lower-body stretches. All seated basic stretching exercises can be adapted to standing exercises. See the corresponding standing exercises in the variations and progression options of the illustrated exercises at the end of chapter 7. Your participants will receive greater balance benefits with the standing exercises, particularly exercises involving a one-legged stand (indicated by a balance icon).

From E. Best-Martini and K.A. Jones-DiGenova, 2014, *Exercise for frail elders*, 2nd ed. (Champaign, IL: Human Kinetics).

from seated to standing exercises, the benefits of standing exercises, when seated exercises are preferred over standing exercises, and the advantages of teaching seated and standing exercises simultaneously.

As the fitness leader, you will be thoughtfully guiding participants to stand or sit during class. We recommend that anyone who cannot safely stand continue with the seated warm-up exercises. Participants with minor balance problems should perform only those standing exercises that leave one hand available to hold on to the back of a sturdy chair for support.

ROM exercises that use two hands should be performed only by participants who are steady on their feet. Focus on fall prevention during standing exercise by having a chair directly centered closely behind all participants so that they can sit down easily if necessary. Remember that participants can have day-to-day variation in their balance ability.

Following are instructions for leading the basic standing warm-ups in the recommended order: (*a*) first posture, (*b*) then breathing, (*c*) then ROM exercises, and (*d*) finally stretching after the body is warmed up.

Table 4.4   The Strategic Eight Stretches: Seated or Standing[a]

Basic stretching exercises[a]	Target body parts and muscles stretched	Functional benefits
7.3 Swan	Chest (pectoralis major) Shoulders (deltoids) Front upper arms (biceps)	Posture, balance, more lung capacity, reaching backward (e.g., personal hygiene, wiping)
7.5 Zipper Stretch	Back of upper arms (triceps) Back (latissimus dorsi)	Reaching upward (e.g., upper shelf), scratching back, bathing, hair washing and brushing, dressing, hooking bra, cleaning
7.7 Spinal Twist	Torso (abdominals, spinal erectors)	Looking behind (e.g., driving), getting in and out of car, passing an item (i.e., a plate), cleaning, loading and unloading dishwasher and dryer
7.8 Tib Touches	Back of thighs (hamstrings) Back (spinal erectors)	Posture, walking, grooming (e.g., toenails), dressing, tying shoes, gardening, housekeeping (e.g., making bed, loading and unloading dishwasher and dryer); improved static and dynamic standing balance
7.9 Quad Stretch	Front thighs (quadriceps) Shins (tibialis anterior)	Posture, walking; improved static and dynamic standing balance
7.10 Splits	Inner thighs (hip adductors)	Bathing, getting in and out of car
7.11 Outer-Thigh Stretch	Outer hips and thighs (hip abductors)	Crossing the legs, dancing requiring crossover steps
7.12 Calf Stretch	Calves (gastrocnemius, soleus)	Balance, walking (prevents shuffling)

[a]All seated basic stretching exercises can be adapted to standing exercises. See the corresponding standing exercises in the variations and progression options of the illustrated exercises at the end of chapter 7. Your participants will receive greater balance benefits with the standing exercises, particularly exercises involving a one-legged stand (indicated by a balance icon).

From E. Best-Martini and K.A. Jones-DiGenova, 2014, *Exercise for frail elders*, 2nd ed. (Champaign, IL: Human Kinetics).

Standing Posture-Awareness Exercise

Teach good standing posture to those who are doing standing exercises to get them in the habit of exercising with good posture. See "Instructions for Good Standing Posture." A primary objective of the posture exercise is to find the natural curves of the spine (see figure 4.2) when standing as erect as possible.

The position of the pelvis is a key to good posture. Teach your participants the Standing Pelvic Tilt part of exercise 4.21, which moves the pelvis forward and backward so that par-ticipants can bring their pelvis toward and ultimately into alignment and find the natural lumbar (lower-back) curve. Refer to the varia-tion and progression options of exercise 4.21 for the standing pelvic tilt. Allow extra time for participants to practice the pelvic tilt in class and give them some "homeplay" to practice it at home (when timely).

Motivate participants to maintain this improved posture throughout the class and throughout the day. You may copy "Instruc-tions for Good Standing Posture" to refer to during class. You may also enlarge figure 4.2 to use as a visual aid for your class.

Instructions for Good Standing Posture

Verbally explain and physically demonstrate the following exercise. Refer to the surround-ing paragraphs for important information for leading this exercise.

1. **Hands**: *Relax your hands by your sides or on the back of a chair for support.*[a]

2. **Feet**: *Place your feet about hip-distance apart and point your toes forward or slightly outward and symmetrical, if that's more comfortable.*

3. **Knees**: *Do not lock your knees; keep them "soft" but not bent ("Ease at the knees").*

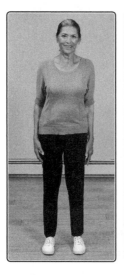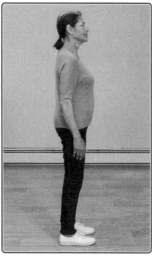

4. **Hips**: *Stand erect. Place one hand behind you and feel the curve of your lower back. Place the other hand on your hips or top of the pelvis, guiding it forward and backward (called a pelvic tilt) until you find a natural curve in your lower back.*

5. **Chest**: *Take a big breath; feel your abdomen, ribs, and chest expand; and feel your chest lift upward. Maintain that lifted feeling.*

6. **Shoulders**: *Shrug and then relax your shoulders while maintaining erect posture (see Shoulder Shrugs, exercise 4.11). Repeat as needed.*

7. **Head and neck**: *Look straight ahead and slightly retract or glide your chin inward and backward.*

Teaching tip: Check each participant for good standing posture. Repeat any step as needed.
Visualization exercises: To help maintain good posture, lead participants in these visualiza-tion activities:

1. *"Imagine a string attached to the top of your head, pulling gently upward. Your torso is lengthening with ease into good posture."*

2. *"Imagine something tall, beautiful, and inspiring like a tree or statue. Allow the uplift-ing image to help you stand tall."*

[a]Suggest that your participants use the top of the back of their chair as a ballet bar. This can be an uplifting image.

From E. Best-Martini and K.A. Jones-DiGenova, 2014, *Exercise for frail elders,* 2nd ed. (Champaign, IL: Human Kinetics).

Standing Three-Part Deep-Breathing Exercise

The instructions for the three-part deep-breathing exercise can be done seated or standing. In general, a seated position is safer and more conducive to relaxing than standing. But when participants do not have balance issues, they can benefit by practicing deep breathing while standing so that they can relax anywhere, any time. As with all components of a functional fitness program, when standing is a safe and suitable option, give your participants a choice to sit or stand and encourage them to sit any time during the class when necessary. Reiterate the general safety precaution: "Stop deep breathing and sit if you feel fatigued, lightheaded, or dizzy."

Standing Joint Range-of-Motion Exercises

When it is safe for a participant to stand and he or she feels ready, the standing ROM exercises will provide additional benefits, such as improved static balance, improved functional mobility and ability to perform daily activities that require standing, and maintained or even increased independence.

The 24 standing ROM exercises, like the seated ones, are a comprehensive set of 6 lower-body exercises and 18 upper-body exercises that target the major joints of the body. Introduce these variations and progression options of the basic seated ROM exercises (presented at the end of the chapter) after you get to know your participant's strengths and current limitations while observing them learn the seated exercises, which eliminate the risk for falling while standing. When a participant has developed good technique with the seated ROM exercises and you have determined that it is safe, encourage standing exercise for the extra benefits that they provide.

Standing Stretching Exercises

The seated stretching exercises can be adapted as standing exercises. Teach standing stretching exercises after the ROM exercises, when your participants are warmed up. Two sets of warm-up stretching exercises for you to choose from appear in table 4.3, The Minimal Five Stretching Exercises, and table 4.4, The Strategic Eight Stretches, both of which are shorter than the comprehensive set of 12 stretching exercises shown in chapter 7. All the stretching exercises are illustrated and described in chapter 7, which also gives safety tips and variations and progression options for each stretch. You may copy tables 4.3 and 4.4 for use during class.

VARIATIONS AND PROGRESSION

The variations and progression options (VPOs) for each of the 24 basic ROM exercises enable you to be creative and progressive with your exercise program to serve the needs of a class full of people from frail to fit. See the exercise instructions at the end of this chapter for these options. Introduce the VPOs after your participants have learned the basic seated ROM exercises, with the exception of the easier options. When your class is ready for a greater challenge, teach variations of one or more of the basic ROM exercises. For example, if your class particularly enjoys the Seated Shoulder Rotation (exercise 4.9), you can add a variation such as shoulder rotation with straight-arm circles. One of countless possibilities is to introduce one new ROM variation for each target joint, each class, each week, or whenever it fits for the pace of a class. After teaching a ROM variation, you can later reintroduce the basic exercise, alternate the basic version and the variations, or teach both the basic exercise and its variations during the same class. For many other ideas for varying and progressing your class, see chapter 8.

In general you can vary a ROM exercise by

- progressing from smaller to larger movements to explore the potential strain free and pain free joint ROM,
- varying the rate (going a little faster or slower),
- varying the rhythm,

- using music (but keeping the movements smooth and not too fast), and

- standing.

Each basic seated ROM exercise has a standing alternative, the primary progression option when it is safe for a participant to stand.

SUMMARY

Always start with a warm-up before exercise for at least 10 minutes to ease the transition from rest to exercise and to help prevent muscle and joint injury. An ideal warm-up for frail elders and adults with special needs includes good posture, deep breathing, ROM, and stretching exercises. This chapter presented guidelines, safety precautions, and explicit teaching instructions for warm-up exercises that enable you to lead a constructive and enjoyable warm-up session. Instructions and illustrations of range-of-motion exercises follow the review questions.

REVIEW QUESTIONS

1. A general recommendation to reduce the risk of hip dislocation for participants with hip replacement is to avoid the following movements (*circle only one*):
    a. turning the leg inward
    b. turning the leg outward
    c. crossing the legs
    d. hip flexion of more than 90 degrees
    e. all of the above
    f. *a, c,* and *d* only

2. Anyone with any trouble controlling neck movement, particularly those with multiple sclerosis and Parkinson's disease, should avoid _____ ROM exercises.

3. Spinal flexion (bending forward at the waist) is contraindicated for individuals with osteoporosis because it increases the risk of _____ fractures.

4. The purpose of a warm-up segment is to (*circle only one*)
    a. increase blood flow to the exercising muscles
    b. raise deep muscle temperature
    c. loosen up muscles and joints and increase joint ROM and function
    d. help prevent muscle and joint injury
    e. all of the above
    f. *a, c,* and *d* only

5. A primary objective of the posture exercise (whether seated or standing) is to find the natural curves of the spine, also known as a _____ spine.

6. The three-part deep-breathing exercise can help improve _____ _____, which can help participants concentrate better on your instructions and thus avoid injury.

7. Hold warm-up stretches for approximately _____ seconds. (During the cool-down, do more stretches and hold them for 15 to 30 seconds.)

8. You can vary a ROM exercise by (*circle only one*):

    a. progressing from smaller to larger movements (to explore the potential strain-free and pain-free joint ROM)

    b. varying the rate (going a little faster or slower)

    c. varying the rhythm

    d. using music (but keeping the movements smooth and not too fast)

    e. all of the above

    f. *a, c,* and *d* only

ILLUSTRATED INSTRUCTION

Exercises 4.1 to 4.6 are lower-body ROM exercises, and exercises 4.7 to 4.24 are for the upper body. The exercise and safety tips and variations and progression options (VPOs) apply to both seated and standing exercises unless otherwise specified. Make sure that participants maintain good posture while performing these exercises.

Good Seated and Standing Posture

Be sure to refer to the instructions for good seated and standing posture found earlier in this chapter and remind participants of them often as you do each exercise.

Seated Up-and-Down Leg March

TARGET JOINT—Hips

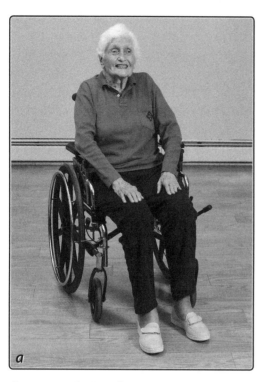

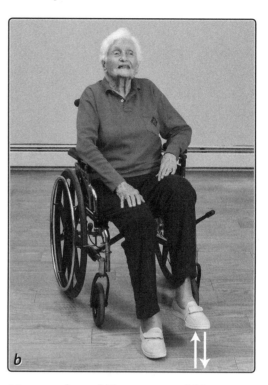

Start and Finish Position

1. Good seated posture.
2. Hands in a comfortable position.

Upward and Downward Movement

3. Lift one foot off the floor.
4. Then put it back down.
5. Alternate legs (march).
6. Perform three to eight repetitions per leg.

 Exercise and Safety Tips

- Lift legs only as high as comfortable while maintaining erect posture.

- Those with a hip fracture or replacement should avoid lifting the leg higher than a 90-degree angle at the hip joint in a seated or standing position.

Variations and Progression Options

- *Easier:* Start by lifting the legs slightly, keeping the toes on the floor. Slowly progress higher.
- *Challenger:* Move feet forward and backward while marching.
- *Challenger (Combo):* Swing arms while marching.

- *In-between:* Perform leg marching between other ROM exercises.
- Standing Up-and-Down Leg March (involves a brief one-legged stand).

Seated Out-and-In Leg March

TARGET JOINT—Hips

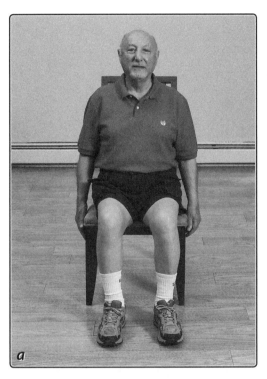

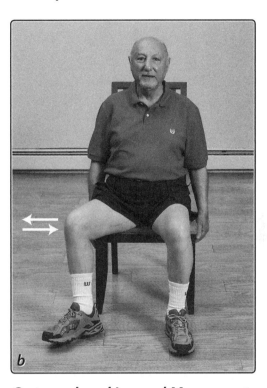

Start and Finish Position

1. Good seated posture.
2. Hands in a comfortable position.

Outward and Inward Movement

3. Lift one leg out to the side.
4. Then move it back to the center.
5. Alternate legs (march).
6. Perform three to eight repetitions per leg.

! *Exercise and Safety Tips*

- Keep each foot directly below each knee.
- Those with a hip fracture or replacement should avoid lifting the leg higher than a 90-degree angle at the hip joint in a seated and standing position.

Variations and Progression Options

- *Easier:* Slide the foot on the floor rather than lift the leg. For the next step, lift the legs slightly.
- *Easier:* Move the leg out to the side 1 to 3 inches (2.5 to 7.5 cm).
- *Challenger:* Progress to higher movements.

- *Combo:* Swing arms while marching.
- *In-between:* Perform leg marching between other ROM exercises.
- *Standing Out-and-In Leg March* (involves a brief one-legged stand).

Seated Hip Rotation

TARGET JOINT—Hips

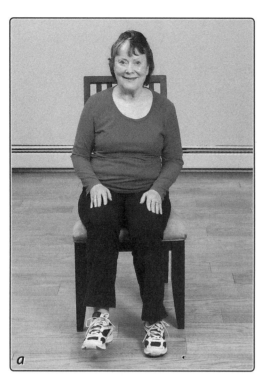

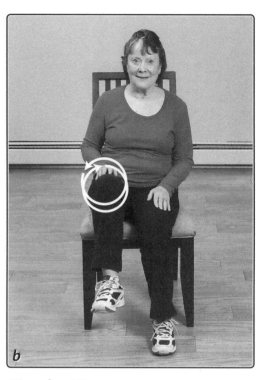

Start and Finish Position

1. Good seated posture.
2. Hands in a comfortable position.
3. Lift the foot 1 to 2 inches (2.5 to 5 cm) off the floor.

Circular Movement

4. Make circles with one knee in one direction. Move the knee up, out, down, and in.
5. Perform three to eight repetitions.
6. Rest the foot on the floor.
7. Repeat in the opposite direction.
8. Repeat steps 3 to 7 with the other leg.

 ### Exercise and Safety Tips

- Start with small circles.

- Those with a hip fracture or replacement should avoid lifting the leg higher than a 90-degree angle at the hip joint in a seated and standing position.

Variations and Progression Options

- *Easier:* Support the rotating leg with one or both hands (when needed); progress to unsupported rotations.
- *Easier:* Keep the toes on the floor instead of lifting them.
- *Challenger:* Skip step 6 for as many reps as comfortable.
- *Challenger:* Progress to larger circles. Be creative with circle sizes.

- *Challenger:* Lift the foot 3 inches (7.5 cm) or more off the floor.
- *Standing Hip Rotation* (involves a one-legged stand): Standing on one leg, raise the other leg slightly off the floor to the front. Keeping both legs straight, make circles with the raised leg so that the foot moves in a small circle (move only the hip joint).

Seated Best Foot Forward and Backward

TARGET JOINT—Knees

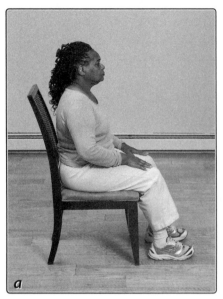 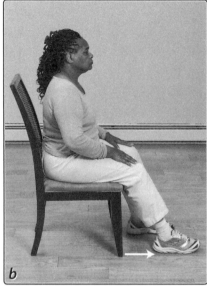 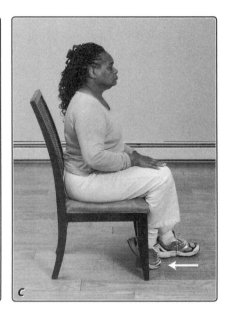

Start and Finish Position

1. Good seated posture.
2. Hands in a comfortable position.

Forward and Backward Movement

3. Step forward with one foot.
4. Then glide the foot backward under the chair.
5. Perform three to eight repetitions.
6. Repeat with the other leg.

 ### Exercise and Safety Tips

- Modification: If chairs have bars prohibiting legs from going under seat, bring the foot back as far as possible.

Variations and Progression Options

- *Foot tap:* Do a gentle heel tap or toe tap forward.
- *Foot tap:* Alternate heel tap and toe tap.

- *Standing Best Foot Forward and Backward* (involves a brief one-legged stand).

Seated Toe Point and Flex

TARGET JOINT—Ankles

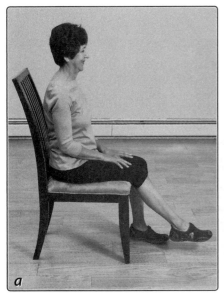
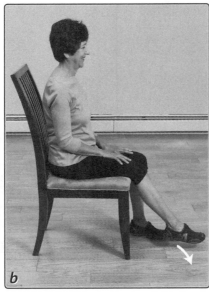
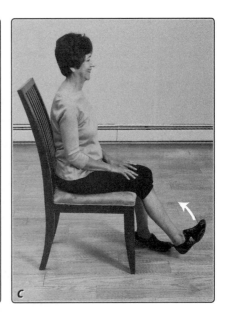

Start and Finish Position

1. Good seated posture.

2. Hands in a comfortable position.

3. Slide one foot forward as far as comfortable.

4. Lift the same foot 1 to 2 inches (2.5 to 5 cm) off the floor.

Downward and Upward Movement

5. Point toes and flex ankle.

6. Perform three to eight repetitions.

7. Repeat with the other leg.

! Exercise and Safety Tips

- If performed standing, hold on to a secure support.

- Avoid locking the knee of the supporting leg during Standing Toe Point and Flex.

Variations and Progression Options

- *Easier:* Rest the heel on the floor while performing Seated Toe Point and Flex.

- *Challenger:* Lift the foot 3 inches (7.5 cm) or more off the floor.

- *Standing Toe Point and Flex* (involves a one-legged stand).

- *Standing Crane Pose* (involves a one-legged stand). Stand like a crane, establish balance, and then add Toe Point and Flex.

- *Prop:* Hold a ball in the hands in front of the chest and overhead for an extra balance challenge.

Seated Butterfly Wings

TARGET JOINT—Shoulders

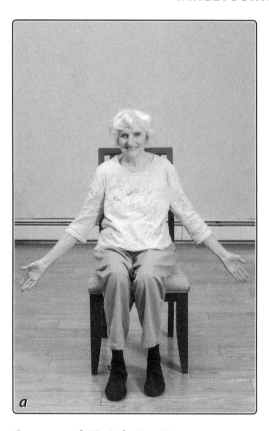

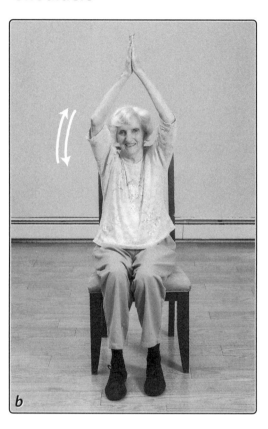

Start and Finish Position

1. Good seated posture.
2. Hold the arms straight at the sides and face the palms forward.

Upward and Downward Movement

3. Raise the arms toward the ceiling as far as comfortable.
4. Slowly lower the arms back to the starting position.
5. Perform three to eight repetitions.

! Exercise and Safety Tips

- Initially, hold on to a support with one hand and lift one arm at a time during Standing Butterfly Wings. Those without balance problems may progress to lifting both arms simultaneously.

Variations and Progression Options

- *Hand positions:* Be creative with the hands. For example, face the palms up on the upward motion and down on the downward motion.

- *Standing Butterfly Wings.*

Seated Shoulder Rotation

TARGET JOINT—Shoulders

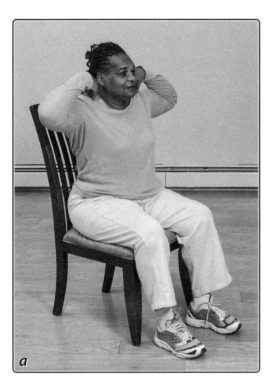

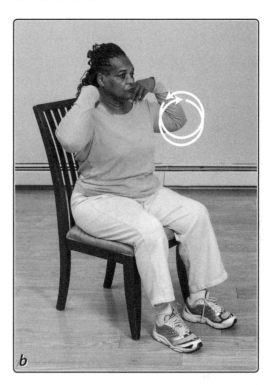

Start and Finish Position

1. Good seated posture.
2. Fingertips on the shoulders.
3. Elbows out to the sides.

Circular Movement

4. Make circles with the elbows.
5. Perform three to eight repetitions.
6. Repeat in the other direction.

! Exercise and Safety Tips

- Focus on lifting and opening the chest while rotating the shoulders.
- Initially, hold on to a secure support with one hand and rotate one arm at a time during Standing Shoulder Rotations. Those without balance problems may progress to rotating both arms simultaneously.

Variations and Progression Options

- *Easier:* Rotate the shoulders with arms straight at the sides.
- *Arm position:* Rotate straight arms at various levels, such as slightly below shoulder level.
- *Circle sizes:* Be creative with circle sizes.
- *Standing Shoulder Rotations.*

Seated Stir the Soup

TARGET JOINT—Shoulders

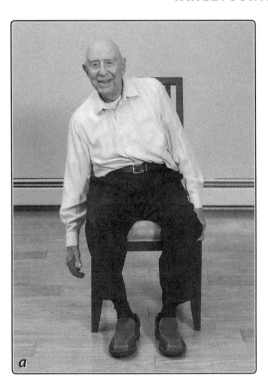 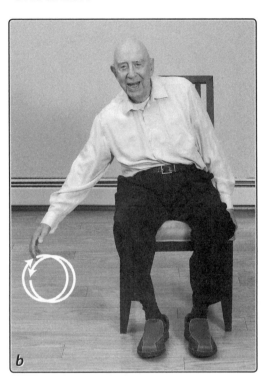

Start and Finish Position

1. Good seated posture.
2. Hold the side of a chair with one arm.
3. Lean toward the opposite side.
4. Hold the free arm straight at the side.

Circular Movement

5. Swing the free arm in a circular motion.
6. Perform three to eight repetitions.
7. Repeat in the other direction.
8. Repeat on the other side.

Exercise and Safety Tips

- Hold on to the chair seat or arm to prevent falling during Seated Stir the Soup.

- Gently shake the arm before performing Seated Stir the Soup to help release residual stiffness so that the arm can freely swing.

Variations and Progression Options

- *Circle sizes:* Be creative with circle sizes.
- *Stir different patterns:* For example, use numbers, letters, or words.

- *Standing Stir the Soup.*

Seated Shoulder Shrugs

TARGET JOINT—Shoulders

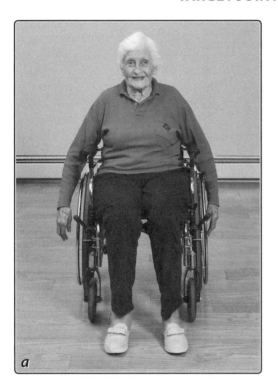 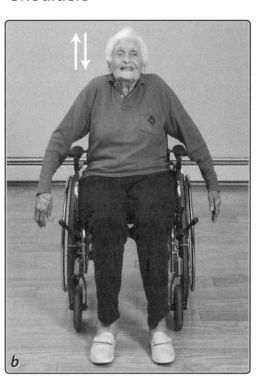

Start and Finish Position

1. Good seated posture.
2. Hold arms straight at the sides and face palms inward.

Upward and Downward Movement

3. Lift both shoulders toward the ears.
4. Slowly return to the starting position.
5. Perform three to eight repetitions.

! Exercise and Safety Tips

- Lower the shoulders smoothly.

Variations and Progression Options

- *Easier:* Start by lifting the shoulders only 1 inch (2.5 cm); then lift them progressively higher.

- *Combo (breath):* Coordinate step 3 with an inhale and step 4 with an exhale.
- *Standing Shoulder Shrugs.*

Seated Rowing

TARGET JOINT—Shoulders and elbows

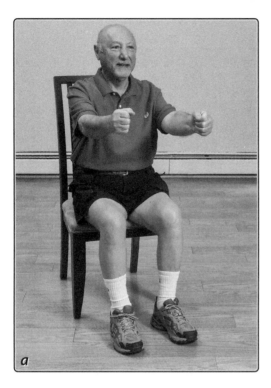 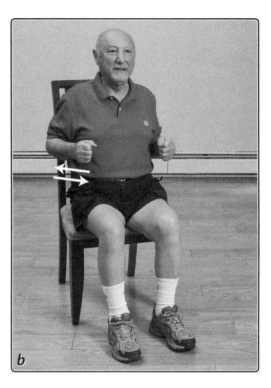

Start and Finish Position

1. Good seated posture.
2. Hold arms straight out in front, slightly below shoulder level.
3. Face palms inward.

Backward and Forward Movement

4. Pull arms backward in a rowing motion.
5. Squeeze the shoulder blades together.
6. Perform three to eight repetitions.

 Exercise and Safety Tips

- Keep the shoulders down.
- Move the elbows straight backward, not to the side.
- On the backward rowing motion, gently squeeze the shoulder blades together by drawing the elbows toward one another behind your back.

- Until participants are proficient at 4.21, Pelvic Tilt and Back Arch (Challenger), warm up the back in a vertical position using 4.12, Rowing, or 4.13, Close the Window, before turning or bending the trunk sideways.

Variations and Progression Options

- *Easier:* Slide hands along the thighs.
- *Easier:* Arms can be held lower than in photograph *a*.
- *Hand position:* Row with an underhand or overhand grip.
- *Hand position:* Row with less or more distance between the hands.
- *Sitting position:* Sit toward the middle of the chair so that the elbows clear the back of the chair, if safe for the participant.
- *Standing Rowing.*

Seated Close the Window

TARGET JOINT—Shoulders and elbows

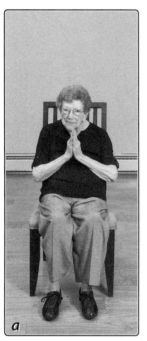 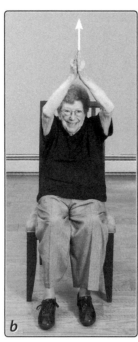 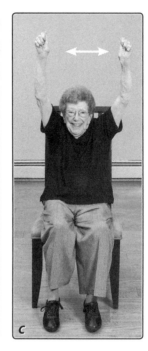 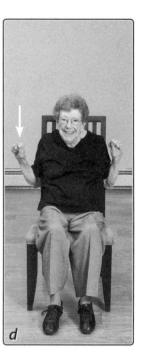

Start and Finish Position

1. Good seated posture.
2. Hands in prayer position (palms together in front of the chest and fingers pointing upward).

Upward and Downward Movement

3. Lift the arms upward as far as comfortable.
4. Open the hands and grasp an imaginary window frame.
5. Pull down the window.
6. Return to the starting position.
7. Perform three to eight repetitions.

! Exercise and Safety Tips

- Stroke: Those recovering from stroke can usually move through a greater ROM on the affected side by clasping their hands instead of pressing their palms together.

- Until participants are proficient at 4.21, Pelvic Tilt and Back Arch (Challenger), warm up the back in a vertical position using 4.12, Rowing, or 4.13, Close the Window, before turning or bending the trunk sideways.

Variations and Progression Options

- *Easier:* Open a low window. Keep the hands below the head. Gradually raise the hands higher over time (within strain-free and pain-free ROM).

- *Elbows in back pockets:* Try to put the elbows in the back pockets (pressing elbows downward and backward) when closing the imaginary window.
- *Standing Close the Window.*

Seated Wrist Flexion and Extension

TARGET JOINT—Wrists

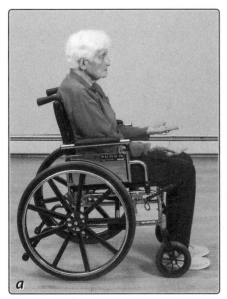 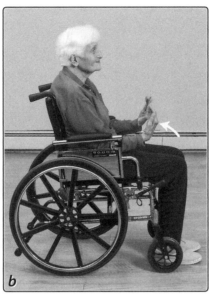 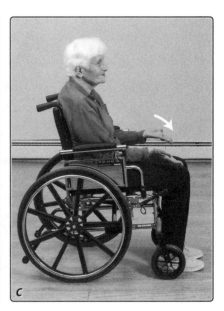

Start and Finish Position

1. Good seated posture.
2. Upper arms by the sides.
3. Forearms parallel with lap, palms up.

Upward and Downward Movement

4. Flex wrists.
5. Extend wrists.
6. Perform three to eight repetitions.

! Exercise and Safety Tips

- If the arms get tired at a 90-degree angle, lower the arms by the sides and continue flexing and extending.

Variations and Progression Options

- *Hand position:* Palms down or facing each other.
- *Arm position:* Hold arms in different positions, from straight overhead to straight at the sides.

- *Standing Wrist Flexion and Extension.*

Seated Wrist Rotations

TARGET JOINT—Wrists

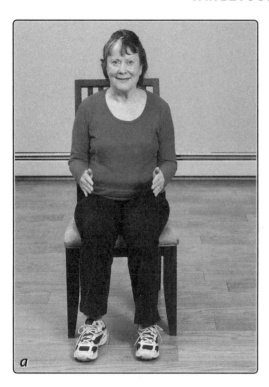

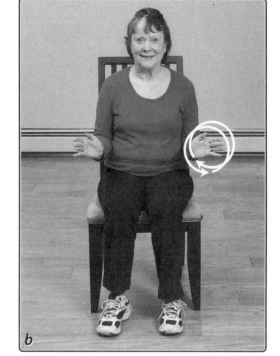

Start and Finish Position

1. Good seated posture.
2. Upper arms by the sides.
3. Forearms parallel with lap.
4. Palms facing inward.

Circular Movement

5. Make circles with the wrist in one direction. Move the wrists up, out, down, and in.
6. Perform three to eight repetitions.
7. Repeat in the opposite direction.

! Exercise and Safety Tips

- If the arms get tired at a 90-degree angle, rest the arms by the sides and continue wrist rotations.

Variations and Progression Options

- *Hand position:* Palms down or facing each other.
- *Arm position:* Hold the arms in different positions, from straight overhead to straight at the sides.
- *Circle sizes:* Be creative with circle sizes.
- *Standing Wrist Rotations.*

Seated Hands Open and Closed

TARGET JOINT—Fingers

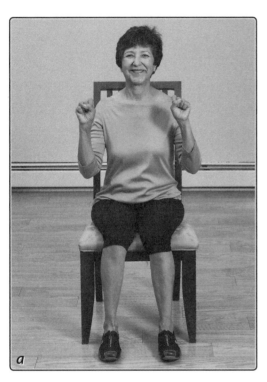 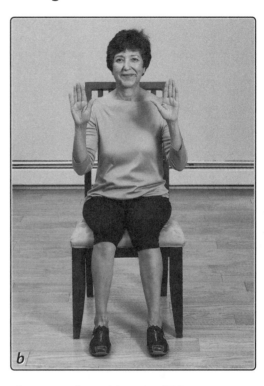

Start and Finish Position

1. Good seated posture.
2. Arms in "stick 'em up" position (palms facing forward near the shoulders), elbows by the sides.
3. Make fists.

Outward and Inward Movement

4. Open fists.
5. Close fists.
6. Perform three to eight repetitions.

! Exercise and Safety Tips

- Remind those who have difficulty moving their hands to go at their own pace and stay within their strain-free and pain-free range of motion.

Variations and Progression Options

- *Hand positions:* Open and close hands randomly in different places, like fireworks exploding throughout the sky.
- *Standing Hands Open and Closed.*

Seated Sun Rays

TARGET JOINT—Fingers

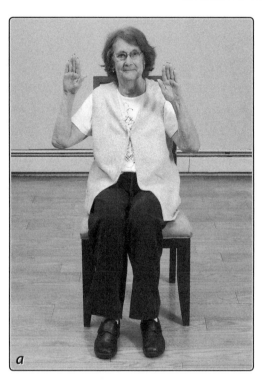 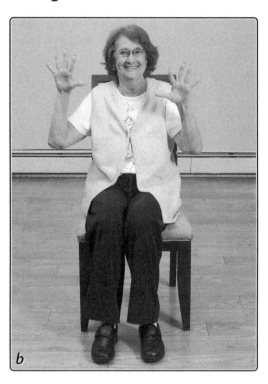

Start and Finish Position

1. Good seated posture.
2. Arms in "stick 'em up" position (palms facing forward near the shoulders), elbows by the sides.
3. Fingers together.

Outward and Inward Movement

4. Spread fingers apart.
5. Then move them back together.
6. Perform three to eight repetitions.

! Exercise and Safety Tips

- Remind those who have difficulty moving their hands to go at their own pace and stay within their strain-free and pain-free range of motion.

Variations and Progression Options

- *Hand positions:* Move hands up and down while spreading fingers, like rays of the rising and setting sun.
- *Standing Sun Rays.*

- *Visualization:* Be creative with other images, such as moon rays.

Seated Piano Playing

TARGET JOINT—Fingers

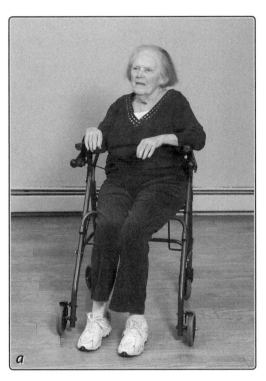

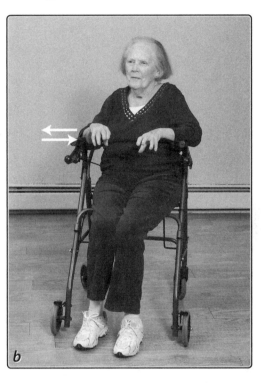

Start and Finish Position

1. Good seated posture.
2. Upper arms by the sides.
3. Forearms parallel with lap, palms down.

Outward and Inward Movement

4. Move the fingers and arms as if playing a piano.
5. Perform three to eight repetitions.

! Exercise and Safety Tips

- Remind those who have difficulty moving their hands to go at their own pace and stay within their strain-free and pain-free range of motion.

- If the arms get tired at a 90-degree angle, lower the arms to the lap and continue Seated Piano Playing.

Variations and Progression Options

- *Standing Piano Playing.*
- *Visualization:* Imagine a wider keyboard as the hands move wider from side to side.

- *Visualization:* Be creative with other images, such as raindrops (with the hands moving in an up and down direction).

Seated Chin to Chest ("Yes")

TARGET JOINT—Cervical spine (neck)

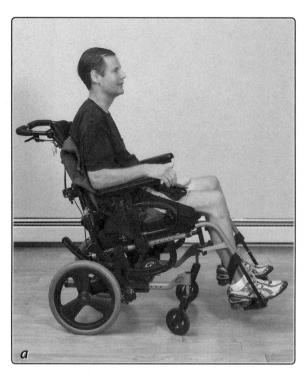

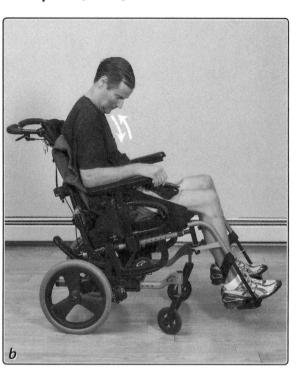

Start and Finish Position

1. Good seated posture.
2. Hands in a comfortable position.

Downward and Upward Movement

3. Slowly lower the chin toward the chest.
4. Slowly lift the head back to the starting position.
5. Perform three to eight repetitions.

 Exercise and Safety Tips

- Do not hyperextend the neck; move the head slowly.

Variations and Progression Options

- *Combo:* Hold the arms straight by the sides, flex the palms, and then press downward (as in exercise 7.2).

- *Combo (standing):* Interlace the fingers behind the back and press downward (as in standing exercise 7.1).
- *Standing Chin to Chest.*

Seated Chin to Shoulder

TARGET JOINT—Cervical spine (neck)

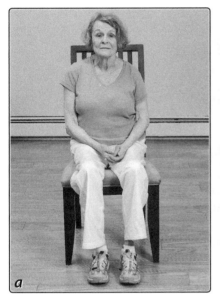 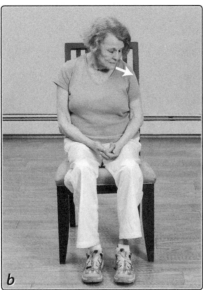 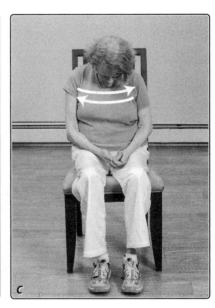

a *b* *c*

Start and Finish Position

1. Good seated posture.
2. Hands in a comfortable position.

Outward and Inward Movement

3. Lower the chin toward the shoulder.
4. Rotate the chin to the chest.
5. Continue rotating toward the other shoulder.
6. Rotate the chin back to the chest.
7. Continue rotating back to the first shoulder.
8. Perform three to eight repetitions.

! Exercise and Safety Tips

- Move the head slowly and smoothly.

Variations and Progression Options

- *Combo:* Combine Chin to Shoulder with interlacing fingers behind the back and press downward.

- *Combo:* Combine Chin to Shoulder with looking at the floor, making a half circle in the front from shoulder to shoulder.
- *Standing Chin to Shoulder.*

Seated Pelvic Tilt and Back Arch (Challenger)

TARGET JOINT—Spine

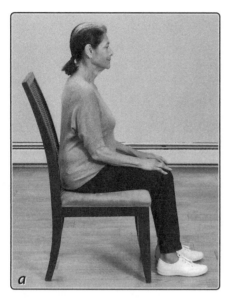

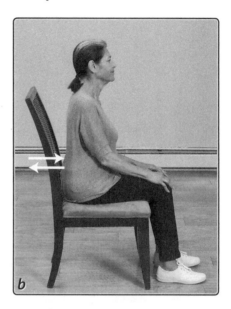

Start and Finish Position

1. Good seated posture.
2. Hands on lap or top of hip bones.

Backward and Forward Movement

3. Press the lower back toward or into the chair back (keeping the torso erect).
4. Come back to the neutral position.
5. Gently arch the back. Keep the shoulders down and back and the chest open.
6. Return to the neutral position.
7. Perform three to eight repetitions.

! Exercise and Safety Tips

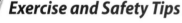

- Review the natural curves of the spine (see figure 4.2) with participants.
- Osteoporosis precaution: Do not slouch or collapse the torso (avoid forward flexion movement of the torso) when pushing the lower back toward or into the back of the chair. This precaution is recommended for all older adults.
- Do not hyperextend the neck when the back is arched. Look forward, not up.

Variations and Progression Options

- *Easier:* First, concentrate on doing a pelvic tilt. Put the hands on the hips and feel the pelvis moving backward and forward. When participants are comfortable with the pelvic tilt, extend the forward tilt to the top of the head, a gentle back arch. Keep the chin level with the floor.
- *Standing Pelvic Tilt and Back Arch (Challenger).*
- *Visualization:* Imagine a string on top of the head being pulled upward, elongating the spine, and a string extending from the belly button that when gently pulled makes the back arch.

Seated Side Reach

TARGET JOINT—Spine

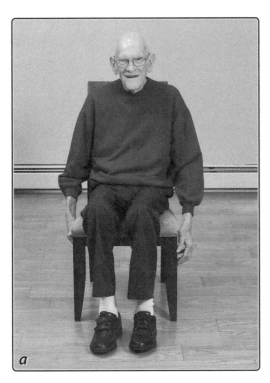 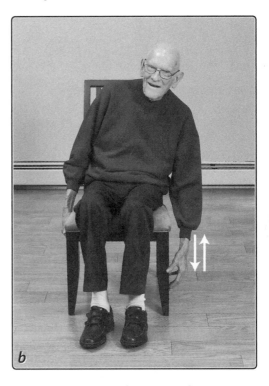

a *b*

Start and Finish Position

1. Good seated posture.
2. Hold the side of the chair with one hand.
3. Hold the opposite arm straight at the side with the palm facing in.

Downward and Upward Movement

4. Lower the hand toward the floor.
5. Return to the starting position.
6. Perform three to eight repetitions.
7. Repeat on the other side.

! Exercise and Safety Tips

- Warm up the back in a vertical position (as in exercise 4.21, Pelvic Tilt and Back Arch [Challenger]; 4.12, Rowing; 4.13, Close the Window) before turning or bending the trunk sideways.

- Hold on to the arm or seat of the chair for support during Seated Side Reach.
- Do not bend the neck. Keep the neck and spine in a neutral position.
- Osteoporosis: Avoid twisting movements, particularly in combination with stooping.

Variations and Progression Options

- *Arm position:* Reach up with one arm overhead.
- *Challenger (arms):* Reach up with both arms overhead.

- *Standing Side Reach.*

131

Seated Torso Rotation

TARGET JOINT—Spine

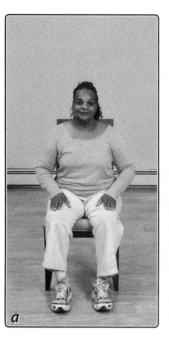 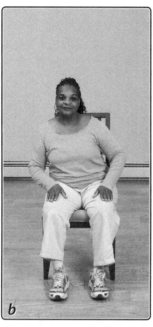 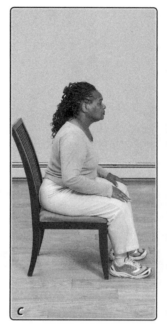 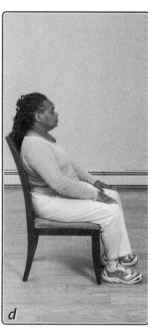

a   b   c   d

Start and Finish Position

1. Good seated posture.
2. Palms on the thighs.

Circular Movement

3. Lean to one side.
4. Then lean forward from the hips.
5. Then lean toward the other side (not shown).
6. Then lean slightly backward from the hips.
7. Return to the starting position.
8. Perform three to eight repetitions.
9. Repeat in the other direction.

 Exercise and Safety Tips

- Warm up the back in a vertical position (as in exercise 4.21, Pelvic Tilt and Back Arch [Challenger]; 4.12, Rowing; 4.13, Close the Window) before turning or bending the trunk sideways.
- Rest the palms on the thighs when leaning forward in Seated Torso Rotation.
- Move the head, neck, and spine as one unit.
- Do not hyperextend (overarch) the lower back when leaning backward.

- Those with hip fracture or replacement should perform only small rotations (avoid leaning forward) to prevent hip flexion of more than 90 degrees.
- Those with osteoporosis should avoid twisting movements, particularly in combination with stooping.

Variations and Progression Options

- *Circle size:* Start with small circles and progress to larger ones. Be creative with circle sizes.
- *Standing Torso Rotation.*
- 🧍 *Center of Gravity Awareness:* While participants are rotating the torso, cue them to be aware of their center of gravity (Bryant and Green 2009, 534). "Notice how your muscles tighten in the front, sides, and back as you move out of vertical alignment (good seated posture)."
- *Prop:* Hold a ball in the hands to the front, side, or overhead for an extra balance challenge.

Seated Twists

TARGET JOINT—Spine

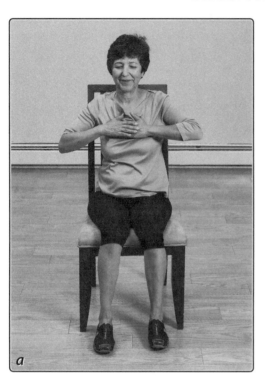

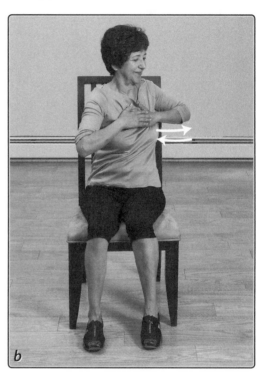

Start and Finish Position

1. Good seated posture.
2. Place palms on the chest, one hand on top of the other.
3. Hold the elbows out.

Twisting Movement

4. Twist the torso, moving one elbow backward and the other forward.
5. Keep the shoulders down.
6. Return to the starting position.
7. Perform three to eight repetitions.
8. Repeat in the opposite direction.

 Exercise and Safety Tips

- Warm up the back in a vertical position (as in exercise 4.21, Pelvic Tilt and Back Arch [Challenger]; 4.12, Rowing; 4.13, Close the Window) before turning or bending the trunk sideways.
- If the back of the chair is in the way, scoot forward in the chair, if this is comfortable.

- Perform twists slowly and smoothly through a comfortable range of motion.
- Do not twist the head or neck. Keep the chin aligned with the breastbone.
- Those with osteoporosis should avoid twisting movements, particularly in combination with stooping.

Variations and Progression Options

- *Easier:* Lower elbows if shoulders or arms get tired.
- *Easier:* Alternating sides may be easier for some participants.
- *Hand position:* Place hands in prayer position, resting on the sternum (breastbone).

- *Standing Twists.*
- *Visualization:* "Imagine a golden [*or let participants choose their color*] string attached to the top of your head, pulling gently upward. Your torso is lengthening with ease into good posture."

CHAPTER

5

Resistance Training

I joined a health spa recently. They had a sign
for "Free Weights." So I took a couple.

∞

—*Scott Wood*

LEARNING OBJECTIVES

After completing this chapter, you will have the tools to

- debunk some common myths about weight training and discuss the benefits;
- lead a safe and effective resistance training component of an exercise session in an individual or group setting;
- design a creative and progressive session using 12 functional resistance exercises with variations and progression options for each exercise;
- apply vital safety precautions and guidelines for teaching resistance training and using weights, bands, and tubes; and
- focus on fall prevention by personalizing your instruction of seated and standing resistance exercises for a class of people with varying fitness levels and one or more special needs.

Resistance training (also called strength training, resistive training, weight training, or weightlifting) "is exercise that causes muscles to work or hold against an applied force or weight" (ACSM 2009b, 1511). This chapter will prepare you for teaching safe and effective resistance training for frail elders and adults with special needs. After debunking common myths about resistance training, this chapter includes safety precautions for a variety of special needs and guidelines for exercise selection, sequence, intensity, and frequency, among other things. A program for basic seated exercises is discussed, followed by the same for basic standing exercises. At the end of the chapter, you will find photos and instructions for 12 resistance-training exercises—5 upper-body and 7 lower-body functional exercises that target the major muscles of the body.

A major benefit of resistance training is preventing or even reversing the usual decline in muscle mass, strength, and functional ability of older adults (Heyward 2010; Takeshima et al. 2007). As participants increase their strength,

137

they are better able to do daily activities requiring strength, such as getting up from a chair, climbing stairs, lifting a grandchild, and so on. The well-rounded functional resistance-training program provided in this chapter, in accordance with evidence-based guidelines, has many other benefits (with regular attendance and participation) including improved posture, balance, and health-related biomarkers (i.e., body composition, blood glucose levels, insulin sensitivity, and blood pressure) (ACSM 2011, 1342).

You can target key muscles used for balance. Both seated and standing resistance exercises can help to improve balance by increasing muscular strength and endurance (Heyward 2010; Hess and Woollacott 2005). Remember to incorporate other functional balance exercises to promote optimal balance benefits (Reid and Fielding 2012; Bovre 2010; Heyward 2010, 309; Rose 2010; Orr et al. 2008; Scott 2008; Shigematsu et al. 2008; Takeshima et al. 2007). This aspect will be discussed further in chapter 8.

MYTHS

Before offering resistance training to your participants, you may want to debunk some common myths about weight training (table 5.1) and discuss its benefits (see functional benefits of table 5.3 and appendix B1, "Benefits of Physical Activity for Older Persons"). This discussion can motivate prospective participants to attend your class and your regular participants not to play hooky. Participants' motivation and regular attendance are key to program success. You may copy tables 5.1, 5.3, and appendix B1 for easy reference and handouts.

SAFETY PRECAUTIONS

Resistance training is safe for frail elders and adults with special needs if appropriate exercise guidelines and precautions are observed. The following general safety precautions and spe-

cific safety precautions for those with special needs can help you lead safe resistance training and keep your participants injury free. You are welcome to photocopy "General Safety Precautions Checklist for Resistance Training."

These general resistance-training safety precautions for older adults also apply to those with special needs. The following specific safety precautions will increase the safety and effectiveness of your exercise program for those with special needs.

Specific Safety Precautions for Those With Special Needs

Following are some specific safety precautions for leading resistance exercises for people with specific needs, particularly when they are beyond an early or mild stage. Therefore, these precautions may not apply to every person with a particular condition. For example, a person with mild symptoms of arthritis may have few limitations with resistance exercises, whereas severe symptoms may prohibit resistance training. Also, remember that an individual's performance ability can vary from day to day. See chapter 1 to learn more about common special needs. For further information see the category "Fitness, Wellness, and Special Needs" in "Suggested Resources."

Alzheimer's Disease and Related Dementias

- Do not use rigid free weights (hand-held weights, such as dumbbells or canned foods), which can cause injury if dropped. Safer alternatives are wrist weights or an improvised weight such as a 1-pound (.45 kg) bag of beans in a sock.
- Because confused or disoriented participants may be unable to rate perceived exertion dependably, be especially vigilant of their response to resistance training.
- Some resistance exercises require the instructor to be extra watchful with participants who may not remember

Table 5.1 Common Myths and Facts About Resistance Training

Myth	Fact
"You have to be in shape first."	Generally, the more out of shape you are, the more you can benefit from resistance training.
"I don't need resistance training because I do aerobics."	Aerobic exercise is great for cardiovascular fitness, but resistance training for muscular strength and endurance rounds out an exercise program.
"Weight training is for men."	Women of all ages as well as men can benefit significantly from resistance-training programs.
"I don't want to develop large, bulky muscles." (women)	Most women's genetic makeup prevents them from developing the large muscles that men can acquire when using weights.
"Weight training requires heavy barbells and other special equipment."	Lighter and less expensive weights can work just as effectively as heavy barbells and other special equipment.
"No pain, no gain."	"Train, don't strain" or "No pain, you gain" is a more sensible approach to resistance training.
"Weight training is hard on the joints."	Sensible resistance exercise can improve joint strength.
"It takes too much time."	All you need is one set of 8 to 12 repetitions of 8 to 10 exercises that condition the major muscle groups, at least twice a week.
"It won't help me lose excess fat weight."	An increase in muscle mass increases your metabolism, which makes it easier to lose fat weight.
"When you quit resistance training, your muscle turns to fat."	The result of detraining is muscle loss. If you keep eating as much as you were during training but don't burn it off with exercise, you will gain fat.
"It takes more willpower and discipline than I have."	One of the many benefits you can gain from resistance training is more energy for daily activities such as exercise class.
"I'm too old to lift weights."	People in their 90s, including nursing home residents, can weight-train safely and increase muscle strength significantly.

From E. Best-Martini and K.A. Jones-DiGenova, 2014, *Exercise for frail elders*, 2nd ed. (Champaign, IL: Human Kinetics).

directions or pose a risk of copying others who are doing an exercise that is contraindicated for their condition. Have those participants sit near you in clear sight. If they have other special needs, ensure that they follow the specific safety precautions for those needs.

• When leading resistance training, if an exercise is performed on one side and then the other, slowly move uninterruptedly from one side to the other. For example, give a visual and verbal cue such as by saying, "Switch sides." Then, after you see them change sides,

GENERAL SAFETY PRECAUTIONS CHECKLIST FOR RESISTANCE TRAINING

☐ Follow the physician's special recommendations and comments for a participant on the "Statement of Medical Clearance for Exercise" (appendix A2) and remind the participant to follow them as well.

☐ Always warm up for at least 10 minutes beforehand and cool down for at least 10 minutes after resistance training.

☐ Focus on fall prevention. During standing exercise have a chair centered closely behind all participants so that they can sit down easily if needed. Remember that participants can have day-to-day variation with their balance ability. When participants are seated make sure that they are safely positioned in their chairs.

☐ Additionally, weight machines can be advantageous for those with upper-body stability and balance issues (Rahl 2010, 224).

☐ Demonstrate all resistance-training exercises in a slow, controlled manner.

☐ Avoid jerking or thrusting weights into position, which can cause injuries.

☐ Instruct your participants not to hold their breath while lifting because doing so increases chest pressure, which may restrict blood return to the heart and markedly elevate blood pressure. Also, breath holding can increase intra-abdominal pressure and cause a hernia.

☐ Do not grip hand weights too tightly. Use a relaxed grip.

☐ Keep wrists in a neutral position (straight) during all upper-body resistance exercises.

☐ Lift arms and legs only as high as comfortable while maintaining erect posture. Participants with hip replacements should avoid resistance exercises that involve hip flexion (decreasing hip joint angle, such as by lifting the thigh toward the upright torso beyond parallel with the floor) of more than 90 degrees.

☐ Avoid hyperextending joints—locking or extending beyond the normal ROM—particularly the elbow and knee. In a straight or standing position, keep the joints soft, not bent.

☐ While performing lower-body resistance exercises, always keep one foot on the floor for stability to maintain good posture and protect the back.

☐ If participants experience strain or pain in or near a joint when using weights, have them stop the exercise. For further information, refer to the section "Modifying the Exercises" in chapter 8 and figure 2.4.

☐ Do not overtrain. Mild muscle soreness lasting up to a few days is normal after resistance training, but exhaustion, sore joints, and unpleasant muscle soreness are signs of overtraining.

☐ Use the same amount of weight on each side for the upper- and lower-body resistance exercises to promote symmetry of the right and left sides of the body, unless instructed otherwise by a qualified professional, such as a physical or occupational therapist.

☐ Remove leg weights before walking around. Walking with leg weights can increase risk of falling.

☐ When the weights are not being used, place them in a safe place, perhaps under participants' chairs, so that no one will trip over them.

☐ Prevent participants' falling forward and a possible increase in cranial pressure by instructing them not to lower their heads below parallel with the floor when bending forward, as when picking up or putting down weights.

☐ Ask participants how they felt after the previous class and make appropriate modifications in the next session to prevent overtraining.

From E. Best-Martini and K.A. Jones-DiGenova, 2014, *Exercise for frail elders,* 2nd ed. (Champaign, IL: Human Kinetics).

continue relevant cueing. This approach helps those with memory issues remember what side they just trained.

Arthritis

- Short, frequent exercise sessions are better tolerated than long, less frequent ones. For example, instead of combining resistance training and aerobics into a 1-hour class on Monday, Wednesday, and Friday, people with arthritis might respond more favorably to shorter, more frequent classes, such as resistance training on Monday and Thursday and aerobics on Tuesday, Wednesday, and Friday or Saturday. Two days of resistance training per week are generally better tolerated than 3. If shorter, more frequent classes are not feasible, people with arthritis may take as many breaks as necessary with longer exercise classes.

- Gradually build up to 8 to 10 repetitions with slight or light resistance (Arthritis Foundation 2009) (an RPE of 2), keeping the resistance below the participant's discomfort threshold. When a participant responds favorably, progress carefully (refer to "Progressing Your Exercise Class" in chapter 8). The Arthritis Foundation (2009, 102) cautions the instructor that multiple repetitions of resistance exercises may cause joint flare-ups.

- If an isotonic resistance exercise (exercise involving contractions against resistance with joint movement, such as standard free-weight training shown in exercises 5.1 through 5.12 in this chapter) causes pain to any joint, decrease the workload or adjust the exercise technique, body position, or speed of the movement. If pain persists, consult the physician or physical therapist.

- Mild isometric resistance exercises (exercise involving contractions against resistance in a stationary position with no joint movement) can strengthen the joint and surrounding muscles while reducing the chance of increasing inflammation. Isometric exercises are less likely to cause inflammation than isotonic exercises are. For further information, refer to the section "Resistance Bands and Isometric Exercises" in "Suggested Resources."

- When a joint is significantly inflamed, rest or significantly modify the program to include only isometric strengthening and gentle ROM exercises (Rahl 2010). A participant can experiment with doing a few repetitions, such as 1 to 3 to begin with (Arthritis Foundation 2009) without weights within a strain-free and pain-free ROM. In the in-between-time when other participants are performing up to 12 to 15 reps, suggest an exercise that the participant can enjoy and benefit from, such as three-part deep breathing. When appropriate, slow and smooth ROM exercises (still with fewer repetitions) may be a beneficial alternative.

- After acute inflammation has subsided, encourage the participant to resume resistance training cautiously to benefit the joints. Well-conditioned muscles are necessary for joint stability and function and may decrease the impact load on the joints (Rahl 2010, 182, 188).

Cerebrovascular Accident (CVA, Stroke)

- See also the safety precautions for those with coronary artery disease (heart disease).

- Providing clear resistance-training instructions is extremely important to participants who have experienced stroke. If a participant has paralysis on the right side, focus on leading exercises mainly by demonstration, using few verbal instructions. If there is paralysis on the left side, rely more on verbal instructions, using fewer gestures (American Senior Fitness Association 2012c).

Chronic Obstructive Pulmonary Disease (COPD)

- Avoid sustained isometrics, holding the breath, heavy weight training, and holding any weight overhead for more than a few seconds to prevent straining the respiratory and cardiovascular systems.

- Avoid hard or heavy resistance (an RPE of 5 or more) without medical clearance, especially for those on long-term steroid medication who are susceptible to muscle or tendon rupture (AACVPR 2011, 46).

- Additionally, chronic steroid use has a side effect of bone density reduction and increased risk of compression fracture (AACVPR 2011, 45; Biskobing 2002). In these cases, the specific safety precautions for osteoporosis apply.

Coronary Artery Disease (Heart Disease)

- Cardiac patients should not resistance-train if they have any of the following conditions: unstable angina, uncon-trolled hypertension, uncontrolled dysrhythmias, recent history of congestive heart failure (that has not been evaluated and effectively treated), severe valvular disease, or left ventricular outflow obstruction (AACVPR 2006, 86–87).

- For cardiac patients without contraindications (mentioned earlier), mild to moderate (approximately 50 percent of the maximal voluntary contraction according to AACVPR 2006, 76) resistance training can provide a safe and effective method for improving muscular strength and endurance (ACSM 2009a).

- Avoid actions that excessively raise blood pressure (see the special precautions for COPD and hypertension).

- Stop exercising at the first signs or symptoms of overexertion or cardiac complications, particularly *a*bnormal heart rhythm, unusual shortness of *b*reath, *c*hest discomfort, or *d*izziness (notice the mnemonic *ABCD*).

Depression

- Lifting heavier weights may be more effective for reducing depression. We recommend using heavier weight (more than 8 pounds, or 3.6 kg) only for those with medical clearance, when working with the participant one on one or in a small class, and when heavy lifting does not compromise the participant's enjoyment.

- If safe and appropriate for the participant, slightly increase the resistance when 11 repetitions (rather than 12 to 15) are completed with good technique in at least two consecutive workouts. If the response to this increase is positive, consider increasing the resistance again when the participant can complete 10 repetitions without strain in at least two successive sessions. Avoid lifting weights that are too heavy by having the participant perform at least 8 repetitions of a resistance exercise.

Diabetes

- Resistance exercise is recommended three times per week (on nonconsecutive days) using moderate or heavy weights for optimal gains in strength and insulin action (ACSM and ADA 2010, 2291) for people with type 2 diabetes. Support participants with type 2 diabetes, who may have other special needs, in gradually progressing in the direction of this goal.

- Participants with diabetic complications may require modifications, such as less resistance intensity, lighter gripping, avoiding isometric contractions, and avoiding exercising to the point of exhaustion (Rahl 2010, 213; ACSM 2010; ACSM and ADA 2010).

Frailty

- Begin frail elders with about four resistance exercises performed at low intensity (start with no weight and progress to .5 pound [.2 kg]). As their strength increases, encourage them to do more exercises and gradually lift more weight.

- Ankle and wrist weights are handy for frail elders.

- Build up to resistance training three times per week.

- Regular, safe resistance training to promote muscular strength and endurance is significant to the goal of restoring function, as well as possible, for frail people. Encourage regular class attendance and acknowledge small steps forward to help them feel good along the road to functional fitness.

- Address other possible special needs associated with their frailty, such as osteoporosis.

Hip Fracture or Replacement

- The physician who gives medical clearance (see appendix A2, "Statement of Medical Clearance for Exercise" form) will determine when a participant is ready after surgery and physical therapy to start a class that includes resistance training.

- Participants may need to work with their physical therapists to modify the resistance exercises.

- Avoid resistance exercises that involve internal rotation (turning the leg inward), hip adduction that crosses the midline of the body (crossing the legs), and hip flexion (decreasing hip joint angle, such as by lifting the thigh toward the upright torso beyond parallel with the floor) of more than 90 degrees to prevent the risk of hip dislocation, unless the participant has written clearance from his or her physician indicating that those specific movements are not contraindicated. Otherwise, participants in chairs that allow their knees to be lower than their hips and who are able to follow directions (see the earlier section "Alzheimer's Disease and Related Dementias") can be asked to raise their feet (one at a time) 1 inch (2.5 cm) or less off the floor for the Seated Hip Flexion (exercise 5.6). During Modified Chair Stands (exercise 5.12), instruct participants to keep their torsos as erect as possible (to lean forward as little as possible). For the Standing Hip Abduction and Adduction (exercise 5.7), they should bring the leg only to the midline of the body (not crossing one leg in front of the other).

Hypertension

- In general, moderate resistance training is beneficial and safe, when hypertension is controlled (Bryant and Green 2009, 192).

- Avoid any exercises that can excessively raise blood pressure, such as lifting heavy weights (an RPE of 5, "hard," or more), performing sustained isometric muscular contractions, doing excessive overhead arm exercise, gripping the exercise accessories or equipment too hard, doing strong-grip exercises using hard rubber balls, and holding the breath.

- Encourage participants to progress gradually into a regular aerobic endurance exercise program in addition to resistance training according to evidence-based guidelines for optimally lowering blood pressure (ACSM 2004a, 545).

Multiple Sclerosis and Parkinson's Disease

- Have participants with Parkinson's disease and multiple sclerosis use light weights (0.5–3 pounds, or 0.2–1.4 kg), if safe and well tolerated (Rahl 2010, 228; ACSM 2009a, 355).
- For some people, such as those with mild symptoms, heavier weights may be beneficial.
- The National Center on Physical Activity and Disability (NCPAD) (2009a) recommends equalizing the strength of opposing muscles for those with MS, which is applicable for all participants (refer to the section "Upper-Body Weights, Bands, and Tubes" in this chapter for more information about opposing muscles).
- Alternate between resistance and aerobic training in successive classes (Rahl 2010, 232; NCPAD 2009a).

Osteoporosis

- With physician consent, start with body weight, lifting the arms and legs without additional weight, and progress to light forms of resistance, such as low-tension exercise bands, soft putty, sponges, or Nerf balls.
- Gradually progress to light (.5 pound [.2 kg], if available, or 1 pound [.45 kg]) handheld or wrist weights and slowly and cautiously increase by increments of .5 to 1 pound (.2 to .45 kg), as tolerated.

- Participants at risk for osteoporosis, such as those with osteopenia ("low bone mineral mass," Heyward 2010, 15) can build up to moderate- to high-intensity resistance to maintain or possibly build bones. Those with osteoporosis (especially milder conditions) may be able to use moderate resistance, but not heavy to avoid injury (ACSM 2010, 257–258; Rahl 2010, 195).
- If symptoms such as pain or reduced function arise from weights, recommend rest and medical evaluation before resuming resistance training with body weight only. If the participant gets a medical evaluation, give him or her another "Statement of Medical Clearance for Exercise" form (appendix A2) and write in a request for specific weight recommendations.
- Avoid resistance exercises that involve spinal flexion, particularly in combination with stooping, which increases the risk of vertebral fractures (ACSM 2009a, 275). During the Chair Stand (exercise 5.12), maintain the natural curves of the spine by moving the head, neck, and spine as one unit throughout the exercise.
- A helpful visualization to promote good seated or standing posture is to have participants imagine a string attached to the top of the head, pulling gently upward.

Sensory Losses

- Use visual cues as often as possible, such as demonstration of the resistance exercises, for participants with hearing loss.
- Describe resistance exercises precisely and directly to participants with visual impairment.

! Safety Tip For safe and effective resistance training for older adults, carefully follow the safety precautions and the following evidence-based guidelines.

GUIDELINES

Several prominent organizations have developed guidelines for safe and effective resistance training, including the American College of Sports Medicine (2011, 2010, 2009b), the American Council on Exercise (Bryant and Green 2010), the American Senior Fitness Association (2012a, b, c), the National Strength and Conditioning Association (Baechle and Earle 2008), and the U.S. Department of Health and Human Services (USDHHS 2008b). Table 5.2 synthesizes resistance-training guidelines that are appropriate for older adults. The recommendations for resistance training in this chapter are based on these evidence-based guidelines, although additional recommendations are presented for a population with special needs. You may make a copy of table 5.2 for easy reference and as an educational handout for your participants. Refer to the earlier section "Specific Safety Precautions for Those With Special Needs" for adapting the following general guidelines to meet your participant's special needs.

The following sections present more detailed information about the guidelines to minimize injury and maximize the benefits of resistance training for frail elders and adults with special needs.

! Safety Tip First, teach good seated posture with back support. Then gradually and on an individual basis build up participants to sitting erect without back support to strengthen the core, or postural, muscles.

Exercise Selection

A well-designed resistance training class includes an initial warm-up period (see chapter 4), a minimum of eight resistance exercises for the major muscles groups, and a final cool-down period (see chapter 7). This chapter provides five upper-body and seven lower-body basic resistance exercises that condition the major muscle groups of the body (identified in table 5.3). Participants can strengthen the postural, or core, muscles (including the abdominals) isometrically by performing resistance exercises sitting erect and not leaning against the back of the chair. But, first make sure they are able to exercise with good seated posture (see instructions in chapter 4) with back support. Then gradually build up participants to sitting erect without back support, with those who are capable. Teach the basic seated resistance exercises first before progressing to standing exercises (see "Instructions for Good Standing Posture" in chapter 4). Also, refer to "Core and Core Stability" in chapter 2 and table 2.3 for seated and standing core exercises.

Exercise Sequence

Follow the given order of the exercises, which goes from larger to smaller muscle groups. This order is recommended for intensive resistance training and is an ideal foundation for beginner-level training. You may teach either the upper-body or lower-body resistance exercises first and then the other to add variety and to find out what works better for your class. When introducing resistance exercises you can start with just upper-body or lower-body exercises and gradually progress from there. Also, you can start with a few of the 5 upper-body or 7 lower-body resistance exercises and carefully build up to performing all 12.

Intensity

Initially, teach the resistance exercises without weights. Participants will be encouraged to learn that lifting the weight of their arms and legs alone is beneficial. When they have learned the exercises, begin with light weights, such as 1 pound (.45 kg). In the section "Basic Seated Resistance Exercises," you will learn how to teach the exercises without weights and the essentials of introducing weights.

How much weight a person lifts depends on several factors, such as his or her special needs,

Table 5.2   General Resistance-Training Guidelines for Older Adults

Exercise selection	Choose at least eight safe exercises that condition the major muscle groups of the body.
Exercise sequence	During light resistance training, move from head to toe or from toe to head. During light or intensive resistance training, move from larger to smaller muscle groups and do postural muscles last.
Intensity (amount of weight or resistance)	Initially, perform about 8 repetitions and then carefully build up to 12 to 15, at an exertion level perceived as "very slight" to "slight" (an RPE of 1 to 2). Progress slowly to "somewhat hard" (an RPE of 4) when a person is ready and has learned good technique.
Frequency	Resistance-train two to three times per week on nonconsecutive days when doing a full-body workout.
Repetitions	Perform 8 to 15 repetitions in a row per set. Begin with about 8 repetitions.
Range of motion	Exercise through the full, strain-free and pain-free range of joint movement without hyperextending.
Speed	Perform slow, smooth movement. Take 3 seconds to lift or push a weight into place and take another 3 seconds to return the weight to the start and finish position.
Sets	Perform one to three sets (a separate bout of an exercise) per exercise.
Rest periods between sets	Wait at least 1 to 2 minutes between sets of 8 to 15 repetitions.
Rest periods between exercises	The rest period can be longer (up to 1 minute) if heavier resistance is used and can be shortened or eliminated with lighter resistance, as the individual's tolerance to exercise increases over time.
Rest periods between workouts	Allow 48 to 72 hours of rest between full-body workouts.
Progression and maintenance	After participants learn to perform the 12 basic seated resistance exercises with body weight and good technique, progress slowly. Gradually increase resistance by increments of 1 pound (.45 kg) or less. Reduce repetitions to 8; progress gradually to 12 to 15 repetitions at the heavier weight. Alternatively, add a second set of 8 repetitions and gradually progress to 15. When participants reach long-term resistance-training goals, encourage lifetime maintenance.

From E. Best-Martini and K.A. Jones-DiGenova, 2014, *Exercise for frail elders*, 2nd ed. (Champaign, IL: Human Kinetics).

goals, motivation, exercise tolerance, and so on. When starting with weights, perform 8 to 15 repetitions at an exertion level perceived as "very slight" to "slight" (an RPE of 1 to 2). You can use the RPE scale to help participants find an appropriate training intensity. After participants learn good technique, gradually progress to 4 ("somewhat hard") on the RPE scale, when appropriate. "Somewhat hard" should be challenging but not involve any strain or pain.

! *Safety Tip* After participants learn good resistance training technique, slowly and safely progress to weights and resistance bands or tubes that are challenging but do not produce any strain or pain.

Table 5.3 Basic Resistance and Balance Exercises: Seated or Standing[a]

Target body parts and muscles	Exercise	Functional benefits
UPPER-BODY RESISTANCE EXERCISES		
Chest (pectoralis major) Back of upper arms (triceps) Shoulders (deltoids)	*5.1 Chest Press	Pushing a door open, pushing a drawer closed, pushing up from a lying position
Back (latissimus dorsi, trapezius) Front of upper arms (biceps) Shoulders (deltoids)	*5.2 Two-Arm Row	Pulling a door or drawer open, posture
Shoulders (deltoids) Back of upper arms (triceps)	*5.3 Overhead Press	Lifting (especially overhead)
Front of upper arms (biceps)	5.4 Biceps Curl	Lifting, pulling
Back of upper arms (triceps)	5.5 Triceps Extension (Challenger)	Pushing, pressing up from seated or lying position
LOWER-BODY RESISTANCE EXERCISES		
Front hips and thighs (hip flexors)	*5.6 Hip Flexion	Stair climbing, posture; improved static and dynamic standing balance
Outer hips and thighs (hip abductors) Inner thighs (hip adductors)	*5.7 Hip Abduction and Adduction	Hip rotation (lateral or medial), pelvic stabilization, posture, walking; improved static and dynamic standing balance
Back of thighs (hamstrings)	5.8 Knee Flexion	Stand from sitting, stair climbing, walking (foot clearance); improved static and dynamic standing balance
Front of thighs (quadriceps)	5.9 Knee Extension	Stand from sitting, stair climbing, walking (forward progression and stability); improved static and dynamic standing balance
Shins (tibialis anterior)	*5.10 Toe Raises	Walking (foot clearance)
Calves (gastrocnemius, soleus)	*5.11 Heel Raises	Walking (push off); improved static and dynamic standing balance
Thighs (quadriceps, hamstrings) Buttocks (gluteals)	*5.12 Chair Stands (Challenger)	Stand from sitting, stair climbing, walking (forward progression and stability)

[a]All seated basic resistance and balance exercises have a corresponding standing exercise. See variations and progression options in the illustrated exercises at the end of the chapter. Your participants will receive greater balance benefits with the standing exercises, particularly exercises involving a one-legged stand (indicated by a balance icon).

*The eight exercises preceded by an asterisk are recommended for a shorter program (see table 8.8, Eight-Exercise Resistance-Training Component).

Adapted, by permission, from S. McKelvey, 2003, *Functional fitness for older adults training manual* (San Diego, CA: Aging and Independent Services), 7. © Kim A. Jones-DiGenova.

From E. Best-Martini and K.A. Jones-DiGenova, 2014, *Exercise for frail elders,* 2nd ed. (Champaign, IL: Human Kinetics).

Frequency

We recommend that you initially schedule resistance training 2 days per week on nonconsecutive days. After your participants respond favorably to resistance training for several months, try three times per week. This schedule increases the chance that your participants can make it to class at least two times per week. Especially encourage frail elders and others with sedentary lifestyles to attend class three times per week. On the other hand, praise beginners for just coming to your class anytime (this can just be a warm smile acknowledging their presence). Encourage regular participation, when it is timely for an individual or for her or his support person (i.e., caregiver).

Repetitions

In general, 8 to 15 repetitions per set of each resistance exercise is recommended for older adults. Repetitions, often shortened to *reps*, is the number of times an exercise is performed within a set; one repetition is a complete movement of an exercise. A set is a separate bout of an exercise—for example, 8 reps might make up a set. After the initial phase of learning the resistance exercises without weights, help each participant select a weight that she or he can lift 8 times comfortably, without strain. Carefully work up to 12 to 15 repetitions per set. Doing 15 repetitions makes it easier to progress to a heavier weight. When a participant reaches 12 to 15 repetitions comfortably, increase the weight and decrease the repetitions back to 8. If some participants are doing fewer repetitions than others are, they must wait for the others to complete the extra repetitions. Therefore, with a class we suggest a maximum of 12 repetitions to minimize the waiting time of those doing fewer repetitions. When working one on one or when appropriate with older, deconditioned, or frail people who are beginning resistance training, experiment with a higher number of repetitions (i.e., 10 to 20) and lower resistance (i.e., very light to light intensity) (ACSM 2011, 1343; Evans 1999).

Use positive terms such as *challenging, happily worked*, and so on when describing the feeling to aim for at the last repetition. Avoid conventional terms such as *fatigue* or *muscular failure* that can have negative connotations or are inappropriate for the frail elder population.

Range of Motion

When the entire range of motion (ROM) is covered during an exercise, the value of the exercise is maximized and flexibility is maintained or possibly improved (Baechle and Earle 2008). Remind your participants to perform the resistance exercises through their full strain-free and pain-free range of motion (the maximum range of joint movement that does not elicit discomfort or pain) without hyperextending or locking their joints. For a constructive adaptation to resistance training, participants should feel the exercises in their muscles and not in their joints.

 Safety Tip Instruct participants to perform the resistance exercises through their full strain-free and pain-free ROM without hyperextending or locking their joints (when in a straight position), especially the elbow and knee.

Speed

Take 3 full seconds to lift or push a weight or resistance band into place and take another 3 full seconds to lower the weight while resisting gravity or to release a band back to the starting position. The count for resistance training is slow (e.g., "1, 1, 1, up, 1, 1, 1, down; 2, 2, 2, up, . . ."). Refer to table 3.3 and the surrounding discussion of counting in chapter 3. Have participants count aloud while learning resistance exercises to reinforce slow movement and make sure that they are not holding their breath.

Sets

One to three sets (a separate bout of an exercise) of 8 to 15 repetitions per exercise is a general recommendation for muscular strength and endurance training. Start with one set. Resistance-training programs using single sets rather than multiple sets are recommended for middle-aged and older beginner exercisers. Single-set programs (in accordance with evidence-based guidelines) are effective in improving muscular strength and endurance, result in less injury or soreness, and take less time (AACVPR 2006, 87). People who are beginning resistance training, in particular, "may significantly improve muscle strength and size" with a single-set program (ACSM 2011, 1336, 1343). When multiple-sets are indicated, you can perform different resistance exercises that target the same muscle group or repeat the same resistance exercise. When repeating the same exercise, we recommend using a variation of that exercise to train the muscle and joints in different ways, to reduce the risk of overuse injury, and to spice up the routine (refer to the variations and progression options in the illustrated instructions sections of chapters 4 through 7). Remember that it is better to do one set slowly with good technique than to do two or three sets quickly, increasing the risk of injury.

When working with adults with frailty and other special needs, you may start with just a few repetitions for the second set and gradually build up to 12 to 15. This approach also applies when progressing to a third or fourth set. Another option for a gentle transition for increasing sets is to use a lighter weight or even no weight (in some cases) for the new set. As you progress your class, a person having difficulty keeping up can have an experience of moving forward by doing the new set (of a few reps) without weights.

Rest Periods Between Sets, Exercises, and Workouts

Have participants wait 1 to 2 minutes before doing a second or third set of 8 to 15 repetitions. Between sets they can perform another resistance exercise that targets another muscle group. If the class needs a short breather from resistance exercises, try three-part deep breathing (chapter 4), a range-of-motion exercise (chapter 4), or a stretching exercise (chapter 7). In general, give longer rest periods between exercises with heavier resistance. Shorten or eliminate rest periods between different exercises of lighter resistance as participants' tolerance to exercise improves. Finally, schedule resistance training so that your participants have 48 to 72 hours of rest between full-body workouts "to optimally promote the cellular and molecular adaptations that stimulate muscle hypertrophy"(increase of muscle size) and associated gains in strength (ACSM 2011,1343). Ideally, schedule a resistance training class that meets 2 days per week with 72 hours between classes (e.g., on Monday and Thursday) and a class that meets 3 days per week with 48 hours between classes (e.g., on Monday, Wednesday, and Friday [Saturday would also work well]).

! Safety Tip For optimal recovery and potential muscular strength and endurance benefits from resistance training, schedule the recommended two to three sessions per week with 48 to 72 hours of rest between full-body workouts.

Progression and Maintenance

You can move forward with the resistance-training component in numerous ways to promote muscular strength and endurance. After participants have learned good technique and are comfortable with the 12 basic seated resistance exercises, you can slowly progress in one of the following ways. Remember to increase only one variable at a time.

- **Standing exercises**. Participants who are able to stand safely can slowly progress to the standing variations of the basic seated resistance exercises. See other variations and progression options in the illustrated exercises at the end of this chapter.

• **Frequency**. Days per week can be increased by one session at a time up to three, on nonconsecutive days when doing a full-body workout.

Alternatively, when participants can easily complete 12 to 15 repetitions of a resistance exercise, they may progress in one of the following ways:

• **Sets**. Add a second set of 8 repetitions and gradually progress to 12 to 15. Less weight can be used for the second set. See the variations and progression options in exercises 5.1 to 5.12 for ideas for varying the second set.

• **Intensity**. Slightly increase the amount of weight (ideally, by 1 pound [.45 kg] or less) and drop back to 8 repetitions. With resistance bands or tubes, increase to a firmer band of slightly more resistance. Gradually progress to a maximum of 12 to 15 repetitions at the heavier resistance.

• **Resistance**. Use "two for one" (use two different weights or bands for one set). Use the next heaviest weight or band for one or a few reps and then go back to the lower resistance for the remainder of the set. Gradually progress to the heavier resistance for a full set.

• **Range of motion**. Start with a narrower ROM—for example, when you increase the resistance—for some or all of the reps. Then gradually increase to a full ROM for the exercise, always staying within strain-free and pain-free ROM.

• **Resting between repetitions**. Do not rest between reps. Start with a few reps and safely progress to a full set. For example, with exercise 5.6, Seated Hip Flexion, do not rest the foot on the floor between reps. With resistance bands and tubes, maintain resistance on the band (keep taut) between reps.

When possible, work with participants' physicians, physical therapists, or other health care professionals to set and modify resistance-training goals and determine how far to progress. We recommend using dumbbells weighing between 1 and 10 pounds (.45 and 4.5 kg) and having participants increase their weights in 1-pound (.45 kg) increments or less. Generally, in a class setting with frail elders and adults with special needs, using weights heavier than 10 pounds (4.5 kg) is not safe or feasible. A safe goal for people with dementia or advanced osteoporosis may be to use 1-pound weights for both the upper- and lower-body exercises. On the other hand, someone with a hip replacement might not be able to use any additional weight for lower-body resistance exercises but may eventually reach 10 pounds for the upper-body exercises.

At some point a participant will cease progressing and begin simply to maintain his or her current level of resistance training, depending on his or her goals, motivation, physical and mental ability, physician's recommendations, and available equipment. A worthwhile goal is to attain the level of strength and endurance required for activities of daily living (termed *functional fitness*) that are important to the participant. For example, if a person has not attained his or her goal of walking up and down the stairs in the home three times per day, the lower-body weights, reps, or sets could be increased (safely, one at a time!) when the participant is ready. But if the person has attained his or her goal of being able to transfer or get out of a wheelchair or chair more easily, he or she may want to maintain their training program with upper-body weights.

When a participant has attained a goal, reevaluate her or his functional fitness goals related to muscular strength and endurance before beginning maintenance with resistance training. This can be a good time to encourage further progress (when appropriate) based on the guidelines for resistance training provided in this section. Individualized resistance-training goals that require maintaining with certain resistance exercises and progressing with others can generally be achieved more easily with one-on-one training. Although significant muscular strength and endurance progress can potentially be made with each participant in a class setting, some people cannot realize their resistance-training goals in a class setting. In such cases, you may want to suggest that they join a local fitness facility or hire a qualified personal trainer.

A key to success in resistance training is recording participants' attendance and progress. The "Fitness Training Log" in appendix B5, which you may copy, enables you and your participants to track weight and repetitions of each resistance exercise. At least once per month, make time at the beginning or end of class to evaluate the resistance-training log with each participant. In the meantime, encourage participants to let you know how they are doing so that you can suggest or make (with those who need more assistance) appropriate adjustments.

Other Training Techniques

In addition to planning and adjusting the components of resistance training, such as intensity, frequency, reps, and sets, be sure to incorporate these guidelines:

- Teach participants to maintain good seated or standing posture when performing resistance exercises.
- Before participants perform each exercise, instruct them to stabilize their shoulders by moving them up, back, and down and to keep their shoulders down throughout each exercise.
- Instruct participants to focus on or feel the major muscles that are being exercised.
- Encourage participants to breathe continuously throughout every repetition. Prevent breath holding by one of these methods:
  1. Have participants count aloud with each repetition (particularly with beginners and larger classes). Par-

ticipants cannot hold their breath if they are speaking.
  2. Have participants practice optimal breathing after they learn to perform the resistance exercises slowly and safely while counting. For optimal breathing, they breathe out as they lift or push the weight or band and breathe in as they return it to the starting position. This breathing pattern feels natural after it is practiced for a while.

- You may integrate a posture, breathing, ROM, or stretching (see chapters 4 and 7) exercise between resistance exercises. With stretching and ROM, pick an exercise that loosens up the body part just worked. For example, after a Chest Press (exercise 5.1), which works the chest and shoulders, try a Shoulder Rotation (exercise 4.9), which loosens up the chest and shoulders.
- Stretch each muscle group after strength training. See the stretching exercises in chapter 7.
- Guide a participant returning to resistance training after a significant time off to start at about half of his or her usual training intensity and then gradually increase the resistance.

! Safety Tip To prevent injury and promote enjoyment of resistance training, teach participants to listen to their body and focus on or feel the major muscles that are being used.

Before introducing resistance training, lay a strong foundation by teaching your participants safe and constructive biomechanics. See appendix B3, "Cueing for Safe and Constructive Biomechanics During Exercise and Activities of Daily Living (ADL)." Although you will be essentially using the cueing in appendix B3 while leading resistance exercises, doing a complete review of appendix B3 can be beneficial when you have a new student or when a significant break has occurred between classes. You may photocopy appendix B3 as a teaching aid and handout for your participants. Remind your participants to use the safe and constructive biomechanics that they learn in your class outside of class with activities of daily living (ADL).

BASIC SEATED RESISTANCE EXERCISES

The 12 basic seated resistance exercises (see table 5.3) are a comprehensive set of 5 upper-body and 7 lower-body functional exercises that target the major muscles of the body. Teach the basic seated resistance exercises first, to eliminate the risk of falling as you get to know your participants' strengths and current limitations, before teaching the standing resistance exercises. Also, introduce the two challenger exercises (5.5, Seated Triceps Extension and 5.12, Modified Chair Stands) after participants have learned the other basic seated exercises (for more information about challenger exercises, see chapter 8). The Modified Chair Stand (Challenger) is included with the seated exercises as a means of progression from the sitting to the standing exercises. Participants who are able to stand safely can slowly progress to the basic standing resistance and balance exercises.

The number of resistance exercises that you teach in an exercise session and the order in which you teach them can vary. An easy approach is to follow the given order of exercises, 5.1 to 5.12, from upper to lower body. For variety, you can lead the lower-body exercises first and then the upper-body exercises or alternate lower- and upper-body exercises (in the given order), which can be an easier way to start for frail and deconditioned participants. The eight exercises marked by an asterisk in table 5.3, which involve the major muscles, are recommended for a shorter program, for easing into the full program, or when time is insufficient to do the 12 exercises. For a gentle

introduction to strength training, you can start with one or two resistance exercises after a 15- to 20-minute warm-up segment (see table 8.7 for how to schedule and time a beginner exercise class) and gradually build up to the shorter program of 8 or the full program of 12. As the time of the resistance segment increases, gradually reduce the warm-up to about 10 minutes (see table 8.5 for an outline of a 45- to 60-minute resistance training class).

Teach your participants the target body parts, major muscles, and functional benefit of each resistance exercise given in table 5.3. Frail elders can be inspired by hearing how these exercises can enhance their activities of daily living. In addition, a good memory exercise is to learn the body parts and major muscles (also called prime mover muscles, the muscles primarily responsible for performing a specific movement) targeted by each resistance exercise (see appendix B2, "Muscles of the Human Body"). This knowledge can help participants focus on feeling the body part or muscles that they are strengthening, an important practice for safe and effective resistance training. For easy reference, you may make a copy of table 5.3 and appendix B2, which are useful handouts for participants.

Start Without Weights

Many older adults require an initial training period to get into shape before lifting a weight. For instance, beginners with a low level of fitness (also, participants who are resuming weight training after an injury or prolonged illness) can perform the arm and leg movements without resistance equipment. This technique is called body-weight exercise. The weight of the arms and legs themselves provides sufficient resistance while doing the exercises, particularly for those who have led a sedentary lifestyle.

Whether a participant is out of shape or not, another good reason for initially teaching resistance training exercises without weights is to prevent injuries while participants are learning proper technique. Also, you can begin with a few resistance exercises, such as just lower-body exercises, for the first week or so. Upper-body exercises can be introduced after the participants are comfortable with the lower-body exercises. Begin with one set of 8 repetitions of each exercise. Cue participants to listen to their bodies. Create a noncompetitive, relaxed atmosphere so that participants will feel comfortable doing less when necessary. Defer introducing free weights until your participants can perform 12 repetitions without weights with good technique.

Introducing Weights

After they learn the basic seated resistance exercises without weights, your participants can start using weights (also called hand weights, free weights, or dumbbells) that are 1 pound (.45 kg) or lighter to prevent undue soreness or injury (Bryant and Green 2009, 193). How do you know when participants are ready to use weights?

- They have learned good exercise technique using just their body weight.
- They can comfortably do 12 repetitions of each exercise.

Reassure participants who are unable to perform 12 repetitions using just their body weight for resistance that they will slowly but surely get stronger. Participants with a higher initial level of fitness can start using weights sooner. Some people may never progress beyond a small weight (e.g., a person with advanced Alzheimer's disease in a large class setting), whereas others may progress safely to a heavier weight within a few weeks. Make sure that a participant who is using a resistive device (all forms of resistance other than just body weight) is able to do at least 8 repetitions of each exercise. If he or she cannot, decrease the resistance until the participant can do at least 8 repetitions. Resistance programs of 8 to 15 reps per exercise that emphasize muscular strength and endurance are safer (less risky for injuries) than programs that use fewer than 8 reps per

exercise and emphasize strength (using higher weights) and muscle hypertrophy.

Upper-Body Weights, Bands, and Tubes

When participants are ready to use weights, provide a minimum of two pairs of upper-body weights: a lighter weight and a heavier weight. In general, lighter weights and resistances are used for singe-joint exercises (one joint moves throughout the ROM of a resistance exercise, recruiting less muscle mass than multijoint exercises do), such as exercise 5.5, Triceps Extension and exercise 5.4, Biceps Curl. In contrast, heavier weights and resistances are used for multijoint exercises (two or more joints move throughout the ROM of a resistance exercise "recruiting multiple muscle groups" [ACSM 2011, 1343]), such as Chest Press (exercise 5.1), Two-Arm Row (exercise 5.2), Overhead Press (exercise 5.3), and Chair Stands (exercise 5.12). Table 5.4 can help you pick two weights for each person. Start with just a lighter pair of weights, 1 pound (.45 kg) or less. Progress to a lighter and heavier pair of 1 and 2 pounds (.45 and .9 kg) when a participant is ready. To prevent muscular imbalances, avoid large discrepancies in weight lifted by opposing muscle groups (muscles that produce the opposite joint movement), such as chest and back, or biceps and triceps.

Bear in mind that you may need to adjust the general weight recommendations in table 5.4 for individual participants. Day-to-day variations in weightlifting ability are common. For instance, if a participant suffered from insomnia the night before class, he or she may not be able to lift as much as usual. Additionally, if your class is large, if you do not have assistance, or if it would be unsafe for participants to reach down to switch weights, have participants use only one pair of weights for all the upper-body exercises or use resistance bands or tubes.

Exercise 5.1, Chest Press, and exercise 5.2, Two-Arm Row, show how to use a band or tube with multijoint exercises that ultimately

Table 5.4 Guidelines for Choosing Upper-Body Weights

Each row of lighter and heavier weights represents an appropriate weight range. For example, if a 3-pound (1.4 kg) weight can be used for an exercise that calls for lighter weight, use 5 pounds (2.3 kg) for heavier-weight exercises.

Lighter weights	Heavier weights	Use lighter resistance with these exercises	Use heavier resistance with these exercises
1 pound (0.45 kg)	2 pounds (0.9 kg)	• Chest Press with weights[b]	• Chest Press with bands or tube
2 pounds (0.9 kg)	3 pounds (1.4 kg)	• Two-Arm Row with weights[b]	• Two-Arm Row with band or tube
3 pounds (1.4 kg)	5 pounds (2.3 kg)	• Triceps Extension	• Overhead Press
4 pounds[a] (1.8 kg)	6 pounds[a] (2.7 kg)	• Biceps Curl	• Chair Stands
5 pounds (2.3 kg)	7 or 8 pounds[a] (3.2 or 3.6 kg)		
6 pounds[a] (2.7 kg)	9 pounds[a] (4.1 kg)		
7 pounds[a] (3.2 kg)	10 pounds (4.5 kg)		
8 pounds (3.6 kg)	10 or 12 pounds (4.5 or 5.4 kg)		

[a]If you use cast-iron weights in your class, ignore the 4-, 6-, 7-, and 9-pound weight options; these weights are not available in cast iron.

[b]Performing the Chest Press and Two-Arm Row in an upright position, seated or standing, puts greater demand on the smaller shoulder muscles if weights are used. Therefore, we recommend using a lighter weight for these exercises. When using resistance bands or tubes, which are not influenced by gravity or body position, bands of heavier resistance can be used for these exercises.

Chair Stands, a lower-body exercise, can be done with hand weights when participants are ready to make the exercise more challenging (see exercise 5.12).

From E. Best-Martini and K.A. Jones-DiGenova, 2014, *Exercise for frail elders,* 2nd ed. (Champaign, IL: Human Kinetics). Adapted, by permission, from S. McKelvey, 2003, *Functional fitness for older adults training manual* (San Diego, CA: Aging and Independent Services), 17-18. © Kim A. Jones-DiGenova.

require "heavier" resistance, which is not practical in a seated or standing position with hand weights. Hand weights put greater demand on the smaller shoulder muscles than the other major muscles that these two exercises target. When using resistance bands or tubes, which are not influenced by gravity or body position, bands of heavier resistance can be used for these exercises. Nonetheless, guide participants who use bands or tubes for the Chest Press and Two-Arm Row to start with light resistance and gradually progress to "heavier" resistance. If you want to use bands or tubes for more than these two exercises, see "Resistance Bands and Isometric Exercises" in "Suggested Resources."

Consider safety and the special needs of your participants when selecting exercise equipment for resistance training. For example, participants who have problems holding on to a dumbbell can use wrist weights or weights with handles. Resistance bands and tubes can be a good choice for participants who cannot safely handle weights. They can also be more effective than free weights for the seated and standing Chest Press and Two-Arm Row exercises.

Lower-Body Weights

Use the same weight for all lower-body exercises. Varying the amount of weight is time consuming and unnecessary—a cumbersome process of taking a leg weight off, adding weight, and then putting it back on—in a class with people who require assistance. Leg weights can be more expensive than hand weights, but participants can make do with one weight by switching it from one leg to the other, although doing so will increase the time spent for the lower-body resistance exercises. Participants who are unable to switch a single leg weight from leg to leg need weights for both legs, unless you or an assistant can help with attaching and removing the weights. For classes with consistent members, you may want to label leg weights with participants' names to keep track of the weight lifted by each individual.

BASIC STANDING RESISTANCE AND BALANCE EXERCISES

All of the exercises listed previously in table 5.3—5 upper-body and 7 lower-body functional exercises—can also be done standing. Introduce these variations and progression options of the 12 basic seated resistance exercises (presented in the illustrated instruction section) after you get to know participants' strengths and current limitations while observing them learn the seated exercises, which reduce the risk of falling. When a participant has developed good technique with the seated resistance exercises and you have determined that he or she can perform standing exercise safely, encourage the person to do so for the extra benefits that standing exercises provide. We recommend that anyone who cannot safely stand continue with the seated resistance exercises. Any participant with minor balance problems may perform only those standing exercises that leave a hand available to hold on to a secure support. Standing exercises that require two hands, such as exercise 5.1, Chest Press, and exercise 5.2, Two-Arm Row, should be performed only by participants who are steady on their feet.

Standing Upper-Body Resistance Exercises

In the variations and progression options of the seated upper-body resistance exercises at the end of this chapter, you will find the standing upper-body resistance exercises. The five seated upper-body resistance exercises can be performed in a standing position. But because these exercises involve both hands for holding onto free weights, bands, or tubes, we recommend that the upper-body resistance exercises be performed seated if a participant has any balance issues, especially in a classroom setting. When leading classes or even when working one on one with someone with balance challenges, first concentrate on developing strength and general fitness while the participant is seated before performing standing upper-body resistance exercises.

Standing Lower-Body Resistance and Balance Exercises

In the variations and progression options of the seated lower-body resistance exercises at the end of this chapter you will find the standing lower-body resistance and balance exercises. The seven seated lower-body resistance exercises can be performed in a standing position. An advantage of the standing lower-body exercises over the upper-body resistance exercises is that both hands are free to hold on to a support, such as a sturdy chair. Therefore, we recommend that you introduce the standing lower-body exercises first, before introducing the standing upper-body resistance exercises. As participants learn the standing lower-body exercises, instruct them to hold on firmly to a secure support, such as the back of a steady chair or railing.

To promote balance, instruct participants to follow steps 1 through 6 at their own pace (besides applying to the lower-body resistance exercises, these steps apply to appropriate ROM, aerobic, and stretching exercises when safe and comfortable for a participant):

1. Hold on firmly with two hands to a secure support.
2. Hold on gently with two hands.
3. Hold on firmly with one hand.
4. Hold on gently with one hand.
5. Hold on gently with four fingers, then three, then two, then one.
6. Do not hold on but hold one or two hands out directly over the support. If participants lose their balance, they can readily regrasp the support.

Move on to step 2 after participants have learned the exercises well, because it is easier to learn a standing exercise while holding on to a support. Those who are ready can slowly progress through the steps. Step 6 is only for those who are steady on their feet, and being in a position to grasp a support is a good safety habit for them to develop. If participants are unsteady during an exercise, help them find the grip that enables them to feel steady on their feet and perform the exercise comfortably. This support progression can also be applied when appropriate to standing range-of-motion (chapter 4), aerobic (chapter 6), and stretching exercises (chapter 7).

VARIATIONS AND PROGRESSION

The variations and progression options (VPOs) for each of the 12 basic seated resistance exercises enable you to be creative and progressive with a functional fitness program to fit the needs of a class full of people with an array of special needs. Refer to the illustrated exercises at the end of this chapter for these options. Introduce one or more of the VPOs after your participants have learned the basic seated resistance exercises, with the exception of the easier

options. The easier options are modifications of the basic exercises for a participant who needs an easier exercise to begin with.

Extensive progression with resistance training may be limited with some classes (e.g., a large class without an assistant in a long-term care setting), but varying the basic seated resistance exercises can benefit and add spice to any class. Conversely, other classes may outgrow the seated exercises and be able to do a standing resistance workout (with the option of sitting when needed). Each basic seated resistance exercise has a standing alternative, an important means of progression when it is safe for a participant to stand. See chapter 8 for guidance in choosing seated versus standing exercise and the benefits of standing. Notice this symbol, which comes before the standing exercises that deliver more significant balance benefits and involve a one-legged stand.

The more you learn about the resistance exercises and the more you learn about your participants' current strengths and challenges, the more skillful you will be at varying and progressing their exercise programs. For example, because back muscles are prone to weakness, especially with disuse as people age, it can be worthwhile (when participants are ready) to do one set of the basic Seated Two-Arm Row (exercise 5.2) and another set with an underhand grip or overhand grip variation. For many other ideas for varying and progressing your class, see chapter 8, including "Duration of Resistance Training."

SUMMARY

A common myth is that seniors are too old to lift weights. In general, frail elders and adults with special needs can benefit markedly from appropriate resistance training. This chapter gives you guidelines, safety precautions, and thorough teaching instructions for leading resistance exercises.

Following the safety precautions for resistance training helps to keep participants injury free. For example, keep blood pressure down by avoiding excessive amounts of overhead exercise, breath holding, and isometric exercises. The guidelines for beneficial results are to provide two to three sessions per week on nonconsecutive days, a minimum of eight safe exercises that condition the major muscle groups of the body, and one to three sets of 8 to 15 repetitions of each exercise. Begin with the basic seated resistance exercises without weights. When participants have learned the exercises, begin with light weights and progress slowly. Participants who regularly resistance-train in your class can potentially have spectacular results, improving their health, fitness, and performance of daily tasks.

REVIEW QUESTIONS

1. List three benefits of a well-rounded resistance-training program.
2. What are two methods for preventing breath holding while resistance training?
3. What is the value of mentioning the major muscles targeted when teaching each resistance exercise?
4. Match the resistance exercise with the target body parts and major muscles:
   - Seated and standing upper-body resistance exercises

     ___ 5.1 Chest Press

     ___ 5.2 Two-Arm Row

     ___ 5.3 Overhead Press

     ___ 5.4 Biceps Curl

     ___ 5.5 Triceps Extension

     a. back of upper arms (triceps)

     b. shoulders (deltoids), back of upper arms (triceps)

     c. front of upper arms (biceps)

     d. chest (pectoralis major), back of upper arms (triceps), shoulders (deltoids)

     e. back (latissimus dorsi, trapezius), front of upper arms (biceps), shoulders (deltoid)

   - Seated and standing lower-body resistance exercises

     ___ 5.6 Hip Flexion

     ___ 5.7 Hip Abduction and Adduction

     ___ 5.8 Knee Flexion

     ___ 5.9 Knee Extension

     ___ 5.10 Toe Raises

     ___ 5.11 Heel Raises

     ___ 5.12 Chair Stands

     f. outer hips and thighs (hip abductors), inner thighs (hip adductors)

     g. back of thighs (hamstrings)

     h. calves (gastrocnemius, soleus)

     i. thighs (quadriceps, hamstrings), buttocks (gluteals)

     j. shins (tibialis anterior)

     k. front of thighs (quadriceps)

     l. front hips and thighs (hip flexors)

5. Stop exercising at the first signs or symptoms of overexertion or cardiac complication, particularly

  • abnormal_____ _____

  • shortness of _____

  • chest_____

  • d_____

6. Begin frail elders with about _____ resistance exercises performed at a low intensity (start with _____ weight and then .5 pound [.2 kg]).

7. To prevent an excessive increase of blood pressure, avoid the following while exercising (circle only one):

  a. heavy weight lifting (an RPE of 5, "hard," or more)

  b. sustained isometric muscular contractions

  c. excessive overhead arm exercise

  d. gripping the exercise accessories or equipment too hard

  e. strong grip exercises using hard rubber balls

  f. holding the breath

  g. all of the above

  h. *a*, *b*, and *f* only

8. Postpone introducing free weights with the resistance-training exercises until your participants can perform _____ repetitions with good technique without resistance (using just the weight of their limbs).

ILLUSTRATED INSTRUCTION

Exercises 5.1 to 5.5 are upper-body resistance exercises, and exercises 5.6 to 5.12 are lower-body resistance exercises. The exercise and safety tips and variations and progression options apply to both seated and standing exercises unless otherwise specified. The standing exercises and other variations and progression options that need further explanation are accompanied by a photograph and description. Before leading resistance training, review the following for a clear understanding of cueing exercises 5.1 to 5.12:

1. "Instructions for Good Seated Posture" and "Instructions for Good Standing Posture" in chapter 4

2. "Step 1: Demonstrate and Describe" in chapter 3 for a review on counting and breathing

3. The section "Repetitions" in this chapter

Before initiating the resistance training component, we recommend that you strengthen your understanding of resistance training by carefully reading this entire chapter and learning the answers to the review questions. Also, if you are a beginner fitness leader or would like to refine your teaching skills, review the three-step instructional process in chapter 3.

Good Seated and Standing Posture

Be sure to refer to the instructions for good seated and standing posture in chapter 4 and remind participants of them often as you do each exercise.

Seated Chest Press

TARGET MUSCLES—Chest (pectoralis major), back of upper arms (triceps), shoulders (deltoids)

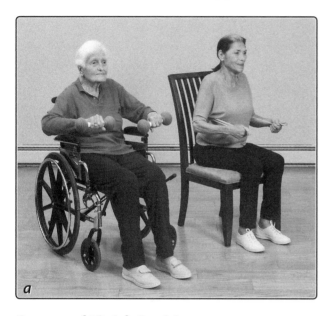

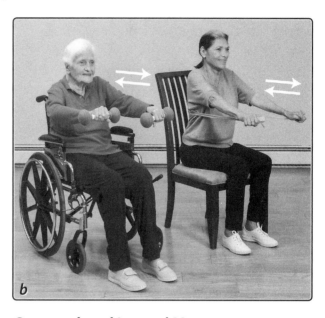

Start and Finish Position

1. Good seated posture.
2. Upper arms by the sides.
3. Hold weights, band, or tube with palms facing downward (see VPOs, *Hand position*) at the level of the lower chest.
4. Hold wrists straight.

Outward and Inward Movement

5. On the outward movement, count, "1, 1, 1, out," or exhale.
6. On the inward movement, count, "1, 1, 1, in," or inhale (return to start and finish position).
7. Move only the elbow and shoulder joint.
8. Perform 8 to 15 repetitions.

! Exercise and Safety Tips

- Stabilize the shoulders (move them up, back, and down) before starting. Keep the shoulders down.
- Keep the wrists neutral (straight) during all upper-body resistance exercises, particularly when using bands and tubes.

Variations and Progression Options

- *Easier:* The upper arms may be held at a lower level if a participant experiences shoulder strain, pain, or fatigue, or just for variety.
- *Challenger (Combo):* Chest Press combined with scapular retraction (squeezing shoulder blades together). Draw the elbows backward toward each other.

(continued)

Seated Chest Press   *(continued)*

Variations and Progression Options   *(continued)*

- *Hand position:* Face palms inward or upward. Palms can start in one position and smoothly rotate to another—for example, from inward to downward (as seen in the model on the right).

- *Arm position:* Keep hands close to each other, shoulder-distance apart, or somewhere in between throughout the ROM.

- *Standing Chest Press.*

- *Prop:* Use a resistance band or tube for a more effective chest and triceps exercise. See "Resistance bands" in appendix B4, "Exercise Equipment."

Seated Two-Arm Row

TARGET MUSCLES—Back (latissimus dorsi, trapezius),
front of upper arms (biceps), shoulders (deltoids)

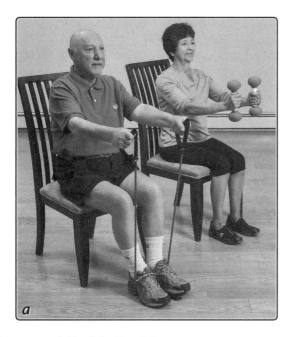 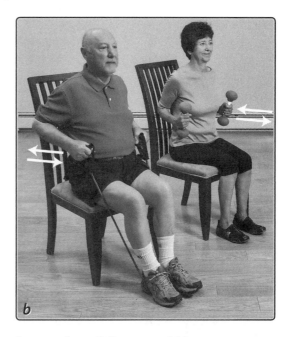

Start and Finish Position

1. Good seated posture.
2. Arms straight out in front, slightly below shoulder level.
3. Hold weights, band, or tube with palms facing inward.

Inward and Outward Movement

4. On the inward movement, count, "1, 1, 1, in," or exhale.
5. On the outward movement, count, "1, 1, 1, out," or inhale (return to start and finish position).
6. Move only the elbow and shoulder joint.
7. Perform 8 to 15 repetitions.

❗ Exercise and Safety Tips

- Stabilize the shoulders (move them up, back, and down) before starting. Keep them down.
- Move the elbows straight backward, not to the side.
- Scapular retraction (for strengthening the rhomboid muscles): On the backward rowing motion, gently squeeze the shoulder blades together by drawing the elbows toward one another behind your back, if the chair is not in the way (see "Seated position" in VPO).
- Keep the wrists straight during all upper-body resistance exercises, particularly when using bands and tubes.
- With the Standing Two-Arm Row, place a chair directly behind the participant in case the band breaks or the participant loses his or her balance.

(continued)

Variations and Progression Options

- *Easier:* Slide hands along thighs.
- *Easier:* Arms can be held at a lower level than photograph *a*.
- *Hand position:* Row with an underhand or overhand grip.
- *Arm position:* Row with less or more distance between hands.
- *Seated position:* Sit toward middle of chair so that elbows clear back of chair to emphasize strengthening the rhomboid muscles, if safe for participant (see the exercise and safety tips).
- *Standing Two-Arm Row* (see photographs *c* and *d* and instructions).
- *Prop:* Use a resistance band or tube for a more effective back and biceps exercise. See appendix B4, "Exercise Equipment," and "Resistance Bands and Isometric Exercises" in "Suggested Resources" for information and resources.

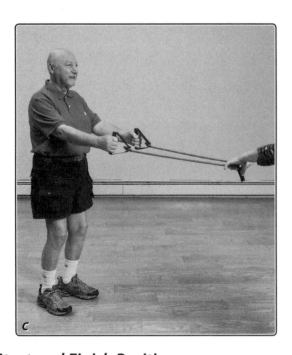

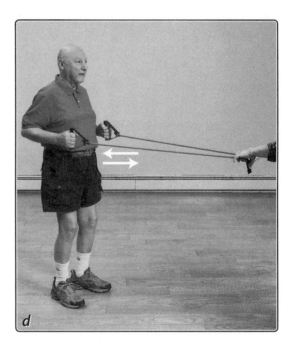

Start and Finish Position

1. Good standing posture.
2. Arms straight out in front, slightly below shoulder level.
3. Palms (with band) facing inward.

Inward and Outward Movement

4. Same as Seated Two-Arm Row.

Seated Overhead Press

TARGET MUSCLES—Shoulders (deltoids), back of upper arms (triceps)

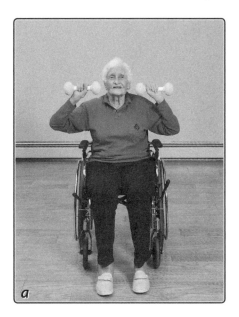

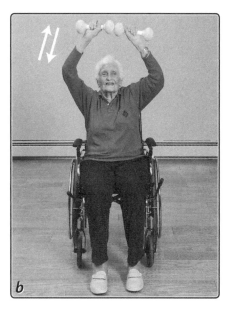

Start and Finish Position

1. Good seated posture.
2. Hold weights at shoulder level.
3. Palms facing forward.

Upward and Downward Movement

4. On the upward movement, count, "1, 1, 1, up," or exhale.
5. On the downward movement, count, "1, 1, 1, down," or inhale (return to start and finish position).
6. Move only the shoulder and elbow joint.
7. Perform 8 to 15 repetitions.

! Exercise and Safety Tips

- Lift the weights in front of the head, as if lifting an object onto a high shelf.
- Modification: If a participant experiences any strain or pain in the shoulder joints when doing the Overhead Press, instruct him or her to not lift the weights as high (see the easier options that follow).

Variations and Progression Options

- *Easier (Underhead Press):* Instruct participants to lift the upper arms no higher than level with the floor, always within a strain-free and pain-free ROM.
- *Hand position:* Palms face inward or backward.
- *Arm position:* Arms start and finish in front of the torso (arms parallel, palms facing inward), rather than the sides of the torso.
- *Standing Overhead* or *Underhead Press.*

Seated Biceps Curl

TARGET MUSCLES—Front of upper arms (biceps)

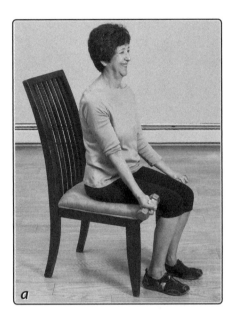

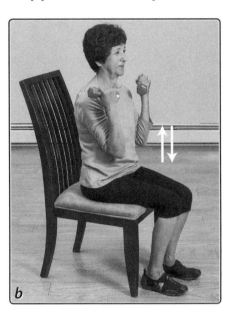

Start and Finish Position

1. Good seated posture.

2. Arms down at sides, upper arms touch sides of torso.

3. Hold weights with palms facing forward.

Upward and Downward Movement

4. On the upward movement, count, "1, 1, 1, up," or exhale.

5. On the downward movement, count, "1, 1, 1, down," or inhale (return to start and finish position).

6. Move only the elbow joint.

7. Perform 8 to 15 repetitions.

! Exercise and Safety Tips

- Stabilize the shoulders (move them up, back, and down) before starting. Keep them down.

- Avoid leaning to one side when performing the Biceps Curl on one side.

- Modification: If the chair has arms, move forward toward the middle of the chair if it is safe to do so, so that the elbows clear the chair arms.

- Check participants' posture to be sure that they are not leaning backward, especially when they are sitting in the middle of their chairs or standing.

Variations and Progression Options

- *Easier:* Perform Biceps Curl with one arm at a time.

- *Hand position:* Perform Biceps Curl with palms facing each other (inward) throughout the exercise, a Hammer Curl.

- *Hand position:* Perform Biceps Curl with palms facing backward (in the starting position), a "French" Curl. Participants can rename it.

- *Standing Biceps Curl* or *Standing Hammer Curl.*

Seated Triceps Extension (Challenger)

TARGET MUSCLES—Back of upper arms (triceps)

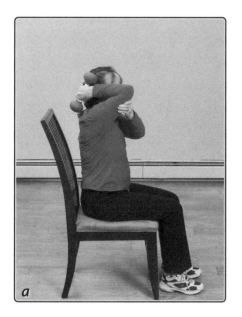 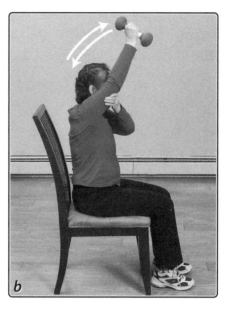

Start and Finish Position

1. Good seated posture.
2. Hold the weight with palm facing inward.
3. Lift the upper arm as high as comfortable.
4. Hold back of the upper arm with the opposite hand.

Upward and Downward Movement

5. On the upward movement, count, "1, 1, 1, up," or exhale.
6. On the downward movement, count, "1, 1, 1, down," or inhale (return to start and finish position).
7. Move only the elbow joint.
8. Perform 8 to 15 repetitions.
9. Repeat on the other side.

! Exercise and Safety Tips

- Stabilize the shoulders (move them up, back, and down) before starting. Keep them down.
- Keep the working upper arm as high as possible while maintaining good posture.
- The upper arm (of the working triceps) remains stationary throughout the Triceps Extension.
- Palm faces inward to keep the weight away from the head.

Variations and Progression Options

- *Stretch (Triceps:)* See exercise 7.5, Zipper Stretch, in chapter 7 before doing the Triceps Extension or between sets. As triceps flexibility increases, participants will be able to lift their arms higher for a more comfortable and effective Triceps Extension.
- *Standing Triceps Extension.*

Seated Hip Flexion

TARGET MUSCLES—Front hips and thighs (hip flexors)

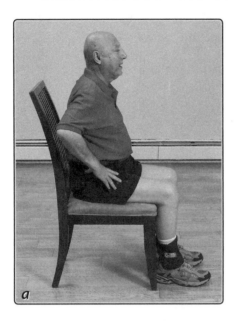

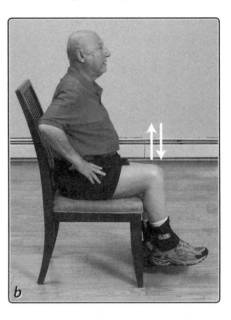

Start and Finish Position

1. Good seated posture.
2. Hands on hips.

Upward and Downward Movement

3. On the upward movement, count, "1, 1, 1, up," or exhale.
4. On the downward movement, count, "1, 1, 1, down," or inhale (return to start and finish position).
5. Move only the hip joint.
6. Perform 8 to 15 repetitions.
7. Repeat on the other side.

! Exercise and Safety Tips

- Hip fracture or replacement: Avoid lifting the leg higher than a 90-degree angle at the hip joint in a seated or standing position.
- Lift the legs only as high as comfortable while maintaining erect posture.
- Feel the hip flexors working.

Variations and Progression Options

- *Easier:* Perform hip flexion with the toe remaining on the floor.
- *Easier:* Perform hip flexion within a narrower ROM or put a foot on the floor between repetitions.
- *Challenger:* Do not put a foot on the floor
- between reps. Start with a few and safely build up to all.
- *Challenger:* Lift the leg higher. Start with a few and carefully build up to all.
- 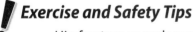 *Standing Hip Flexion* (involves a one-legged stand).

Seated Hip Abduction and Adduction

TARGET MUSCLES—Outer hips and thighs (hip abductors), inner thighs (hip adductors)

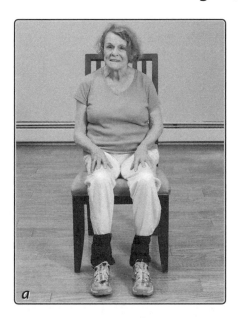

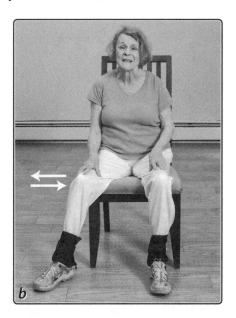

Start and Finish Position

1. Good seated posture.
2. Hands in a comfortable position.

Outward and Inward Movement

3. On the outward movement, count, "1, 1, 1, out," or exhale.
4. On the inward movement, count, "1, 1, 1, in," or inhale (return to start and finish position).
5. Move only the hip joint.
6. Perform 8 to 15 repetitions.
7. Repeat on the other side.

❗ Exercise and Safety Tips

- When seated, keep each foot directly below each knee. When standing, keep the toes of the moving foot pointed straight ahead.
- When adducting the leg (inward movement) while standing, cross the midline of the body as far as comfortable, keeping the torso stationary.

- Those with a hip fracture or replacement should avoid flexing the hip more than 90 degrees, as in the functional variation (see VPO). Do not cross the midline in the standing variation (see "Hip Fracture or Replacement" earlier in this chapter).

(continued)

Variations and Progression Options

- *Easier:* Slide the foot on the floor for some or all repetitions.
- *Functional variation:* Lift the leg while abducting and adducting in seated position, similar to the motion of lifting a leg in and out of a car.

- *Standing Hip Abduction and Adduction*: Involves a one-legged stand (see photographs *c* and *d* and instructions).

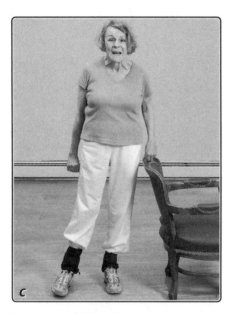

Start and Finish Position

1. Good standing posture.
2. Hold on to a secure support with one hand.

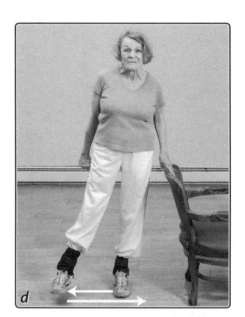

Outward and Inward Movement

3. Same as Seated Hip Abduction and Adduction.
4. On the inward movement, the moving leg crosses the midline.

Seated Knee Flexion

TARGET MUSCLES—Back of thighs (hamstrings)

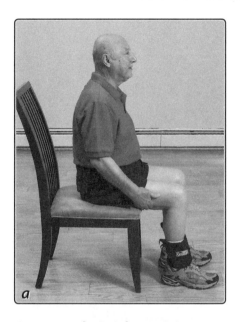 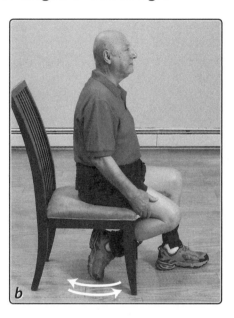

Start and Finish Position

1. Good seated posture.
2. Hands under the thighs.

Upward and Downward Movement

3. On the upward movement, count, "1, 1, 1, up," or exhale.
4. On the downward movement, count, "1, 1, 1, down," or inhale (return to start and finish position).
5. Focus on moving the knee joint.
6. Perform 8 to 15 repetitions.
7. Repeat on the other side.

❗ Exercise and Safety Tips

- Modification: If bars between the front legs of the chairs impede movement, instruct participants to move forward 4 to 6 inches (10 to 15 cm) in their seats if they can do so safely. Instruct them to hold on to the sides or arms of their chairs when sitting forward in their chairs.
- During Standing Knee Flexion, keep the pelvis aligned.

(continued)

Variations and Progression Options

- *Easier:* Do not bring the calf and foot up as high, for some or all repetitions.
- *Easier (standing):* Allow knee of working leg to not be aligned with other knee (as shown in photographs *c* and *d*).

- *Challenger:* Bring the heel up higher but still within a strain-free and pain-free range of motion.
- *Standing Knee Flexion:* Involves a one-legged stand (see photographs *c* and *d* and following instructions).

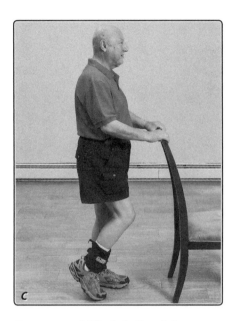

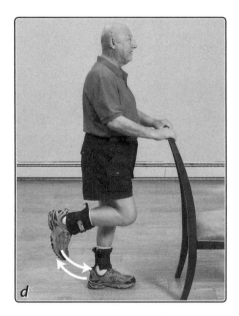

Start and Finish Position

1. Good standing posture.
2. Hands holding on to a secure support.
3. Knees aligned if possible.

Upward and Downward Movement

4. Same as Seated Knee Flexion.

Seated Knee Extension

TARGET MUSCLES—Front of thighs (quadriceps)

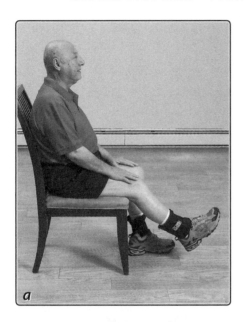
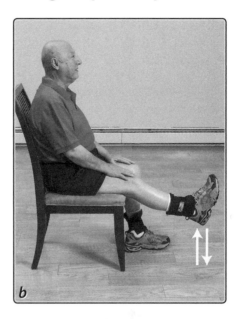

Start and Finish Position

1. Good seated posture.
2. Palms on thighs.
3. Leg slightly bent.

Upward and Downward Movement

4. On the upward movement, count, "1, 1, 1, up," or exhale.
5. On the downward movement, count, "1, 1, 1, down," or inhale (return to start and finish position).
6. Move only the knee joint.
7. Perform 8 to 15 repetitions.
8. Repeat on the other side.

❗ Exercise and Safety Tips

- Feel the quadriceps working.
- Avoid extending the knee through the full range of motion when using leg weights, which can cause the back of the patella (kneecap) to degenerate.
- After initially straightening the leg, lower it 6 inches (15 cm) or less.
- Scoot the buttocks all the way to the back of the chair for maximum back support.
- When standing, the working thigh can be raised less than 90 degrees.

(continued)

Variations and Progression Options

- *Easier:* Start and end each repetition with the heel on the floor and lift the foot 6 inches (15 cm) or less. The knee is bent throughout the exercise.

- *Stretch (Hamstrings):* Perform exercise 7.8, Tib Touches, in chapter 7 before doing the Standing Knee Extension. As they increase their hamstring flexibility, standing participants will be able to lift the thigh higher than 45 degrees.

- *Challenger (Combo):* Plantar flex (point the toes) and then dorsiflex (point toes toward nose) the ankle with each repetition when the leg is straight. Start with a few reps and carefully build up to all.

- *Standing Knee Extension:* Involves a one-legged stand (see photographs *c* and *d* and instructions).

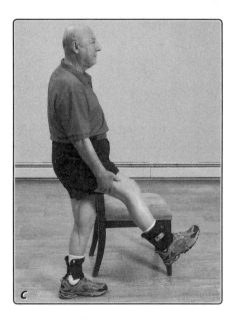

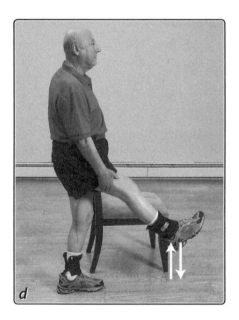

Start and Finish Position

1. Good standing posture.
2. Hold on to a secure support with one hand.
3. One thigh is at 45 degrees.
4. Same leg is slightly bent.
5. Support thigh with hand.

Upward and Downward Movement

6. Same as Seated Knee Extension.

Seated Toe Raises

TARGET MUSCLES—Shins (tibialis anterior)

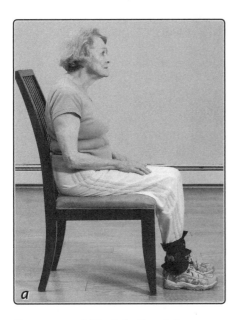 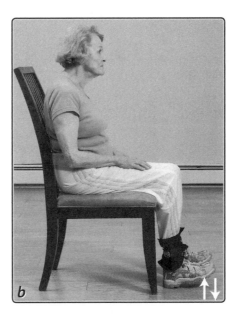

Start and Finish Position

1. Good seated posture.
2. Hands in a comfortable position.

Upward and Downward Movement

3. On the upward movement, count, "1, 1, 1, up," or exhale.
4. On the downward movement, count, "1, 1, 1, down," or inhale (return to start and finish position).
5. Move only the ankle joint.
6. Perform 8 to 15 repetitions.

❗ Exercise and Safety Tips

- Put feet together to make sure that they are symmetrical, rising and lowering together.
- Instruct participants not to rock the whole body back when raising their toes. Cue them to focus on moving only the ankle joint.

Variations and Progression Options

- *Easier:* Put the foot on the floor between repetitions.
- *Challenger:* Do not put the foot on the floor between repetitions. Start with a few and carefully build up to all.
- *Standing Toe Raises:* Raise the toes on both feet at the same time.
- *Prop:* Use a wall to support the upper body during Standing Toe Raises.

Seated Heel Raises

TARGET MUSCLES—Calves (gastrocnemius, soleus)

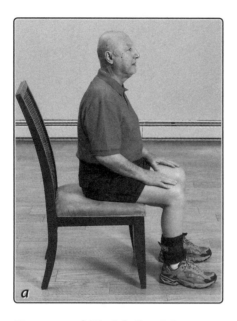

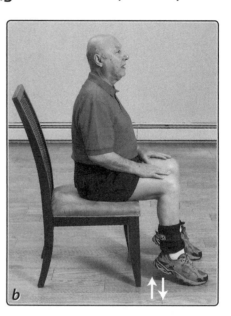

Start and Finish Position

1. Good seated posture.
2. Hands in a comfortable position.

Upward and Downward Movement

3. On the upward movement, count, "1, 1, 1, up," or exhale.
4. On the downward movement, count, "1, 1, 1, down," or inhale (return to start and finish position).
5. Move only the ankle joint.
6. Perform 8 to 15 repetitions.

! Exercise and Safety Tips

- Instruct participants to distribute their weight evenly on the balls of the feet when the heels are lifted.

Variations and Progression Options

- *Easier:* Put heels on the floor between repetitions.
- *Challenger:* Do not put heels on the floor between repetitions. Start with a few and carefully build up to all.
- *Challenger:* Combination of some two- and some one-legged heel raises.

- *Standing Heel Raises:* Raise both heels at the same time.
- 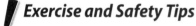 *Standing One-Legged Heel Raises* (involves a one-legged stand).

Modified Chair Stands (Challenger)

TARGET MUSCLES—Thighs (quadriceps, hamstrings) and buttocks (gluteals)

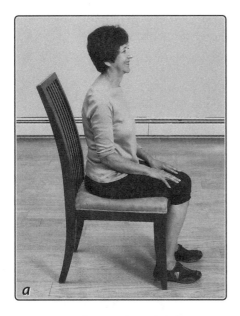

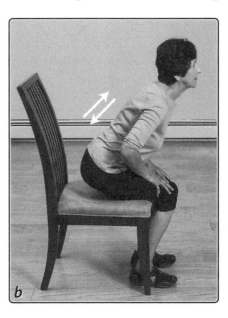

Start and Finish Position

1. Good seated posture.
2. Palms on thighs.
3. Feet hip-width apart.

Upward and Downward Movement

4. On the upward movement, count, "1, 1, 1, up," or exhale.
5. On the downward movement, count, "1, 1, 1, down," or inhale (return to start and finish position).
6. Move only the hip, knee, and ankle joints.
7. Perform 8 to 15 repetitions.

❗ Exercise and Safety Tips

- Maintain a neutral spine (see figure 4.2). Move the head, neck, and spine as one unit.
- Spot (one-on-one facilitation) those with balance problems.
- Keep the shoulders down throughout the exercise.
- Lean forward from the hips and push off the thighs with the hands while standing.
- Start by raising the buttocks 1 inch (2.5 cm) off the chair and then slowly sit back down. Do 8 to 15 repetitions.

- Do not project the knees beyond the toes in any weight-bearing exercise.
- Remind those with knee problems to stay within their strain-free and pain-free range of motion, even if that range is quite limited.
- Those with a hip fracture or replacement should keep the torso as erect as possible (lean forward as little as possible) to avoid hip flexion of more than 90 degrees in a seated or standing position.

(continued)

Variations and Progression Options

- *Easier:* Sit down on a chair between repetitions.

- *Arm position:* Without weights, put the arms in a comfortable position, such as crossed across the chest or reaching forward.

- *Chair Stands (Challenger):* Do not sit down on a chair between repetitions. Start with a few reps and carefully build up to all. See photographs *c* and *d* and instructions.

- *Challenger (With Weights):* Use hand weights when participants are ready to make Chair Stands more challenging (see photographs *c* and *d*).

- *Props:* Push up with the hands using the seat or arms of a chair or wheelchair, a cane, or a walker (with brake on).

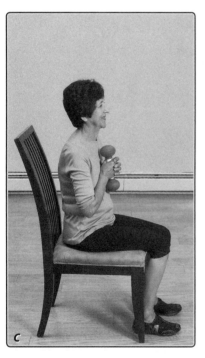 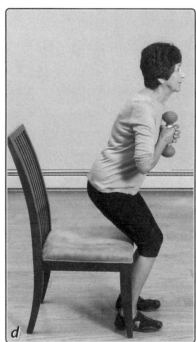 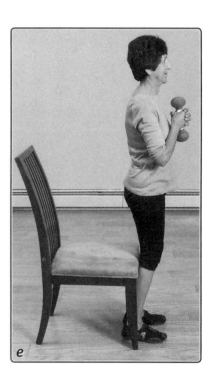

Start and Finish Position

1. Good seated posture.

2. Hold weights with palms facing the chest.

3. Rest hands on the chest.

4. Feet are shoulder-width apart.

Upward and Downward Movement

5. Same as Modified Chair Stands.

Aerobic Training and Dynamic Balance Activities

Janie Clark*

Appropriate aerobic training will yield benefits
including more efficient respiratory and cardiovascular systems
and improved functional level and overall health status.

—*Taylor and Johnson 2008*

LEARNING OBJECTIVES

After completing this chapter, you will have the tools to

- integrate dynamic balance training into exercise programming,
- define the term *aerobic exercise* and distinguish it from activities that do not produce aerobic training effects,
- develop an activity plan that incorporates five key elements needed for successful aerobic exercise programming,
- select aerobic exercises that match participants' ability and can be done while standing or seated, and
- integrate dynamic balance activities into aerobic exercise sessions.

Aerobic exercise (moderate-intensity activity involving large muscle groups using oxygen-supplied energy) is done to increase cardiovascular endurance (also known as aerobic fitness, the ability to take in, transport, and utilize oxygen). Effective aerobic training produces significant improvements in cardiovascular (involving the heart and circulatory system) health.

Well-designed aerobic programming includes dynamic balance activity for maintaining and enhancing a participant's functional level. Balance is the process of controlling the body's center of mass with respect to its base of support, whether the body is stationary or moving (Rose 2010). Static balance refers to that ability while relatively still, such as while quietly standing (Peterson 2004); dynamic balance

*Janie Clark, MA, is an exercise physiologist and is president of the American Senior Fitness Association, New Smyrna Beach, Florida.

refers to that ability while leaning or moving through space (Jones and Rose 2005). Whereas static training strategies (such as standing in place heel to toe while holding and reading aloud from a book) are incompatible with the aerobics segment of a workout, dynamic balance activities can be addressed. Walking, marching, and other aerobic exercise movements performed while standing are inherently supportive of balance. For participants who can safely do so, simply progressing over time from all or mostly chair-seated activity to increased standing activity will be beneficial.

For wheelchair users and any others completely restricted to seated exercise, it is challenging to institute activities specifically designed to promote balance while simultaneously meeting aerobic training criteria. Yet balance is important to that population, especially in terms of transferring to and from bed, wheelchair, and toilet. In fact, combining aerobic conditioning with dynamic balance activity in the chair-seated position can be done in several practical ways.

Be aware of these paradoxes. Static balance does not involve the absence of all skeletal muscle movement; simply standing upright requires active muscular contraction (Rose 2010). Likewise, not all tasks considered dynamic balance activities reach the intensity threshold necessary to produce aerobic training effects. Whether undertaken while standing or seated, many dynamic balance activities must be done somewhat slowly for reasons of safety and effectiveness. If such considerations preclude lively, near-continuous rhythmic movement of the limbs (particularly the legs), your workout will no longer have an aerobics segment. Consequently, such activities belong elsewhere in the workout following sufficient warm-up. That said, it still may be necessary to introduce aerobic training gradually to beginners, perhaps by alternating very light activity with brisker work until participants have built up to performing a sustained aerobic workout.

In exercise program design, every viable occasion to foster balance should be pursued. Therefore, this chapter will point out opportunities to incorporate elements of dynamic balance

training for both ambulatory and seated participants during your aerobic exercise segment. Look for the special balance symbol, which denotes applicable exercises.

Keep in mind that dynamic balance activities are embedded in the aerobic exercise instructions in this chapter. Thus, when the terms *aerobic* and *aerobics* appear in the text, they also refer to any dynamic balance activities included in this chapter.

The five keys to conducting a successful aerobic exercise program for elderly fitness participants include individualization, proper integration of aerobic-training variables, inclusion of essential exercise session components, safety awareness, and creativity. This chapter provides guidance in all these important areas.

• **Individualization**. Elderly participants differ in health and fitness status, skill level, and training tolerance. In this chapter you will learn how to help your aerobics participants pace themselves effectively and how to adapt your program for those who need modifications to perform well.

• **Integration of training variables**. Factors such as intensity, frequency, and duration must be set in a way that permits gradual, progressive training. Using the guidelines provided in this chapter, start with the lower-body movements of the basic seated aerobic exercises. You will learn to add upper-body movements safely and to help certain participants perform the basic standing aerobic exercises. The seated and standing exercises are designed to be taught at the same time so that your exercise class can accommodate people of various performance abilities.

• **Inclusion of essential components**. Your aerobic exercise class should feature three phases: an initial warm-up period of light movement and stretches (see chapter 4), the aerobic exercises, and a cool-down period of light movement followed by stretching (see chapter 7). Table 6.1 provides an overview. A good way to include resistance training in the class is to complete the three phases just described, followed by resistance training and another cool-down period. Warm-up and cool-

Table 6.1 Components of an Aerobic Exercise Session for Older Adults

Component	Includes these exercises	Duration
Warm-up (see chapter 4)	Posture awareness Deep breathing Range-of-motion exercises Easy-paced activities such as slow walking Mild stretching	10–15 minutes
Aerobic exercise	Low- to moderate-intensity rhythmic work using large muscle groups	Time permitting, build up to 30–60 minutes (depending on intensity)
Cool-down (see chapter 7)	Low-intensity aerobic exercises Light, limbering ROM movements Sustained stretching Relaxation	10–15 minutes

down periods include activities performed with aerobically produced energy. Indeed, they may include many of the same exercises as the main aerobic-training component itself, but movements during the aerobic phase of the workout should be performed more energetically and for a longer duration (Clark 2005).

• **Safety awareness.** In functional fitness programming for frail elders and adults with special needs, nothing is more important than safety. Following the detailed safety guidelines provided in this chapter helps keep your aerobics participants injury free. In your day-to-day work, always keep in mind this important advice: "Generally, older persons are more fragile, more susceptible to orthopedic injury and possible cardiovascular problems. Therefore, [aerobic] exercise prescription should emphasize low-moderate intensity exercise, low-impact activity, starting slowly, and gradually progressing in duration and frequency" (Swart, Pollock, and Brechue 1996, 9).

• **Creativity.** Technical programming criteria pertain to the science of aerobic training. Creativity, however, concerns the *art* of aerobic training. The lively nature of aerobic exercise affords participants extraordinary opportunities to enjoy movement to music in a stimulating, motivational environment that promotes continued participation. This chapter provides numerous suggestions on how to incorporate music, variety, and fun into your aerobic exercise program.

SAFETY PRECAUTIONS

Aerobic training can be safe for older adults if appropriate training guidelines and precautions are observed. The following general safety precautions checklist for aerobics and specific safety precautions for those with special needs can help you lead safe aerobic training and keep your participants injury free. You may photocopy "General Safety Precautions Checklist for Aerobics and Dynamic Balance" and "Safety Guidelines Checklist" in chapter 2.

Specific Safety Precautions for Those With Special Needs

In serving frail elders and adults with other special needs, keep in mind that aerobic exercise engages not only the cardiovascular system but also the pulmonary, nervous, and musculoskeletal systems. Follow the appropriate specific safety precautions when leading aerobic training for those with special needs. These precautions may not apply when a participant is in an early or mild stage of a particular condition. See chapter 1 to learn more about common special needs. For further information see "Fitness, Wellness, and Special Needs" in "Suggested Resources."

GENERAL SAFETY PRECAUTIONS CHECKLIST
FOR AEROBICS AND DYNAMIC BALANCE

☐ People who lead aerobic training for frail elderly adults should hold both CPR and first-aid certification.

☐ Before initiating aerobic training, review any special do's and don'ts that the physician has written on the medical clearance form.

☐ Aerobics participants should wear sturdy shoes with adequate arch support and ample cushioning.

☐ Seated participants should be able to place their backs securely against the backs of their chairs or wheelchairs while keeping their feet flat on the floor. If they do not, correct their positioning with pillows or platforms.

☐ Remind seated and standing participants to maintain good posture.

☐ Participants should look forward (not down at their feet), focusing on a point at eye level to facilitate erect posture and balance.

☐ Participants with blindness, extreme frailty, or balance problems that place them at risk of falling should perform only seated aerobic exercise.

☐ Although it is possible to conduct aerobic exercise using balance support devices, the standing versions of the exercises given in this chapter are intended solely for persons capable of participating in a freestanding manner without the use of canes, walkers, railings, chair backs, or other equipment. Even so, they must be closely observed at all times, which may mandate the use of instructor's assistants. Standing participants who begin to appear lightheaded, clumsy, weak, overfatigued, or short of breath or show other slow-down signs must be moved into the chair-seated position. They may then be able to continue activity in a slow, gentle way until renewed; conversely, a rest break or cessation of activity may be indicated.

☐ An exception to the freestanding rule given earlier may apply if the participant has his or her own experienced spotter in a personal training setting or, if in a class setting, the participant has his or her own experienced spotter and can safely take part without curtailing or impeding the group's aerobic and dynamic balance routines. For more details, see "Progressing from Seated to Standing" in chapter 8.

☐ Perform only low-impact activity (exercise that does not significantly jar the joints).

☐ Demonstrate all aerobic exercises in a controlled manner at a moderate speed.

☐ Do not use weights or any type of resistive equipment during aerobic training. Nonresistive accessories, such as scarves, may be used.

☐ Avoid jerking or slinging motions of the limbs. Encourage smooth, rhythmic movement.

☐ Don't overdo it. Aerobic exercise should energize participants, not exhaust them. For example, if arms or legs grow fatigued while working at the suggested elevation, have participants lower them to a more comfortable height at which to perform the motions.

☐ Remind participants to pace themselves.

☐ Instruct your participants never to hold their breath during aerobic exercise. They need a steady supply of oxygen to produce the energy necessary to sustain continuous movement. Have participants sing along with familiar workout tunes. Counting aloud is another good practice. During the prolonged performance of a single exercise, ask people open-ended questions. Participants cannot hold their breath when vocalizing.

☐ In addition to using ratings of perceived exertion (RPE; discussed later in this chapter), always observe your participants closely during aerobic exercise. Stay alert for warning signs such as labored breathing.

☐ Even more than other forms of exercise, aerobic training requires thorough warm-up and cool-down periods, especially for elderly participants. Most cardiac complications that occur during exercise arise at the beginning or end of workouts. Warming up is vital because the heart and circulation need sufficient transition time to accommodate the increased oxygen demands of aerobic exercise. The cool-down prevents potentially dangerous blood pooling in the lower extremities and lowers the risk of arrhythmia (abnormal heart rhythm). In aerobic training, warm up and cool down for a minimum of 10 to 15 minutes. Begin the aerobics class warm-up with low-intensity limbering movements, proceed to light calisthenics and other easy-paced activities such as slow walking, and conclude with mild stretching. Begin the aerobics class cool-down with low-intensity aerobic exercise, proceed to lighter limbering movements, and conclude with sustained stretches (American Senior Fitness Association 2012c).

☐ In aerobics classes for frail elderly participants, an entirely noncompetitive atmosphere should be maintained.

☐ Because aerobic exercise promotes sweating, be sure to provide participants with opportunities for fluid replacement. Make water available before, during, and after aerobic training.

☐ Participants should not perform aerobic exercise with an elevated body temperature. They should wait until body temperature has been normal again for 24 hours and then gradually resume activity.

☐ When returning from a layoff, participants should resume aerobic training at a perceived exertion rating of 3 or less and then gradually build back up to an RPE of 3 to 4.

From E. Best-Martini and K.A. Jones-DiGenova, 2014, *Exercise for frail elders*, 2nd ed. (Champaign, IL: Human Kinetics).

Alzheimer's Disease and Related Dementias

• Participants with cognitive impairments may not perform well when asked to learn numerous dance exercise moves; an aerobics program based mainly on walking can be especially beneficial for them (American Senior Fitness Association 2012a).

• Because confused or disoriented participants may not be able to rate their exertion reliably, your constant and unfailing observation is essential.

Arthritis

• Thorough warm-up and cool-down periods are especially critical for aerobics participants with arthritis. Their joints need extra time to prepare for and recover from extended periods of continuous activity.

• If a participant experiences a flare-up of arthritis, modify or suspend exercise activity but aerobic training should be resumed (in a gradual manner, if necessary) as soon as the participant is able (Clark 2012a).

Cerebrovascular Accident (Stroke)

- See also the safety precautions for those with coronary artery disease (heart disease).

- Providing clear instructions is extremely important to aerobics participants who have experienced stroke. If a participant has paralysis on the right side, focus on leading exercises mainly by demonstration, using few verbal instructions. If paralysis is on the left side, rely more on verbal instructions, using fewer gestures (American Senior Fitness Association 2012c).

Chronic Obstructive Pulmonary Disease

- Thorough warm-up and cool-down periods are especially critical for aerobics participants with COPD. Their lungs and cardiovascular systems need extra time to adapt to changes in exertion level.

- All older adults should perform only modest amounts of overhead arm work, but such movements should be even more limited for those who have COPD. In people with COPD, excessive overhead work unduly raises ventilatory demand (the amount of air that must be breathed in and out to satisfy the body's need for oxygen and to dispose of carbon dioxide waste).

- Here are three methods that can help prevent breathlessness during aerobic training:

  1. Alternate energetic training periods with easy training periods during the workout (AACVPR 2011). For example, work briskly for 5 minutes, work lightly for 5 minutes, and continue alternating. Use longer easy periods if needed.

  2. Accumulate the desired duration by performing short bouts of exercise throughout the day (see "Duration" later in this chapter).

  3. Work at an intensity near the lower end of the desirable range (an RPE of 3 instead of an RPE from 3 to 4) but for a longer duration (American Senior Fitness Association 2012c).

- A participant who has an inhaler should use it according to the physician's instructions to prevent or minimize exercise-induced asthma.

Coronary Artery Disease (Heart Disease)

- Thorough warm-up and cool-down periods are especially critical for aerobics participants with heart disease. Their cardiovascular systems need extra time to adapt to changes in exertion level.

- All older adults should perform only modest amounts of overhead arm work, but such movements should be even more limited for those who have heart disease. Excessive overhead work can raise blood pressure.

- A good practice is to monitor pre- and postexercise blood pressure and pulse rate.

Depression

- Because aerobic exercise stimulates the brain to release hormones that foster a sense of well-being, it can be an extremely useful tool in combating depression (Clark 2012a).

- Strive to make your aerobics class an enjoyable event that participants always look forward to. Regular training can significantly reduce depression.

Diabetes

- Keep in mind that many people with diabetes also develop heart disease. See also the precautions for those with coronary artery disease.

- Because weight loss can help control diabetes, appropriate long-term aerobic training can be valuable.

- Be vigilant in watching for symptoms of diabetic emergency. Keep on hand simple carbohydrates that are readily digestible, such as sugar, candy, or fruit juice.

- Make sure that participants with diabetes wear proper socks and shoes. Take special care to avoid injuries to the feet. In people with diabetes, small injuries tend to develop more quickly into serious problems and complications, especially when nerves are diseased or circulation is restricted. At the first sign of any foot problem (e.g., a minor cut), seek medical care (American Senior Fitness Association 2012c).

Frailty

- Regular, safe movement, such as seated low-intensity aerobic exercise, is essential for the goal of restoring function, as best as possible, for frail people. Encourage regular class attendance and a home walking program (if appropriate, recruiting the support of their caregiver). Compliment small steps forward, even if a participant only occasionally comes to class and moves minimally.
- Address other possible special needs associated with their frailty, such as osteoporosis. Refer to "Common Medical Disorders and Special Needs" in chapter 1.

Hip Fracture or Replacement

- Avoid aerobic and dynamic balance exercises that involve internal rotation (turning the leg inward), hip adduction (crossing the legs), and hip flexion that involves lifting the foot higher than slightly off the floor (thigh higher than parallel with the floor)—such as exercises 6.4, Marching in Place; 6.11, Alternate Knee Lifts; and 6.12, Alternate Double Knee Lifts—to prevent the risk of hip dislocation, unless a participant has written clearance from his or her physician indicating that those specific movements are not contraindicated. Substitute exercise 6.3, Walking in Place, keeping the thigh no higher than parallel with the floor.

Hypertension

- See also the precautions for coronary artery disease.

- "Regular aerobic endurance exercise reduces blood pressure in older adults" (ACSM 2004a, 539). Encourage gradual, individualized progression of aerobic training according to evidence-based guidelines, presented later in this chapter.
- Because weight loss helps reduce or control blood pressure, appropriate long-term aerobic training can be valuable.

Multiple Sclerosis and Parkinson's Disease

- The aerobics participant with Parkinson's disease or multiple sclerosis may need extra reminders and encouragement to maintain optimal posture.
- Many people with Parkinson's disease or multiple sclerosis are at high risk of falling. Ask the physician if an affected frail elderly person should remain on an all-seated aerobic exercise program (American Senior Fitness Association 2012a).

Osteoporosis

- When symptoms are minor, walking or low-impact aerobic dance can be undertaken as tolerated and may be beneficial in managing the disease.
- An ambulatory participant can combine seated and standing activities during a single aerobics session to perform successfully.
- When osteoporosis is advanced, standing exercise may not be safe because of increased risk for falling and fracture. In that case, the participant should do only seated aerobics.

Sensory Losses

- People with visual impairments should do structured aerobic training in a seated position. Standing dance activities to music can be enjoyable and beneficial for people with visual impairments, but it is safer to use such activities to promote pleasure, creativity, and range of motion than as a means of aerobic conditioning.

- Provide clear and effective voice cues to people with visual impairment.
- Provide clear and effective demonstration cues to people with hearing loss. Appropriate visual gestures enhance the participant's ability to follow verbal instructions.
- Consider using instrumental music, because it may be easier for participants with hearing loss to follow directions when your voice does not have to compete with vocals in the music (American Senior Fitness Association 2012a; Clark 2012a).

! Safety Tip For safe and effective aerobics for older adults, carefully follow the safety precautions and the following evidence-based guidelines.

GUIDELINES

Several prominent organizations have developed guidelines for safe and effective aerobic training, including the American Senior Fitness Association (2012a, b, c), the American College of Sports Medicine and the American Heart Association (ACSM and AHA 2007), the American College of Sports Medicine (ACSM 2010, 2009a, b), and the U.S. Department of Health and Human Services (USDHHS 2008b). Table 6.2 provides a conservative synthesis of their guidelines, specifically adapted by the American Senior Fitness Association to be appropriate for frail elderly participants. The basic seated and standing aerobic exercises in this chapter are based on these well-researched guidelines. You may make a copy of table 6.2 for easy reference.

Even more than other forms of exercise, participation in aerobic training calls for medical approval. A great exercise science pioneer, Dr. Michael L. Pollock, set the standards for individualizing training protocols (for frequency, intensity, duration, and exercise mode)

for aerobic exercise with elderly participants depending on the participant's exercise test results and any musculoskeletal or other health-related limitations (Swart, Pollock, and Brechue 1996). Your participant's physician is familiar with exercise testing procedures and can administer any indicated laboratory tests during the medical clearance process. After participants have secured medical approval for a gentle program of aerobic conditioning, they can work productively within a set of general guidelines, so long as only activities that prove to be well tolerated are pursued (Clark 2012b).

The following sections offer guidelines to prevent injury and maximize the benefits of aerobic training and dynamic balance activities for frail elders and adults with special needs.

Exercise Selection

The exercise program in this chapter includes 12 basic aerobic and dynamic balance exercises that contribute to cardiovascular health and endurance. These exercises are safe and appropriate for frail elders and adults with special needs who have medical clearance. Teach the basic seated lower-body movements first. Progress to incorporating the corresponding upper-body movements. Participants who are able to do so safely can progress further to standing aerobic exercises.

Other forms of low-impact aerobic conditioning, such as stationary cycling, rowing, treadmill walking, and water activities, also can be considered. Rotating different types of aerobic exercise engages different muscle groups, decreases the odds for overuse injuries, and can increase exercise adherence. In all cases, participants' safety should be the first consideration. Therefore, risks must be anticipated and eliminated in advance (Garber et al. 2011; Swart, Pollock, and Brechue 1996).

Exercise Sequence

If the aerobic training session follows a proper warm-up period, the aerobic exercises in this chapter can be performed in any order that you deem practical. Several considerations are important:

Table 6.2 General Aerobic-Training Guidelines for Older Adults

Exercise selection	At least one safe, low-impact exercise (such as walking) that uses large muscle groups or a combination of such exercises (such as the aerobic program in this chapter)
Exercise sequence	As desired and well tolerated
Training intensity	3–4 on the RPE scale ("moderate" to "somewhat hard")
Training frequency	3–5 days per week
Training duration	Time permitting, build up to 30 continuous minutes of low to moderate work or up to 60 minutes when only very low intensity work is tolerated. If needed, the desired duration can be accumulated by performing short bouts of activity.
Training range of motion	Through the full, strain-free and pain-free range of joint movement without hyperextending (overreaching), except when a reduced range is necessary to control intensity
Training speed	A moderate speed that facilitates rhythmic, controlled movement through a broad range of motion
Number of repetitions	As desired and well tolerated
Rest periods	Rest breaks as necessary, with continuous movement or easy, light activity when possible rather than complete cessation of movement
Progression and maintenance	Gradual, conservative increases in frequency and duration (and, to a lesser extent, intensity); continued long-term training after the desired health and fitness level is reached

From E. Best-Martini and K.A. Jones-DiGenova, 2014, *Exercise for frail elders*, 2nd ed. (Champaign, IL: Human Kinetics).

1. Many people perform their best when the graph of energy expenditure during aerobic exercise is bell shaped. Therefore, begin with easier, lighter movements. Gradually build up to increasingly demanding movements. After peak moves (the most energetic of your workout), move back through less demanding exercises until you return to the easiest and lightest.

2. Depending on how well participants tolerate the bell-shaped model just described, it may be necessary to pace them by interspersing easy, light moves throughout the aerobics session. Individual participants should always be encouraged to pace themselves as needed during group aerobic training.

Intensity

Aerobic exercise intensity (how hard to work) must be controlled for two important reasons:

1. Excessive intensity can lead to cardiovascular complications (ACSM and AHA 2007) and musculoskeletal injuries.

2. On the other hand, insufficient intensity does not produce the desired training effects (Garber et al. 2011; Swart, Pollock, and Brechue 1996).

How can you help participants find that middle ground where their aerobic efforts are both safe and effective? A useful tool for monitoring aerobic exercise intensity is the rating of perceived exertion (RPE) scale (see table 6.3). This scale, based on the participant's feelings of fatigue, provides a subjective guide to his or her response to exercise. A practical RPE scale extending to 10 has been described by a number of reliable sources including the American Council on Exercise (2011), the Cleveland Clinic (2011), the University of Michigan Health Service (2011), and MedicineNet (2011). Generally, a rating from 3 to 4 ("moderate" to "somewhat hard") is a suitable range for improving health and fitness in the elderly.

When using the scale, you need to take into account the participant's overall sense of tiredness. For example, encourage your participants to note the onset of shortness of breath as well as how weary their legs feel. Keep in mind that frail elders maintaining a 3 to 4 rating of perceived exertion will appear less active than highly fit adults working in the same intensity range. To assist your participants, you may wish to display an RPE poster in your activity area. One helpful version features simple cartoon-style facial expressions alongside the numbers to represent degree of intensity (see "Suggested Resources" near the end of this book). Ask your participants to express their RPE frequently during aerobic training. With frail elderly participants, especially beginners, it is not unreasonable to check every few minutes.

Throughout the aerobic exercise session, participants should work at a pace that allows them to breathe naturally and never feel short of breath. They should be able to talk normally at all times. Otherwise, the intensity level is too high and needs to be reduced. When conducting aerobic exercise for frail elderly participants, you should constantly aim for a safe and effective level of effort.

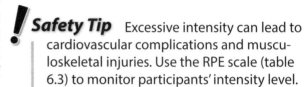

Safety Tip Excessive intensity can lead to cardiovascular complications and musculoskeletal injuries. Use the RPE scale (table 6.3) to monitor participants' intensity level.

Frequency

Initially, schedule aerobic training three times per week (on nonconsecutive days, if possible). After your participants respond favorably to aerobic training for several months, increase the frequency to four and then five times per week. This schedule increases the chance that

Table 6.3   Rating of Perceived Exertion (RPE) Scale

RPE number	Breathing rate/ability to talk	Exertion
1	Resting	Very slight
2	Talking is easy	Slight
3	Talking is easy	Moderate
4	You can talk but with more effort	Somewhat hard
5	You can talk but with more effort	Hard
6	Breathing is challenged/don't want to talk	Hard
7	Breathing is challenged/don't want to talk	Very hard
8	Panting hard/conversation is difficult	Very hard
9	Panting hard/conversation is difficult	Very, very hard
10	Cannot sustain this intensity for too long	Maximal

your participants will make it to class at least three times per week. Encourage beginners to your class to start with 3 days and slowly progress to 5.

Duration

A sound approach is to schedule 10- to 15-minute aerobic exercise sessions initially (preceded and followed by 10- to 15-minute periods of light movement and stretching). Try increasing aerobic exercise duration by 5-minute increments every 4 weeks until participants are performing sustained aerobic exercise for 30 minutes or longer (Clark 2012b; Swart, Pollock, and Brechue 1996). Encourage beginners to your class to pace themselves as necessary and to progress slowly to performing the entire aerobics routine.

Especially at first, duration can be limited by the participant's tolerance. In that case, rest breaks can be interspersed with aerobic exercise periods to accumulate the recommended exercise time. In other words, the recommended duration can be accumulated either in one exercise session or during short activity bouts, such as three 10-minute bouts (ACSM 2011, 1339; Rahl 2010, 125; Bryant and Green 2009, 533; ACSM 2009b, 1511; USDHHS 2008b) throughout the day. If such bouts are undertaken in separate sessions, take care to include adequate warm-up and cool-down periods. This type of intermittent aerobic activity produces health benefits similar to those achieved through continuous movement (Clark 2012a; Coleman et al. 1999; Swart, Pollock, and Brechue 1996).

If time constraints prevent you from scheduling classes that include 30 minutes of aerobic exercise, aerobics sessions from 15 to 20 minutes in duration are also productive. But extending aerobic training to 30 minutes for frail elderly participants is preferable when possible: For a given quantity of work, the intensity and duration of training are inversely related. That is, activities of lower intensity and longer duration provide the same benefits as those of higher intensity and shorter duration. Because low- to moderate-intensity exercise is preferred for frail elderly populations, a longer duration of up to 30 minutes helps to ensure that participants reap maximum benefits. In fact, people who can tolerate only very low intensity work can benefit from durations of up to 60 minutes (Clark 2012b; Swart, Pollock, and Brechue 1996).

Range of Motion

Using fuller ranges of motion (such as higher limb elevations) increases intensity level, whereas using limited ranges reduces it. Fuller ranges contribute more toward preserving mobility than do limited ranges. As participants become fatigued during the course of an aerobic exercise session, they may need to decrease range to maintain an RPE of 3 to 4 ("moderate" or "somewhat hard," not "hard" or "very hard"). Otherwise, remind them to work through their full, strain-free and pain-free range of joint movement without hyperextending their joints (Clark 2012a).

Speed

Aerobic movement that is too fast can cause orthopedic injuries, raise intensity too high, and take the pleasure out of training. Set a rhythmic pace that allows controlled movement through a broad range of motion. If your participants begin flinging their limbs or their form is compromised (e.g., only partial arm reaches when you are teaching fully extended reaches), you should reduce speed. Remind participants that their individual ranges of motion vary and to stay within their strain-free and pain-free range of motion. Well-chosen music during the aerobic exercise session can help set an appropriate pace while adding fun to your workout. Choose musical numbers that your participants enjoy and perhaps remember fondly. Here are some good styles:

- Marches
- Show tunes
- Country
- Gospel
- Ragtime

- Old standards
- Swing
- Popular symphony overtures
- Light pop
- Easy listening
- Calypso and tropical sounds
- Music from around the world

To promote participation and prevent discomfort among participants, always keep the volume conservative.

Many instructors find it convenient to establish the right pace by using tunes with a specific number of beats per minute (BPM). Commercial exercise music marketers offer audiotapes, compact discs, and MP3 downloads labeled with the BPM (see "Suggested Resources" near the end of this book). For active, independent-living older adults, a tempo from 120 to 140 BPM is viable during aerobic exercise. For frail elderly participants, try a range from 110 to 130 BPM or even slower (American Senior Fitness Association 2012b).

Whether or not you select music based on its BPM, remember that the beat of your music must facilitate the three major goals discussed earlier:

1. Rhythmic activity
2. Controlled movement
3. Broad ranges of motion

Safety Tip Aerobic movement that is too fast can cause orthopedic injuries and raise exercise intensity too high. Set a rhythmic pace that allows controlled movement through a broad strain-free and pain-free range of motion.

Number of Repetitions

In aerobic exercise, no rule dictates when to change from one exercise to the next. Indeed, participants can obtain aerobic benefits simply by performing a single aerobic activity (such as walking, cycling, or rowing) at the recom-

mended intensity and duration for the entire exercise session. Therefore, the rate at which you change from one exercise to another should depend on the characteristics of your exercise group. Here are some important considerations:

1. Changing too quickly from one aerobic exercise to the next can overwhelm elderly participants, especially beginners. They should do enough repetitions to master the movement and to experience a sense of confidence in performing it before moving on. Ensuring that participants can follow your workout successfully encourages their continued attendance.

2. As participants perfect their skills, you can change moves more frequently. Varying the aerobic exercises promotes several benefits:
   - Decreased risk of overuse injury
   - Better conditioning of joints and muscles by working them through different angles
   - Improved coordination and balance
   - Mental stimulation, which supports cognitive health
   - Discouraging boredom and increasing interest and enjoyment

3. You can perform a specific exercise, proceed through a series of other moves, and then repeat the original exercise or a variation of it. In fact, you can return to favorite moves often during any single workout session.

Rest Periods

Elderly aerobics participants should be taught and reminded often to pace themselves as needed throughout the exercise session. At times, participants (beginners especially) may feel the need to cease movement completely. But as they grow stronger, encourage them to pace themselves by simply slowing down or substituting lighter, easier movements for a while when they feel tired. Sustaining continuous activity in this way can help build endurance.

Keep in mind that some frail elders tolerate aerobic exercise best when it is measured out in short (5- to 10-minute) bouts of activity throughout the day, as long as they accumulate the total recommended duration.

Progression and Maintenance

Progression can be achieved through gradual, conservative increases in frequency and duration (and, to a lesser extent, intensity). Only one variable at a time should be increased. With this population, progression should be pursued slowly over the course of several months, a year, or even longer if indicated. Frequency can be increased, by one session at a time, from 3 to 5 days per week if well tolerated. Duration can be increased, by a few minutes at a time, from approximately 10 minutes per session to 30 minutes or longer if well tolerated. Intensity can be increased, by small increments, when RPE falls below 3 to 4. For ideas on how to increase aerobic intensity, refer to the section "Variations and Progression" in this chapter. Participants who are able to stand safely can slowly progress to the standing variations of the basic seated aerobic exercises (see variations and progression options in the illustrated instruction section at the end of the chapter).

At some point a participant may cease progressing and begin only to maintain his or her current level of aerobic training, depending on his or her goals, motivation, physical and mental ability, and physician's recommendations. A meaningful goal is to attain the level of cardiovascular endurance required for activities of daily living (termed *functional fitness*) that are important to the participant. For example, if a person has not attained his or her goal of walking a block without sitting down on the walker seat, the duration or frequency (remember, just one at a time!) of the aerobics program can be increased when he or she is ready. When a participant has reached his or her goal, reevaluate his or her functional fit-

ness goals related to cardiovascular endurance before initiating maintenance with aerobic training. This can be a good time to encourage further progress (when appropriate) based on the guidelines for aerobic training provided in this section. Refer to "Suggested Resources" or *Senior Fitness Instructor Training Manual* (American Senior Fitness Association 2012b) for how to test participants' aerobic endurance, a foundation for setting goals. In chapter 8 you will learn more about this topic in the sections "Progressing Your Exercise Class" and "Maintaining Fitness Results."

! Safety Tip Progress your class gradually and conservatively with increases in frequency and duration (and, to a lesser extent, intensity). Increase only one (frequency, duration, or intensity) at a time.

Other Training Techniques

Here is the simplest way to use the exercises in this chapter to lead your initial aerobic workouts:

1. First, follow the given order of the exercises. Make the whole sequence last half the desired duration of your aerobics session and plan the duration of each exercise accordingly. For example, for a 24-minute aerobics session using 12 exercises, perform each exercise for 1 minute for a subtotal of 12 minutes.

2. Then reverse the given order of the exercises, taking the same length of time for each movement. Teaching the given order followed by the reversed order results in an aerobics session of the desired duration with higher-intensity exercises at the midpoint and easier exercises at the beginning and end. With practice and experience, you will learn to vary the exercise sequences while maintaining the appropriate intensity throughout your aerobics class.

3. If the example just given produces an aerobics session too long for your needs,

select fewer exercises and conduct them in the manner described. For example, using 6 or 10 exercises would yield an aerobics session lasting 12 or 20 minutes, respectively. Remember that beginners may need to do shorter sessions at first, building up to longer ones over time.

Develop exercise patterns and combinations, like these:

1. Combine two single exercises into an exercise pattern. For example, perform four Alternate Toe Touches to Front (exercise 6.5), four Alternate Heel Touches to Front (exercise 6.6), and continue repeating the pattern.

2. When participants have mastered the first pattern, teach them a new pattern. For example, perform four Alternate Toe Touches to Sides (exercise 6.7), four Alternate Heel Touches to Sides (exercise 6.8), and continue repeating that pattern.

3. When participants have mastered two patterns, teach them a combination of the two: four Alternate Toe Touches to Front, four Alternate Heel Touches to Front, four Alternate Toe Touches to Sides, and four Alternate Heel Touches to Sides. Repeat the combination for as long as desired.

When each exercise also includes its own specific arm moves, such patterns and combinations of patterns create an appealing dance atmosphere—especially if accompanied by music. Developing numerous patterns and combinations adds variety and excitement to your aerobics class. Also, you can recycle your participants' favorite patterns and combinations by performing them to new musical selections.

Supplement the exercises in this chapter with additional aerobic movements that are consistent with your participants' performance ability. Develop your own new exercises by mixing and matching basic lower-body movements with various upper-body movements.

For ideas, see the box "Developing New Aerobic Exercises." Achieve even more variety by combining your new exercises into patterns and combinations as described earlier. The variety of your aerobic workouts is limited only by your creativity.

When changing from one aerobic exercise to another, cue your participants clearly and well in advance. Initially, conduct smooth transitions by asking your participants to walk in place (or alternate heel lifts for the easiest transition) briefly after each exercise while you demonstrate the next one for them. This method helps ensure their continuous movement throughout the aerobic workout. As you become more expert at cueing and as your participants grow familiar with the exercises, they will be able to move directly from one exercise to another.

BASIC SEATED AEROBIC EXERCISES

As you initially get to know your participants' strengths and current limitations, start your classes with the basic seated aerobic and dynamic balance exercises. Seated exercise eliminates the risk of falling while standing, but you need to make sure that your participants are safely positioned in their seats. Before initiating this component, we recommend that you step up your understanding of aerobic training and dynamic balance activities by carefully reading this entire chapter and learning the answers to the review questions at the end.

The basic aerobic exercises are 12 lower-body aerobic training and dynamic balance activities. These are listed in table 6.4 and can be done seated or standing. The illustrated instruction section at the end of the chapter illustrates and describes these 12 exercises. Teach these lower-body movements first. When your participants are ready to progress and enjoy more variety, add the corresponding upper-body movements listed as variations and progression options in the illustrated instruction section. To introduce additional moves and add further variety to your aerobic and dynamic balance program, refer to the previous discussion. You may copy table 6.4 and "Developing New Aerobic Exercises" for easy reference and handouts for your participants.

Some elderly participants can progress to standing aerobic exercises. Many others in this population, however, need to remain on a seated program, including nonambulatory participants, those with vision losses, those with balance problems that place them at high

Developing New Aerobic Exercises

Create new moves by mixing and matching the arm movements given here with the leg movements of exercises 6.1 to 6.12 (either seated or standing). All these arm movements are compatible with exercise 6.3 (Walking in Place). Identify other good matchups by trying different arm and leg moves together outside class. Then teach new combinations that work well to your participants during class.

Alternately snap fingers and then clap hands together.

Alternately slap the front of the thighs lightly and then clap hands together.

Reach with both arms in any direction (up, down, front, or out to each side).

Alternately reach with both arms in one direction and then another (for example, front and then out to the sides).

Punch with both arms in any direction (up, down, front, or out to each side).

Alternately punch with both arms in one direction and then another (for example, up and then down).

Push with both hands in any direction (up, down, front, or out to each side).

Alternately push with both hands in one direction and then another (for example, up and then front).

Fly like a bird (gently simulate a bird flapping its wings).

Be a movie reviewer (alternately turn thumbs up and then thumbs down).

Be a hitchhiker (alternately thumb a ride in one direction with one arm and then in the opposite direction with the other arm).

Go for a drive (using both hands, simulate turning the steering wheel of a car).

Join the army (alternately salute with one hand and then the other).

Join the circus (simulate the actions of a juggler).

Play ball.

1. *First, simulate pitching the ball alternately with one arm and then the other. Gently pitch both underhand and overhand. Continue for as long as desired.*

2. *Then swing the bat, taking a few swings as a right-handed batter and then a few as a left-handed batter.*

Go swimming.

1. *Simulate the crawl stroke. Continue for as long as desired.*

2. *Simulate the breast (or back or side) stroke. Continue each stroke for as long as desired.*

Play a symphony.

1. *Simulate playing various musical instruments that inspire energetic movements, such as the piano, trombone, violin, harp, accordion, kettle drums, and bongo drums. Continue each for as long as desired.*

2. *Then imitate the actions of an orchestra conductor, moving both arms about dramatically.*

Table 6.4 Basic Aerobic and Dynamic Balance Exercises: Seated or Standing[a]

Exercise
6.1 Alternate Weight Shifts
6.2 Alternate Heel Lifts
6.3 Walking in Place
6.4 Marching in Place
6.5 Alternate Toe Touches to Front
6.6 Alternate Heel Touches to Front
6.7 Alternate Toe Touches to Sides
6.8 Alternate Heel Touches to Sides
6.9 Alternate Step-Touches
6.10 Alternate Kicks
6.11 Alternate Knee Lifts
6.12 Alternate Double Knee Lifts

[a] All seated aerobic and dynamic balance exercises can be adapted to standing exercises. See the corresponding standing exercises in the variations and progression options of the illustrated exercises at the end of the chapter.

From E. Best-Martini and K.A. Jones-DiGenova, 2014, *Exercise for frail elders*, 2nd ed. (Champaign, IL: Human Kinetics).

risk of falling, and frail participants (particularly those with osteoporosis) at high risk of bone fractures.

BASIC STANDING AEROBIC EXERCISES

Seated lower-body aerobic and dynamic balance exercises can be adapted to a standing position. Although dynamic balance training typically is performed in a standing position, participants who need seated routines also can take part in dynamic balance activities. As with the basic seated exercises, teach the lower-body movements first. When your participants are ready to progress and enjoy more variety, add the corresponding upper-body movements listed as variations and progression options in the illustrated instruction section at the end of the chapter. To introduce additional moves and add further variety to your aerobic program,

refer to the earlier section "Other Training Techniques" and the box "Developing New Aerobic Exercises."

Standing aerobic and dynamic balance exercises can replace seated work for qualified participants after they have become proficient with seated methods. During class, some participants can do the seated exercises while others do the standing versions. Also, a single aerobics and dynamic balance session can involve some combination of both seated and standing activity for certain individuals. For people who tolerate standing work well, the more standing aerobic exercises they perform, the better their results will be (Clark 2005). Refer to chapter 8 to find out more about when to implement standing exercises, the benefits of standing exercises, when seated exercises are preferred over standing exercises, and the advantages of teaching both the seated and standing exercises simultaneously.

VARIATIONS AND PROGRESSION

The illustrated aerobics instruction section at the end of the chapter gives variations and progression options for each basic seated aerobic exercise, which you may introduce after your participants have learned the basic seated exercises. As previously mentioned, including different types of aerobic exercise benefits more muscle groups, reduces the risk for overuse injury, and can improve attendance and participation rates by making your class more interesting. Create your own original exercise patterns and combinations by following the instructions provided in "Other Training Techniques" and develop new aerobic movements for your class using the ideas in "Developing New Aerobic Exercises."

Over time, gradual increases in the intensity, frequency, and duration of aerobic activity enable a participant to progress. Following are instructions for manipulating those three training variables.

As participants grow stronger, intensity can be increased gradually within sensible limits. Here are some ways to increase intensity:

- Incorporate upper-body movements along with the basic lower-body movements.
- Work at a faster speed (but always in a controlled manner).
- Work through fuller ranges of motion (lift legs higher, reach arms farther, and generally perform bigger movements).
- Progress from seated to standing activity. Notice this symbol, which identifies the exercises that enhance balance, before the standing exercises.

When increasing the intensity for frail elderly participants, remember that the RPE should never exceed 4. In this population, most progression should be achieved through slow increases in frequency and duration. Gradually, over a period of several months, frequency can be increased from 3 to 5 days per week. Likewise, duration can be increased from about 10 minutes per aerobics session to 30 minutes or longer.

Elderly participants can take up to a year to reach the maintenance stage, the stage when an individual achieves his or her desired level of health or fitness. Practically speaking, most frail elderly participants can be regarded as maintenance candidates when they can well tolerate 30-minute sessions of continuous aerobic activity at an RPE of 3 to 4, 3 to 5 days per week. At this stage, the emphasis shifts from progression to long-term, continued training (see chapter 8).

SUMMARY

Elderly fitness participants stand to gain substantially from well-designed aerobic exercise programs. Because the physical well-being of your participants is paramount, remember to err on the side of safety. By following the guidelines in this chapter, you can employ necessary safeguards without compromising the integrity of your aerobic workout or limiting your participants' fun and enthusiasm. Participants who regularly perform aerobic exercise in your class can experience major benefits, including enhanced performance, fitness, and health. In addition, the experience can be socially rewarding, for both your participants and you!

REVIEW QUESTIONS

1. List and briefly describe five keys to conducting a successful aerobic exercise program for elderly fitness participants:

   a. _____

   b. _____

   c. _____

   d. _____

   e. _____

2. T or F. In general, older adults are more susceptible to orthopedic injury and cardiovascular problems. Therefore, aerobic exercise prescription should emphasize low-impact and low- to moderate-intensity exercise, starting slowly and gradually progressing in duration and frequency.

3. T or F. When using the recommended RPE (rating of perceived exertion) scale, a subjective method of monitoring aerobic exercise intensity, it is not necessary to observe your participants for warning signs, such as labored breathing.

4. What are three different methods that can help prevent breathlessness for participants with COPD during aerobic training?

5. Which of the following statements pertain to people with osteoporosis? (*Circle only one.*)

   a. When symptoms are minor, low-impact aerobic dance or walking (as tolerated) can be beneficial in managing osteoporosis.

   b. An ambulatory participant can benefit from alternating between seated and standing aerobic exercise within one class.

   c. When osteoporosis is advanced, standing exercise may not be safe because of increased risk for falling and fracture.

   d. Only seated exercises are recommended for participants with advanced osteoporosis.

   e. All of the above

   f. *a* and *b* only

6. With the frail elderly population, most progressions with aerobic training should be achieved through slow increases in _____ and _____.

7. Standing in place while reading aloud from a book is an example of a relatively _____ balance training activity.

ILLUSTRATED INSTRUCTION

Exercises 6.1 through 6.12 are seated and standing aerobic and dynamic balance exercises. The exercise and safety tips and variations and progression options apply to both seated and standing exercises unless otherwise specified.

Good Seated and Standing Posture

Be sure to refer to the instructions for good seated and standing posture in chapter 4 and remind participants of them often as you do each exercise.

Seated Alternate Weight Shifts

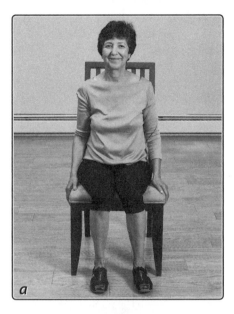

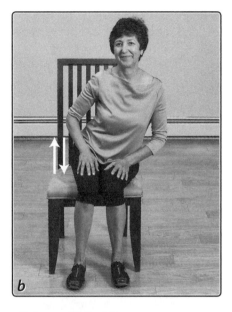

Start and Finish Position

1. Good seated posture.
2. Hands on lap or wheelchair arms.
3. Feet flat on the floor.

Side to Side Movement

4. Lift one buttock slightly off the chair seat.
5. Lower it back onto the chair seat.
6. Lift the other buttock slightly off the chair seat.
7. Lower it back onto the chair seat.

! Exercise and Safety Tips

- Weight shifts should be performed in a deliberate manner at a moderate rate of speed.
- In a chair, gently roll on the buttocks from one side to the other between lifts to shift weight smoothly.
- Be sure that participants maintain erect posture. Some seated participants, in particular, may tend to begin slumping after this exercise gets underway.

- If standing, shift weight from leg to leg instead of from buttock to buttock. Feet should be about shoulder-width apart, and knees should be "soft" (slightly bent, not locked).
- When incorporating the arm motions suggested in "Variations and Progression Options," if participants' arms grow fatigued while working at chest level, they can lower them to a more comfortable height at which to perform the motions.

(continued)

Seated Alternate Weight Shifts   *(continued)*

Variations and Progression Options

- While shifting weight from side to side, perform arm rotations.
- Whether seated or standing, keep both feet flat on floor while learning this exercise. Progress to lifting the heel on the non-weight-bearing side off the floor.
- Over time, certain participants may safely be able to reach the next level of

progression: lifting the entire foot on the non-weight-bearing side slightly off the floor.

- *Standing Alternate Weight Shifts.* Add Arm Rotations (see photographs *c* and *d* and instructions).

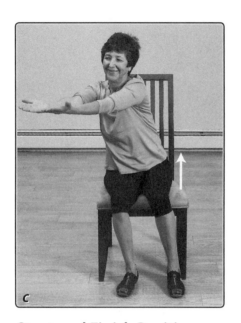

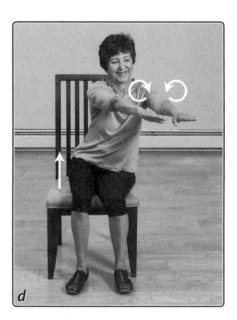

Start and Finish Position

1. Place feet flat on the floor.
2. Extend arms to the front at chest level.
3. Palms face upward.

Movement Phase

4. Begin Alternate Weight Shifts.
5. As weight shifts to one side, rotate arms inward until the palms face downward.
6. As weight shifts to the opposite side, rotate arms outward until the palms face upward.

Seated Alternate Heel Lifts

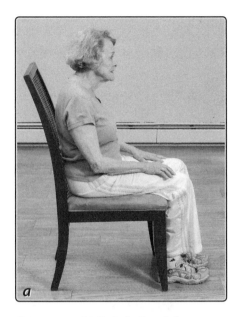

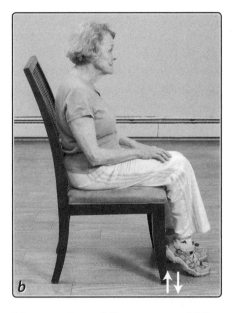

Start and Finish Position

1. Good seated posture.
2. Hands on lap or wheelchair arms.
3. Feet flat on the floor.

Upward and Downward Movement

4. Raise one heel off the floor.
5. Lower it back onto the floor.
6. Raise the other heel off the floor.
7. Lower it back onto the floor.

❗ *Exercise and Safety Tips*

- If feet are positioned too far away from the chair, heel lifts will not be high enough.
- Touch heels to the floor lightly to prevent bruising.
- To optimize aerobic benefits, perform heel lifts as quickly as safely possible.
- If fatigued, participants may reduce speed.
- If participants do not move in time to the musical beat during this (or any other) exercise, do not be disturbed. Simply encourage them to do their best and to enjoy themselves.
- For the standing version, pay special attention to maintaining erect posture; leaning forward during standing heel lifts may compromise balance.

(continued)

Variations and Progression Options

- While performing the lower-body movements, raise both arms slowly up and down while shaking fingers "Charleston style."

- For the seated version only, discontinue the suggested arm motions and place the palms on top of the upper thighs. Do, however, continue performing heel lifts as quickly as safely possible. At the same time, slowly lean forward (bending from the hips and keeping the back straight), hold for a moment, and then slowly return to upright seated posture. In this way, participants may also lean toward the front diagonals and toward the back. Participants with hip replacements should obtain their doctor's approval before performing this move.

- *Standing Alternate Heel Lifts.* Add Charleston fingers (see photographs *c* and *d* and instructions).

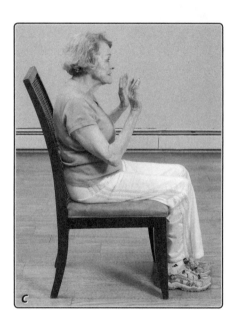

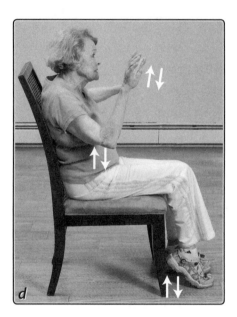

Start and Finish Position

1. Place feet flat on the floor.
2. Bend elbows at the sides.
3. Open hands wide.
4. Palms face front.
5. Fingers point upward.

Movement Phase

6. Begin Alternate Heel Lifts.
7. Shake fingers quickly from side to side.
8. Move arms slowly upward and downward.

Seated Walking in Place

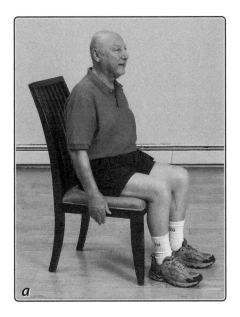

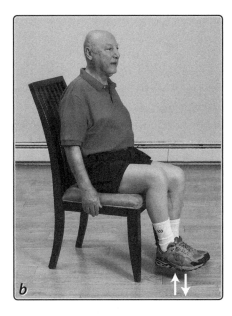

Start and Finish Position

1. Good seated posture.
2. Arms by the sides.
3. Feet flat on the floor.

Upward and Downward Movement

4. Walk in place.

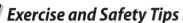

⚠ Exercise and Safety Tips

- Be sure to lower the heel to the floor with each step; walking on the toes does not provide sufficient shock absorption.
- Touch feet to the floor lightly to prevent foot injuries.
- If fatigued, seated participants may substitute Alternate Heel Lifts and standing participants may change to the seated exercise.

- When incorporating the arm motions suggested in "Variations and Progression Options," relax the hands and fingers to encourage circulation.
- When incorporating the suggested arm motions, swing the arms energetically to optimize aerobic benefits.

Variations and Progression Options

- While walking in place, perform Alternate Arm Swings. Start with whichever arm feels more natural.
- 🧍 For the seated version, discontinue the suggested arm motions and place the palms on top of the upper thighs. While sitting tall, continue walking in place with the hips aimed forward. At the same time, slowly rotate the trunk toward side 1, looking back over the shoulder. Hold for a moment and then slowly rotate back to starting position. Repeat toward side 2.

(continued)

Variations and Progression Options *(continued)*

- Some participants may enjoy walking about occasionally, instead of walking in place. Walking laps (in a large circular pattern) works well indoors. Also, participants can take a certain number of steps in one direction and then in a different direction. Note, however, that walking backward can compromise balance in some participants, so it is better to have them walk forward in one direction, give them ample time to turn, and then have them walk forward in the new direction.

- Have standing participants try walking forward on their toes; seated participants can toe-walk in place.

- Have standing participants try walking forward on their heels; seated participants can heel-walk in place.

- Before class, use chalk or tape to mark a straight line on the floor. Have standing participants try to stay on the line while walking forward. As noted earlier in this chapter, participants should look ahead, not down at their feet, during physical activity. Let them slow their walking speed, as necessary, for this exercise. Ensure that each person has enough space to use his or her arms for balance.

- Have standing participants try walking heel to toe. With each step, they place the heel just in front of the toes of the other foot (with heel and toes lightly touching or nearly so). They apply the same safety precautions as those given for line walking, described earlier.

- Form pairs or small groups of three or four standing participants and have them converse while walking laps.

- Have standing participants try taking longer steps along with longer arm swings as they walk about.

- *Standing Walking in Place.* Add Alternate Arm Swings (see photographs *c* and *d* and instructions).

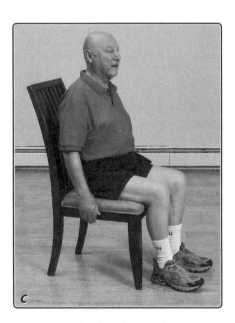

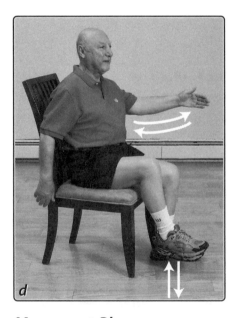

Start and Finish Position

1. Place feet flat on the floor.
2. Extend both arms down at the sides.
3. Relax the arms, hands, and fingers.

Movement Phase

4. Begin Walking in Place.
5. Alternately swing one arm and then the other.
6. Swing once with each step.
7. Swing naturally, forward and backward.

Seated Marching in Place

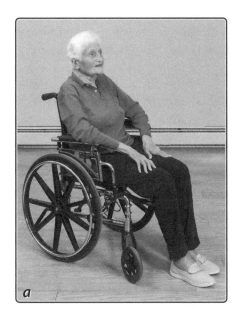

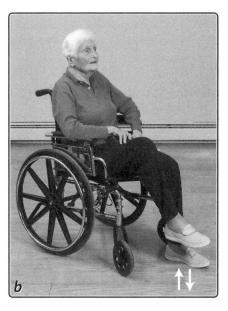

Start and Finish Position

1. Good seated posture.
2. Hands on lap or wheelchair arms.
3. Feet flat on the floor.

Upward and Downward Movement

4. March in place.

! *Exercise and Safety Tips*

- Be sure to lower the heel to the floor with each step; marching on the toes does not provide sufficient shock absorption.
- Touch the feet to the floor lightly to prevent foot injuries.
- If fatigued, seated participants may substitute Walking in Place and standing participants may change to the seated exercise.

- When incorporating the arm motions suggested in "Variations and Progression Options," keep the fists loose to spare the joints of the hands and fingers and to encourage circulation.
- When incorporating the suggested arm motions, swing elbows energetically to optimize aerobic benefits.

Variations and Progression Options

- While marching in place, perform Alternate Elbow Swings. Start with whichever elbow feels more natural.
- For the seated version, discontinue the suggested arm motions and place the palms on top of the upper thighs. Continue marching in place and maintaining erect seated posture. At the same time, slowly raise one extended arm forward to shoulder level, hold for a moment, and then slowly lower it to starting position. With the same arm and in the same manner, repeat to the side. Repeat the exercises using the opposite arm. Then repeat the exercises using both arms.

(continued)

Variations and Progression Options *(continued)*

- 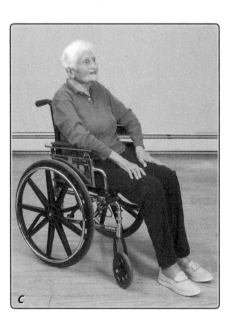 Whether seated or standing, march in place with the feet wide apart for eight steps and then close together for eight steps. Repeat as desired. Over time, participants may be able to progress to four steps wide and four steps together, and perhaps even to two steps wide and two steps together (suggested verbal cue: "Out, out, in, in"). If more readily achievable by participants, conduct this exercise while walking in place instead of marching in place.

- Some participants may enjoy marching about occasionally, instead of marching in place. A combination of marching and walking laps (in a large circular pattern) works well indoors. Also, participants can take a certain number of steps in one direction and then in a different direction. Note, however, that marching backward can compromise balance in some participants, so it is better to have them walk forward in one direction, give them ample time to turn, and then have them walk forward in the new direction.

- Have standing participants pretend to be in a marching band. Have them march forward from one end of room to the other, allow them ample transition time to turn around, and then have them march forward to return to starting position. Over time, teach them to stop marching on your oral cue. Conduct such stops occasionally at various places along the route between the turnaround points and then have them quickly resume marching forward.

- Have standing participants try taking larger steps along with longer elbow swings as they march about.

- *Perform Standing Marching in Place.* Add Alternate Elbow Swings (see photographs *c* and *d* and instructions).

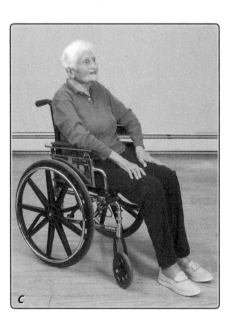

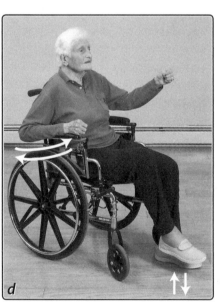

Start and Finish Position

1. Place feet flat on the floor.
2. Bend elbows at the sides.

Movement Phase

3. Begin Marching in Place.
4. Alternately swing one elbow and then the other.
5. Swing once with each step.
6. Swing naturally, forward and backward.

Seated Alternate Toe Touches to Front

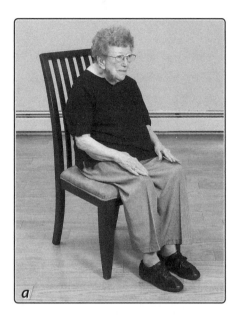

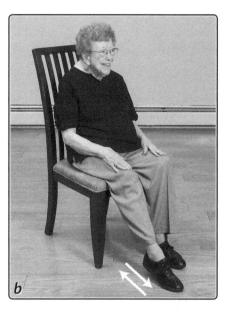

Start and Finish Position

1. Good seated posture.
2. Hands on lap.
3. Feet flat on the floor.

Forward and Backward Movement

4. Move one foot forward and then touch the toes to the floor.
5. Return the foot to starting position.
6. Touch the toes of the other foot to the floor in front.
7. Return the foot to starting position.

! *Exercise and Safety Tips*

- If fatigued, seated participants may substitute Alternate Heel Lifts (exercise 6.2) or Walking in Place (exercise 6.3) and standing participants may change to the seated exercise.
- When incorporating the arm motions suggested in "Variations and Progression Options," avoid slinging the arms outward. Move them in a controlled manner to protect the shoulders and elbows.

- When incorporating the suggested arm motions, people with painful arthritis in their hands should simply touch their hands together rather than clap.
- If standing, participants should protect joints from excessive impact by keeping one foot on the floor at all times. Resist any temptation to perform a jumping version of this exercise.

(continued)

Variations and Progression Options

- While performing the lower-body movements, alternately clap hands together and move arms apart.

- *Standing Alternate Toe Touches to Front.* Add clapping (see photographs *c* and *d* and instructions).

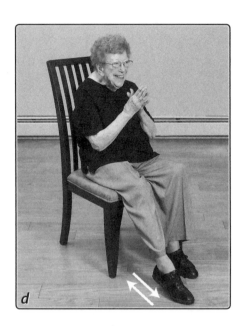

Start and Finish Position

1. Place feet flat on the floor.
2. Bend elbows at the sides.
3. Palms face each other.

Movement Phase

4. Begin Alternate Toe Touches to Front.
5. Clap when toes touch front.
6. Spread arms apart when the feet are together.

Seated Alternate Heel Touches to Front

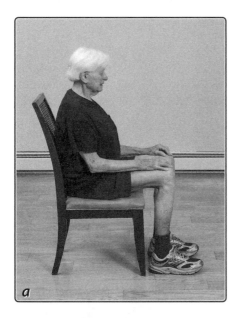

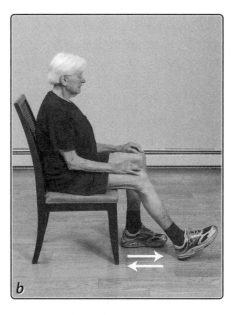

Start and Finish Position

1. Good seated posture.
2. Hands on lap.
3. Feet flat on the floor.

Forward and Backward Movement

4. Touch one heel to the floor in front.
5. Return the foot to starting position.
6. Touch the other heel to the floor in front.
7. Return the foot to starting position.

! Exercise and Safety Tips

- Touch heels to the floor lightly to avoid bruising.
- If fatigued, seated participants may substitute Alternate Heel Lifts (exercise 6.2) or Walking in Place (exercise 6.3) and standing participants may change to the seated exercise.

- When incorporating the arm motions suggested in "Variations and Progression Options," stretch the fingers comfortably.
- If standing, protect joints from excessive impact by keeping one foot on the floor at all times. Resist any temptation to perform a jumping version of this exercise.

Variations and Progression Options

- While performing the lower-body movements, participants should alternately reach one arm and then the other toward the front. They reach with the arm opposite the extended leg.
- This exercise helps prepare participants for more advanced progression options

given in exercises 6.7 and 6.8. When learning this exercise, participants should place their hands on the lap if seated and on the hips with arms akimbo if standing. They perform two Alternate Toe Touches to Front (one touch with each foot) and then two Alternate Heel Touches to Front. Continue repeating.

(continued)

Variations and Progression Options *(continued)*

- Over time, participants may progress to adding arm motions. The simplest method is to push both arms toward the front with each toe and heel touch. Depending on participants' performance levels, you may choose to introduce more challenging arm motions at a future time.

- *Standing Alternate Heel Touches to Front.* Add Alternate Reaches Toward Front (see photographs *c* and *d* and instructions).

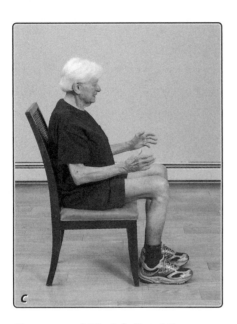

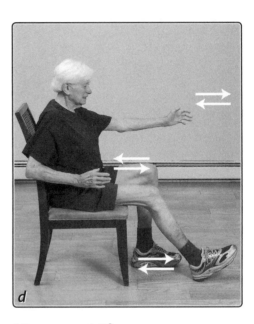

Start and Finish Position

1. Place feet flat on the floor.
2. Bend elbows at the sides.
3. Relax hands and fingers.

Movement Phase

4. Begin Alternate Heel Touches to Front.
5. As each heel touches, reach forward with the opposite arm.
6. Bend elbows at the sides when the feet are together.

Seated Alternate Toe Touches to Sides

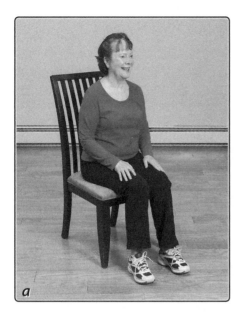

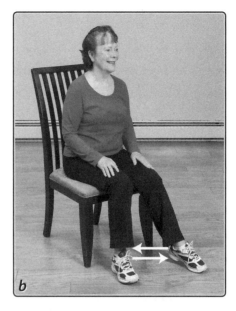

Start and Finish Position

1. Good seated posture.

2. Hands on lap.

3. Both feet flat on the floor.

Outward and Inward Movement

4. Touch toes of one foot to the floor at side.

5. Return foot to starting position.

6. Touch toes of the other foot to the floor at side.

7. Return the foot to starting position.

! Exercise and Safety Tips

- If fatigued, seated participants may substitute Alternate Heel Lifts (exercise 6.2), Walking in Place (exercise 6.3), or Marching in Place (exercise 6.4) and standing participants may change to the seated exercise.

- When incorporating the arm motions suggested in "Variations and Progression Options," if high arm raises are uncomfortable or impossible to perform, participants can simply raise the arms as high as feels natural.

- If standing, participants should protect their joints from excessive impact by keeping one foot on the floor at all times. Resist any temptation to perform a jumping version of this exercise.

(continued)

Variations and Progression Options

• While performing the lower-body movements, add Jumping-Jack Arms. Raise both arms high at the sides as each leg extends. Lower the arms as the leg returns to starting position.

• When learning this exercise, participants should place their hands on the lap if seated and on the hips with arms akimbo if standing. For more directional change and weight shifting, perform two Alternate Toe Touches to Front (one touch with each foot) and then two Alternate Toe Touches to Sides. Continue repeating. Over time, participants may progress to adding arm motions. The simplest method is to push both arms toward the front with each toe touch to the front and then push both toward the sides with each toe touch to the side. Depending on participants' performance levels, you may choose to introduce more challenging arm motions at a future time.

• *Standing Alternate Toe Touches to Sides.* Add Jumping-Jack Arms (see photographs *c* and *d* and instructions).

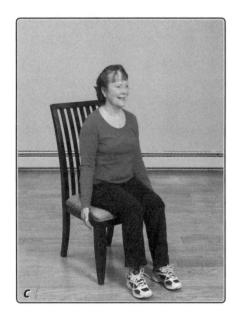

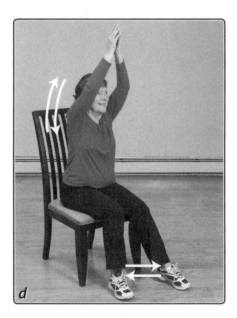

Start and Finish Position

1. Place both feet flat on the floor.
2. Extend arms down at the sides.

Movement Phase

3. Begin Alternate Toe Touches to Sides.
4. As each leg extends, raise both arms.
5. Lower arms when feet are together.

Seated Alternate Heel Touches to Sides

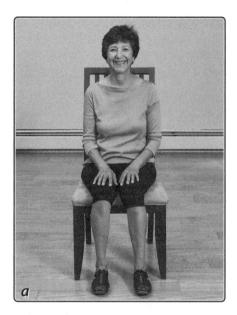

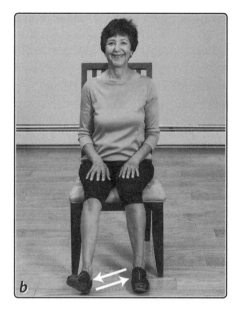

Start and Finish Position

1. Good seated posture.
2. Hands on lap.
3. Feet flat on the floor.

Outward and Inward Movement

4. Touch one heel to the floor at side, as far to the side as comfortable.
5. Return the foot to starting position.
6. Touch the other heel to the floor at side.
7. Return the foot to starting position.

Exercise and Safety Tips

- Touch heels to the floor lightly to prevent bruising.
- If fatigued, seated participants may substitute Alternate Heel Lifts (exercise 6.2), Walking in Place (exercise 6.3), or Marching in Place (exercise 6.4) and standing participants may change to the seated exercise.
- If standing, protect joints from excessive impact by keeping one foot on the floor at all times. Resist any temptation to perform a jumping version of this exercise.

- When standing and extending one leg toward the side, slightly bend the opposite knee to increase range and ease of movement.
- If standing, gently turn the trunk and look to the side as each leg extends to enhance enjoyment and benefits. But if turning causes discomfort or a lightheaded feeling, keep the trunk and head facing forward during limb extensions.

Variations and Progression Options

- While performing the lower-body movements, add Alternate Arm Pushes to Sides. Push both arms toward one side along with the extended leg.

- This exercise helps prepare participants for more advanced progression options given later. When learning this exercise, participants should place their hands

(continued)

Variations and Progression Options   *(continued)*

on the lap if seated and on the hips with arms akimbo if standing. Perform two Alternate Toe Touches to Sides (one touch with each foot) and then two Alternate Heel Touches to Sides. Continue repeating. Over time, participants may progress to adding arm motions. The simplest method is to push both arms toward the sides with each toe and heel touch. Depending on participants' performance levels, you may choose to introduce more challenging arm motions at a future time.

- When learning this exercise, participants should place their hands on the lap if seated and on the hips with arms akimbo if standing. For more directional change and weight shifting, perform two Alternate Heel Touches to Front (one touch with each foot) and then two Alternate Heel Touches to Sides. Continue repeating. Over time, participants may progress to adding arm motions. The simplest method is to push

both arms toward the front with each heel touch to the front and then push both toward the sides with each heel touch to the side. Depending on participants' performance levels, you may choose to introduce more challenging arm motions at a future time.

- 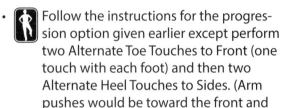 Follow the instructions for the progression option given earlier except perform two Alternate Toe Touches to Front (one touch with each foot) and then two Alternate Heel Touches to Sides. (Arm pushes would be toward the front and sides.)

- Follow the instructions for the progression option given earlier except perform two Alternate Heel Touches to Front (one touch with each foot) and then two Alternate Toe Touches to Sides. (Arm pushes would be toward the front and sides.)

- *Standing Alternate Heel Touches to Sides.* Add Alternate Arm Pushes to Sides (see photographs *c* and *d* and instructions).

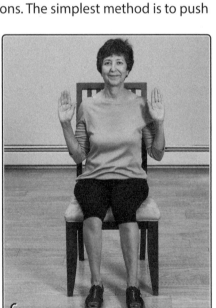

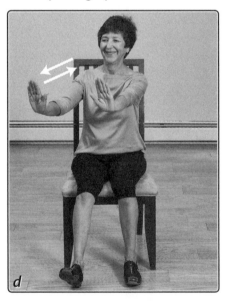

Start and Finish Position

1. Place feet flat on the floor.
2. Hold arms in "stick 'em up" position (palms facing forward near shoulders) and elbows by the sides.
3. Point fingers upward.

Movement Phase

4. Begin Alternate Heel Touches to Sides.
5. As each leg extends, push arms along with it out to the side.
6. Bend elbows at the sides when feet are together.

AEROBIC
E X E R C I S E
6.9

Seated Alternate Step-Touches

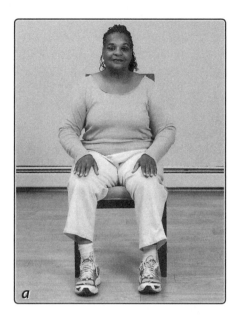

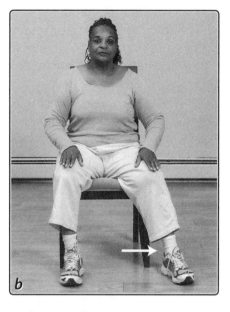

Start and Finish Position

1. Good seated posture.
2. Hands on lap or wheelchair arms.
3. Feet flat on the floor.

Side to Side Movement

4. Step to the outside with the first foot, placing it flat on the floor.
5. Move the second foot in the same direction, touching toes lightly to the floor beside the first foot.
6. Lift the second foot and step to the opposite side, placing it flat on the floor.
7. Move the first foot in the same direction, touching toes lightly to the floor beside the second foot.
8. Continue repeating steps 4 through 7.

❗ Exercise and Safety Tips

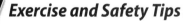

- If fatigued, seated participants may substitute Alternate Heel Lifts (exercise 6.2), Walking in Place (exercise 6.3), or Marching in Place (exercise 6.4) and standing participants may change to the seated exercise.

- 🧍 When conducting this exercise, keep in mind that a step is weight bearing whereas a touch is a non-weight-bearing transitional move in preparation for a directional change. This distinction is especially important if standing.

(continued)

Variations and Progression Options

- To increase intensity when incorporating the suggested arm motions, hold the elbows higher (but not above shoulder level) and extend the arms more fully at the sides.

- While performing Standing Alternate Step-Touches, add Shoulder Touches (see photographs *c* and *d* and instructions).

- Participants may progress to taking two steps toward each side instead of one. To do so, step to the outside with foot 1, touch next to it with foot 2, step to the outside with foot 1, touch next to it with foot 2, and return leading with foot 2. Repeat as desired.

- Eventually, more than two steps toward each side may be performed in the manner just described. If participants are standing, the number of steps is limited only by the amount of space available and participants' performance levels. If seated, taking more steps will necessitate taking smaller steps, so taking more than two steps each way is impractical.

- If standing, certain participants (only those whose balance is not jeopardized by stepping backward) can safely step-touch from front to back as well as from side to side. They should change the lead foot occasionally.

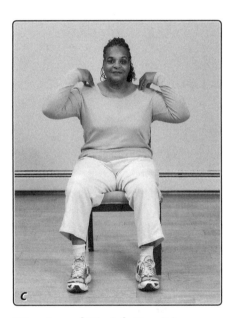

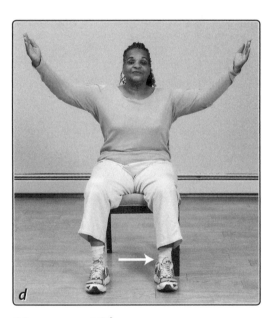

Start and Finish Position

1. Place feet flat on the floor.
2. Hold arms out at the sides and have elbows bent comfortably below shoulder level.
3. Fingertips touch shoulder tops.

Movement Phase

4. Begin Alternate Step-Touches.
5. During steps, open arms at the sides.
6. During toe touches, touch shoulder tops with fingertips.

Seated Alternate Kicks

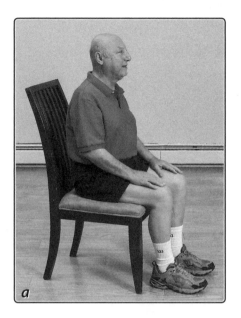

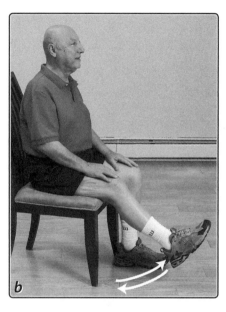

Start and Finish Position

1. Good seated posture.
2. Hands on lap.
3. Both feet flat on the floor.

Upward and Downward Movement

4. Straighten leg.
5. Return foot to starting position.
6. Straighten the other leg.
7. Return foot to starting position.

! Exercise and Safety Tips

- If fatigued, seated participants may substitute Alternate Heel Lifts (exercise 6.2), Walking in Place (exercise 6.3), or Marching in Place (exercise 6.4) and standing participants may change to the seated exercise.
- Avoid flinging the legs during knee extensions. Move legs in a controlled manner to protect the knees (and the hips while standing).
- If standing, protect joints from excessive impact by keeping one foot on the floor at all times. Resist any temptation to perform a jumping version of this exercise.
- Although the lifted leg should be extended when standing, its knee should not be locked (rigidly straightened), which is stressful to the joint.
- If standing, lift the leg to a moderate height; excessively high lifts can cause falls.

Variations and Progression Options

- While performing Alternate Kicks, swing both arms back and forth across the front.
- *Standing Alternate Kicks.* Add Arm Swings Across Front (see photographs *c* and *d* and instructions).

(continued)

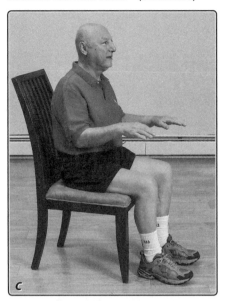

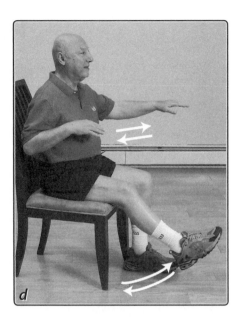

Start and Finish Position

1. Place feet flat on the floor.
2. Bend elbows at the sides.
3. Position hands slightly above lap.
4. Extend fingers.
5. Hold palms face down.

Movement Phase

6. Begin Alternate Kicks.
7. As each leg extends, sweep arms up to the opposite side.
8. Sweep arms low across lap when feet are together.

Seated Alternate Knee Lifts

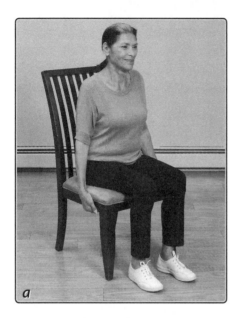

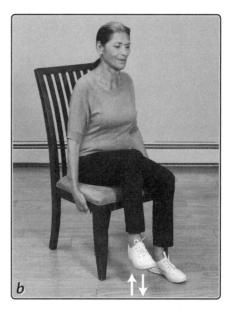

Start and Finish Position

1. Good seated posture.
2. Hands hold side of the chair.
3. Both feet are flat on the floor.

Upward and Downward Movement

4. Raise one knee high to the front.
5. Lower foot back to the floor.
6. Raise the other knee high to the front.
7. Lower foot back to the floor.

! Exercise and Safety Tips

- To prevent foot injuries, avoid stomping on the floor during this exercise.
- If fatigued, seated participants may substitute Alternate Heel Lifts (exercise 6.2), Walking in Place (exercise 6.3), or Marching in Place (exercise 6.4) and standing participants may change to the seated exercise.
- When incorporating the arm motions suggested in "Variations and Progression Options," keep fists loose during punches, never tight.
- To optimize aerobic benefits, raise the knees as high as safely possible when standing, but not so high that balance is compromised or the torso collapses (keep the upper body erect).

Variations and Progression Options

- While performing Alternate Knee Lifts, perform Alternate Punches toward the front. Punch with the arm opposite the lifted knee.
- *Standing Alternate Knee Lifts.* Add Alternate Punches (see photographs *c* and *d* and instructions).
- Whether seated or standing, participants who can safely build up to performing higher knee lifts will more effectively engage the core.

(continued)

Seated Alternate Knee Lifts   *(continued)*

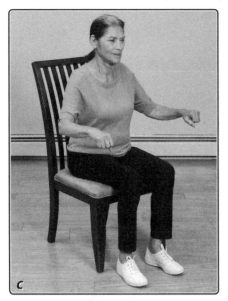

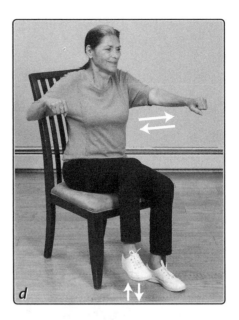

Start and Finish Position

1. Place feet flat on the floor.
2. Bend elbows at the sides.
3. Make loose fists.
4. Hold palms face down.

Movement Phase

5. Begin Alternate Knee Lifts.
6. As each knee lifts, punch forward with the opposite arm.
7. Bend elbows at the sides when feet are together.

AEROBIC EXERCISE 6.12

Seated Alternate Double Knee Lifts

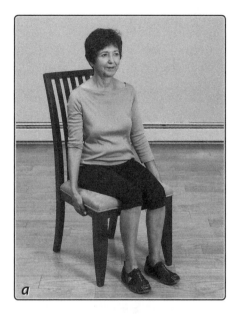

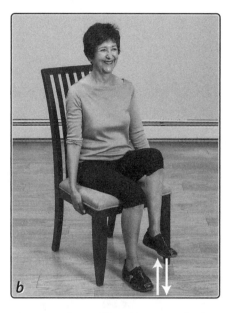

Start and Finish Position

1. Good seated posture.
2. Hands hold side of the chair.
3. Feet are flat on the floor.

Upward and Downward Movement

4. Lift one knee high to the front.
5. Lower foot back to the floor.
6. Lift the same knee high to the front.
7. Lower foot back to the floor.
8. Lift the other knee high to the front.
9. Lower foot back to the floor.
10. Lift the other knee high to the front.
11. Lower foot back to the floor.

! Exercise and Safety Tips

- To prevent foot injuries, avoid stomping on the floor during this exercise.
- If Alternate Double Knee Lifts feel too strenuous, participants may substitute single lifts (exercise 5.9).
- When incorporating the arm motions suggested in "Variations and Progression Options," if pushing arms high overhead is uncomfortable or impossible, simply push as high as feels natural.
- To optimize aerobic benefits, lift knees as high as safely possible when standing, but not so high that balance is compromised or the torso collapses (keep the upper body erect).

(continued)

Variations and Progression Options

- While performing Alternate Double Knee Lifts, perform Upward Arm Pushes.

- An easier lower-body variation is to lower the knee lifts.

- An easier upper-body variation is to lower the "stick 'em up" position.

- *Standing Alternate Double Knee Lifts*. Add Upward Arm Pushes (see photographs *c* and *d* and instructions).

- Whether seated or standing, participants who can safely build up to performing higher double knee lifts will more effectively engage the core.

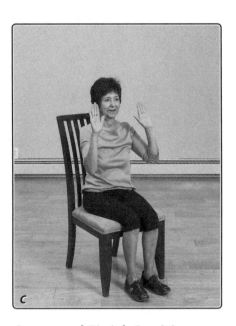

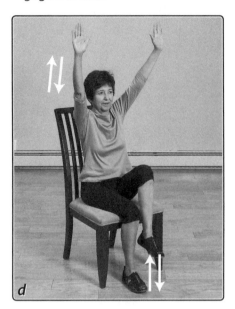

Start and Finish Position

1. Place feet flat on the floor.

2. Arms in "stick 'em up" position (palms facing upward near shoulders) and elbows by the sides.

Movement Phase

3. Begin Alternate Double Knee Lifts.

4. Push both arms upward with each knee lift.

Cool-Down:
Stretching and Relaxation Exercises

Too many people confine their exercise to stretching
the truth, running up bills, sidestepping responsibility,
pushing their luck, and jumping to conclusions.

—Anonymous

LEARNING OBJECTIVES

After completing this chapter, you will have the tools to

- teach a safe and effective cool-down component of an exercise session for frail elders and adults with special needs;
- design a creative and progressive session using 12 functional stretching exercises, many variations and progression options, and relaxation exercises;
- Apply essential safety precautions and guidelines for leading cool-down exercises; and
- focus on fall prevention by personalizing your instruction of seated and standing cool-down exercises for a class of people with varying fitness levels and one or more special needs.

This chapter provides guidelines, safety precautions, and specific teaching instructions for leading a safe and effective cool-down, the final component of an exercise session, in an individual or group setting. Always have your participants cool down to facilitate the transition between exercise and rest and to promote flexibility (the ability to move joints and muscles through their full, normal range of motion) and relaxation. Stopping exercise abruptly creates a risk of irregular heartbeat, dizziness, fainting, and coughing and wheezing for those with asthma and bronchitis. The cool-down after aerobics consists of progressively slower-paced movements that slowly lower the heartrate (low-intensity aerobics, chapter 6) and can include ROM exercises (chapter 4). The cool-down period after any workout is an essential time to concentrate on stretching. This chapter focuses on stretching exercises and includes relaxation exercises appropriate for frail elders and adults with special needs.

Start with the basic seated stretching and balance exercises. Participants who are able to stand safely can carefully progress to the basic standing stretching and balance exercises. The seated and standing exercises are designed to be taught together to accommodate both those who can stand and those who cannot or who prefer to sit. Keep in mind, when referring to the set of seated and standing stretching exercises throughout this chapter, that the concept of balance is implied even if not stated overtly. Improved balance is one benefit of increasing flexibility and joint ROM (ACSM 2011, 1344).

SAFETY PRECAUTIONS

Cool-down exercises are safe for frail elders and adults with special needs when appropriate guidelines and precautions are observed. The following general safety precautions and specific safety precautions for those with special needs can help you lead a safe cool-down and keep your participants injury free. For easy reference, you may photocopy the following "General Safety Precautions Checklist for Stretching" and the general exercise "Safety Guidelines Checklist" in chapter 2.

Specific Safety Precautions for Those With Special Needs

Following are some specific safety precautions for leading the cool-down for those with special needs, particularly those with conditions beyond an early or mild stage. Thus, these precautions may not apply to every person with a particular condition. For example, an individual with mild symptoms of Parkinson's disease may have no limitations on stretching exercises, whereas severe symptoms may cause difficulty with all stretching exercises. Also, remember that a person's performance ability can vary from day to day. See chapter 1 to learn more about common special needs. For further information see "Fitness, Wellness, and Special Needs" in "Suggested Resources."

These general stretching safety precautions for older adults also apply to those with special needs. However, the following specific safety precautions will further the safety and effectiveness of your exercise program for those with special needs.

Alzheimer's Disease and Related Dementias

- Some cool-down exercises require the instructor to be extra vigilant with participants who may not remember directions or pose a risk of copying others who are doing an exercise that is contraindicated for their condition. Have these participants sit near you in clear sight. If they have other special needs, ensure that they follow the specific safety precautions for that special need.

- When leading stretching, if a stretch is performed on one side then the other, slowly flow uninterruptedly from one side to the other. For example, give a visual and verbal cue such as by saying, "Change sides." Then, after you see them change sides, continue relevant cueing. This procedure helps those with memory issues remember what side they just stretched.

Arthritis

- A thorough cool-down is especially important for people with arthritis, whose joints may need extra time to recover from exercise, especially longer sessions.

- Flexibility (stretching and ROM) exercises performed with low-intensity and controlled movements generally do not increase symptoms or pain for those with osteoarthritis, the most common type of arthritis (Rahl 2010, 184).

- Gentle static stretching is recommended once to several times a day, even during acute flare-ups (Rahl 2010, 183, 184). Encourage a safe home program for those who are capable.

GENERAL SAFETY PRECAUTIONS CHECKLIST FOR STRETCHING

☐ Follow the physician's special recommendations and comments for each participant on the "Statement of Medical Clearance for Exercise" (appendix A2) and remind the participant to follow them, as well.

☐ Always leave at least 10 minutes at the end of class for a cool-down period to return safely to a resting state, reduce the incidence of cardiovascular complications, and promote flexibility and relaxation (ACSM 2010; Bryant and Green 2009, 532).

☐ Focus on fall prevention. During standing exercise have a chair centered closely behind all participants so that they can sit down easily if needed. Remember that participants can have day-to-day variation in their balance ability. For those with balance issues, a chair directly in front or one on each side to hold on to can enable some participants to do lower-body standing exercises. When participants are seated, make sure that they are safely positioned in their chairs.

☐ Do not move a joint beyond its strain-free and pain-free range of motion.

☐ Avoid hyperextending or locking any joints when stretching, especially the elbow and knee.

☐ Avoid stretching beyond the body's natural limits. Overstretching weakens joints and increases risk of injury (Picone 2000).

☐ Always keep one foot planted firmly on the floor while stretching the other leg to help prevent lower-back strain.

☐ Remind participants to stop deep breathing and sit if standing if they feel fatigued, light-headed, or dizzy.

☐ Continually encourage your participants to maintain good posture and breathe fully while exercising (and throughout the day). Teach them to not hold their breath, which can increase blood pressure and decrease enjoyment of physical activities.

☐ As always, focus on fun and safety, number one!

Cerebrovascular Accident (CVA, Stroke)

- See also the safety precautions for those with coronary artery disease (heart disease).

- Providing clear cool-down instructions is extremely important to participants who have experienced stroke. If a participant has paralysis on the right side, focus on leading exercises mainly by demonstration, using few verbal instructions. If a participant has paralysis on the left side, rely more on verbal instructions, using fewer gestures (American Senior Fitness Association 2012c).

- The American Senior Fitness Association (2012a) recommends that people with a history of stroke hold neck stretches no longer than 2 to 3 seconds. No longer than 5 seconds is recommended for older adult participants in general.

- Always ensure that participants keep the head above the heart when bending forward because of the danger of increased vascular pressure within the brain and the risk of stroke. We have excluded such stretching exercises from this book. We suggest that stroke survivors, those at risk for stroke, those with uncontrolled proliferative retinopathy (see the section on "Diabetes"), and glaucoma pay particular attention to this precaution when bending forward to tie shoes, pick up weights from the floor, and so on.

Chronic Obstructive Pulmonary Disease

- A thorough cool-down is critical for people with COPD, whose lungs and cardiovascular systems need extra time to adapt to changes in exertion level. For these participants, a cool-down reduces the risk of bronchospasm, arrhythmias, orthostatic hypotension (decrease of blood pressure below normal upon standing from a lying or seated position), and syncopal (fainting) episodes (ACSM 2010; AACVPR 2011, 43).

- Participants should avoid holding their breath with stretching and controlled breathing exercises to prevent straining the respiratory and cardiovascular systems.

Coronary Artery Disease (Heart Disease)

- A careful cool-down is critical for participants with heart disease, whose cardiovascular systems need extra time to adapt to changes in exertion level. For these participants, a cool-down helps "to avoid the decrease in central blood volume that can occur with the abrupt cessation of physical activity" (ACSM and AHA 2007, 893).

Depression

- Throughout class observe participants' facial expression and posture. Notice how they may change favorably in response to constructive exercise.

- End your class on a cheerful note, such as by wholeheartedly thanking participants for coming, telling a tasteful joke, or offering an inspirational quotation.

- After establishing rapport, encourage participants to exercise daily, gradually building up to that goal. You may want to elicit the support of a caregiver or other support person to help encourage the participant outside of class.

Diabetes

- Instruct participants with peripheral vascular disease (PVD, which causes poor circulation to the legs and feet), to which people with diabetes are predisposed, to avoid seated crossed-leg positions in general and when stretching (restricting circulation), as in exercise 7.11, Seated Outer-Thigh Stretch. Refer to the exercise and safety tips for alternatives.

- Instruct participants with uncontrolled proliferative diabetic retinopathy to avoid activities (such as hanging the head below the heart) that increase intraocular pressure and risk of hemorrhage (ACSM and ADA 2010, 2286). Refer to the last point of the section "Cerebrovascular Accident (CVA, Stroke)."

Frailty

- Regular, safe stretching to promote flexibility and joint ROM can be a key contributor to the goal of restoring function, as best as possible, for frail people. Encourage regular class attendance, suggest a home stretching program (recruiting the support of the caregiver, if possible), and compliment small steps forward, even if the participant is coming to class for only a few minutes. Be as flexible as possible to make your class inviting.

- Address other possible special needs associated with their frailty, such as osteoporosis. Refer to "What Is Frailty?" in chapter 1.

Hip Fracture or Replacement

- Avoid stretching exercises that involve internal rotation (turning the leg inward), hip adduction that crosses the midline of the body (crossing the legs), and hip flexion (decreasing hip joint angle by bending forward at the hip or lifting the thigh toward the upright torso) of more than 90 degrees to prevent the risk of hip dislocation, unless a participant has written clearance from his or her physician indicating that those specific movements are not contraindicated. Refer to "Exercise and Safety Tips" for alternatives for those with hip fracture or replacement for exercise 7.8, Seated or Standing Tib Touches, and exercise 7.11, Seated or Standing Outer-Thigh Stretch.

Hypertension

- People with hypertension may be susceptible to rebound hypotension (an abrupt drop in blood pressures soon after exercise) that can result in dizziness and fainting. Therefore, a gradual cool-down from exercise is crucial (Williamson 2011, 239).

- Avoid inverted static stretches (not provided in this book) and holding strenuous stretches (Bryant and Green 2009, 193). Only introduce the Challenger stretches to participants who are able to perform them comfortably, without straining.

- Instruct participants to transition slowly between static stretches (Bryant and Green 2009, 193).

- Give reminders not to hold the breath (including with controlled breathing exercises), which can increase blood pressure.

Multiple Sclerosis and Parkinson's Disease

- Stretching is recommended seven times per week (NCPAD 2009a, b). Encourage a home program for those who are capable on days that you do not offer a class that includes stretching.

- When working one on one with people who have both coordination and flexibility limitations, consider functional flexibility exercises, such as using a stationary bicycle. Such exercises may serve better than standard stretching, especially early in training. Exercise equipment with a fan, such as the Schwinn Airdyne, can be helpful for people with MS who are prone to heat sensitivity (Rahl 2010, 232).

- Anyone with any trouble controlling neck movement should avoid neck stretches because of the increased risk of injury.

Osteoporosis

- Stretching is recommended five to seven times per week.

- Encourage a home program for those who are capable on days that you do not offer a class that includes stretching.

- Avoid stretching exercises that involve spinal flexion, such as exercise 7.8, Tib Touches, particularly in combination with stooping, which increases risk of vertebral fractures. Instruct those who are unable to follow specific directions to do the exercise seated without leaning forward. For participants who are able to follow specific directions emphasize the cue "Bend forward at the hips" and "Maintain a neutral spine (long and lifted) throughout the stretch."

- Avoid spinal bending (exercise 7.6) and twisting (exercise 7.7) (Minne and Pfeifer 2005, 11), particularly in combination with stooping (ACSM 2009a, 275), unless the participant has milder osteoporosis and medical clearance for those movements.

Sensory Losses

- Give a clear demonstration of the cool-down exercises to participants with hearing loss.

- Describe cool-down exercises precisely and directly to participants with visual impairment.

GUIDELINES

"Guidelines for Stretching Exercises" and "Guidelines for Relaxation Exercises" will help you understand the importance of leaving at least 10 minutes at the end of your class for the cool-down. Table 7.1 shows duration of the parts of a 10- to 15-minute cool-down. Notice that the cool-down following aerobics includes low-level aerobics—progressively slower-paced movements that allow the respiration rate, heart rate, and blood pressure to decrease gradually to the preaerobic state. See chapter 6 for aerobic exercises that can be performed slowly at a lower intensity. The cool-down phase after resistance training begins with range-of-motion exercises (see chapter 4) and concentrates on stretching. Range-of-motion exercises performed slowly can ease the transition from resistance training (especially when intensive) to stretching when needed to achieve a gradual lowering of breathing rate, heart rate, and blood pressure. Relaxation exercises are optional after resistance training, aerobics, or a class combining both components. A relaxation exercise, such as deep breathing, can be combined with stretching exercises (when

appropriate). Of course, another option is to schedule more time for relaxation exercises if your participants are interested.

The following guidelines for stretching and relaxation exercises apply to both seated and standing exercises and are intended to minimize injury and maximize the benefits of the cool-down. Refer to the previous section "Specific Safety Precautions for Those With Special Needs" for adapting these general guidelines to meet your participant's special needs.

Guidelines for Stretching Exercises

A well-rounded stretching program can prevent or even reverse the usual decline in flexibility of older adults and improve their posture, balance, and functional ability. As participants' flexibility improves, they can more easily perform daily activities requiring flexibility, such as bathing, grooming, dressing and undressing, reaching, and so on. Several prominent organizations have developed guidelines for stretching, including the American College of Sports Medicine (2011, 2009b), the American Council on Exercise (Bryant and Green 2010), the American Senior Fitness Association (2012a, b, c), the National Strength and Conditioning Association (Baechle and Earle 2008), and the U.S. Department of Health and Human Services (USDHHS 2008b). Table 7.2 synthesizes the stretching guidelines that are appropriate for older adults. The recommen-

Table 7.1   Duration of the Segments of a 10- to 15-Minute Cool-Down[a]

Cool-down exercises	After resistance training	After aerobics and dynamic balance
1. Low-level aerobics	Not applicable	5 minutes
2. Range-of-motion exercises	2 to 3 minutes	0[b] to 1 minute
3. Stretching	8 to 10 minutes	5 to 8 minutes
4. Relaxation	0[b] to 2 minutes	0[b] to 1 minute

[a]Exercises are in the recommended order, and times are approximate.

[b]0 indicates that ROM or relaxation exercises are optional, but they can enhance the cool-down period if time permits.

dations for stretching in this chapter are based on those evidence-based guidelines, although some more conservative recommendations are presented for a population with special needs. You may make a copy of table 7.2 for easy reference and as an educational handout for your participants.

When to Stretch During a Workout

The best time to improve long-term flexibility is at the end of a workout, when muscles are warm and pliable. "Flexibility exercise is most effective when the muscle temperature is elevated through light-to-moderate cardiorespiratory or muscular endurance exercise" (ACSM 2011, 1345). Cool down for a mini-

mum of 10 minutes after resistance training or aerobics, whichever is the last exercise component of your class. See table 7.1 for the durations of the segments of a cool-down for ending a workout after resistance training or aerobics and dynamic balance. The four phases of a cool-down are (1) low-level aerobics, (2) ROM exercises, (3) stretching, and (4) relaxation. An ideal way to promote flexibility is to teach a stretching-only class. In this case, you would warm up for a minimum of 7 minutes (subtracting the initial 1 to 3 minutes of stretching at the end of a typical 10- to 15-minute warm-up) before a luxurious class of stretching to increase circulation, internal body temperature, and joint range of motion.

Table 7.2 General Stretching Guidelines for Older Adults

When to stretch during a workout	Stretch at the end of the warm-up before exercise and after exercise. If you do both resistance training and aerobics in one class, also briefly stretch between those components.
Frequency	Stretch two to seven times per week.
Exercise selection	Stretch the major muscle groups of the body.
Stretching mode	Static stretching is recommended over ballistic stretching.
Intensity (how should a stretch feel)	Stretches should be taken only to the point of tightness or mild intensity, not strain or pain.
Duration (how long to hold a stretch)	10 to 30 seconds, except 5 seconds or less for neck stretches
Repetitions	1 to 4
Speed	Slowly ease in and out of a stretch.
Rest periods between sets of the same stretch	A few seconds or none if the stretches involve changing sides
Rest periods between different stretches	None or a few seconds if a posture, breathing, or ROM exercise (that participants are familiar with) is integrated between stretches with shortened instruction
Progression and maintenance	After participants learn to perform the 12 basic seated stretching exercises with good technique, they can progress slowly by increasing frequency, duration, or repetitions of the stretching exercises; by decreasing rest periods; or by performing the stretches standing (increase only one at a time). When participants reach long-term flexibility goals, encourage lifetime maintenance.

From E. Best-Martini and K.A. Jones-DiGenova, 2014, *Exercise for frail elders*, 2nd ed. (Champaign, IL: Human Kinetics).

Integrate light stretching (for a short time) advantageously throughout an exercise class for an optimal functional fitness program design, such as the following:

1. At the end of the warm-up, before resistance training or aerobics, perform light stretching for 1 to 3 minutes.

2. If you are leading both resistance training and aerobics in one class, with aerobics before resistance training, finish with several minutes of low-intensity aerobic exercise using the legs. Follow this with the minimal five stretching exercises (see table 4.3) before you begin resistance training.

3. If you do resistance exercises before aerobics, end with the minimal five stretches and then perform several minutes of active rhythmic movement (such as slow walking or low-intensity aerobic leg exercises) before starting aerobics. After aerobics, cool down by first lowering the intensity of the aerobic exercise before optional range-of-motion exercises and a longer, final stretching and relaxation segment (see table 7.1).

4. Between resistance exercises, doing a stretch can feel good. For example, after Heel Raises (exercise 5.11), which strengthen the calf muscles, it can feel good to stretch those muscles with the Calf Stretch (exercise 7.12). If you have enough time in the final cool-down stretching, repeat the Calf Stretch, a beneficial functional exercise that increases ankle ROM and can improve gait and balance.

Exercise Selection

The stretching component of your class can range from the minimal five (table 4.3) at the end of your warm-up and the strategic eight (table 4.4) during the cool-down to a class that concentrates on promoting joint ROM, flexibility, and relaxation. Stretching-only classes include an initial warm-up period of light movement (see chapter 4 for ROM exercises and chapter 6 for low-level aerobics), the stretching exercises, and a final period of relaxation (refer to table 8.5, [Model stretching and relaxation class]). The comprehensive stretching routine presented in this chapter includes seven upper-body and five lower-body basic stretches, with many variations and progression options, that target the major muscle groups of the body (as shown in table 7.3). These exercises are safe and appropriate for frail elders and adults with special needs.

For a shorter set of stretching exercises see table 4.3, The Minimal Five Stretching Exercises, or table 4.4, the Strategic Eight Stretches, in chapter 4. These shorter stretching routines are derived from the 12 comprehensive stretching exercises and both include essential stretches for body parts that are notoriously tight for most older adults and that can compromise posture, impair balance, and reduce functional ability. No matter how many stretches you teach, start with the basic seated stretching exercises before incorporating the variations and progression options, with the exception of the easier options, in the illustrated instruction section at the end of the chapter. Participants who are stable on their feet can progress to basic standing stretching exercises.

Stretching Mode

Static (held or sustained) stretching is a simple, effective, and safe method, so long as it is not done too strenuously. Conversely, ballistic stretching—high-force, short-duration bouncing, jerking, or swinging motion—is not recommended because it is less effective than static stretching and carries a greater risk of injuring muscles and connective tissue. The preferred static stretch used in this text is slow and constant. The end, or stretch, position—the position that stretches the muscle to the greatest length—is held without movement for generally 10 to 30 seconds. Refer to "AEIOUs of Leading Static Stretching" later in this chapter.

Intensity

Instruct participants to stretch only to the point of tightness or a pleasant pulling sensation of mild intensity, not to the point of strain or pain. Teach them to slowly stretch as far as possible into this end position. With each stretch, remind participants to breathe, relax, and focus on lengthening (or "letting go of") the muscles involved in the stretch. A stretch should be felt in the muscles, not the joints. Minimize movement of body parts that are not involved in the stretch.

How do you know whether participants are stretching effectively?

- If they do not feel the stretch, they have not gone far enough.
- If they feel the stretch, a mild tightness, they have gone far enough.
- If they feel strain or pain, they have gone too far. In this case, reduce the stretch to eliminate the uncomfortable sensation and to feel a good stretch. If easing up on the stretch does not eliminate the strain or pain, choose another way to modify the stretch if appropriate.

The *A* through *E* mnemonic that follows will help you remember with ease how to modify a stretch (see chapter 8 for further description):

- *A*djust the speed of the movement (move slowly and smoothly in and out of a stretch).
- *B*ody position—check for good posture and proper limb position.
- *C*onsult the physician or physical therapist.
- *D*ecrease the workload by holding a stretch for a shorter duration, performing fewer repetitions, taking longer rest periods, or sitting instead of standing.
- *E*xercise technique—check for safety and effectiveness, such as proper breathing and mindful stretching to the point of mild tightness. See the exercise and safety tips and variations and progression options of the illustrated instruction section for alternate ways of performing a stretch. For example, many of the exercises have an easier option.

When describing how a stretch should feel to your participants, use positive words, such as *pleasant pulling sensation*, to describe the end point rather than *mild discomfort* or other terms with negative connotations. Phrases such as "No gain with pain" (Anderson 2010), "Train, don't strain," and "No pain, you gain" can be fun educational tools. Now could be a good time to review "Good Sensation and Bad Sensation (Pain) During Exercise Class" in chapter 2.

! Safety Tip Teach participants to stretch only to the point of tightness or a gentle pulling sensation of mild intensity, not to the point of strain or pain.

Frequency

Because flexibility and freedom of movement typically decline with age, older adults can benefit greatly from a regular stretching program. Stretching 2 to 3 days per week is considered a maintenance program. For progression, 5 to 7 days per week of stretching are recommended. "Greater gains in joint range of motion are accrued with daily flexibility exercise" (ACSM 2011, 1345). On the days that you do not offer stretching, encourage your participants to stretch on their own (if they are able) after they have learned the stretches in class. The Minimal Five Stretching Exercises (table 4.3) or the other short routine, the Strategic Eight Stretches, table 4.4, are ideal options for an easy, "no excuses," independent program. Ideally, encourage participants to do the comprehensive set of 12 stretches shown in table 7.3 independently, seated or standing, whichever is appropriate for the individual, on most days that they are not in class, especially if they have insufficient joint ROM and flexibility. You may copy these tables for your participants.

Duration

The general recommended duration for a stretch is 10 to 30 seconds, depending on the muscle or muscles being stretched, the person's tolerance, and the time available. Neck stretches, however, should be held for 5 seconds or less (American Senior Fitness Association 2012a).When performing two to four repetitions of a stretch, the goal is to achieve 60 seconds of total stretching time per stretch by adjusting duration and repetitions according to individual needs. For example, 60 seconds per stretch can be met by two bouts of 30 seconds, three bouts of 20 seconds, one bout of 30 seconds and two bouts of 15 seconds, and so on (ACSM 2011; Decoster et al. 2005). When teaching a class that focuses on stretching, experiment with longer-duration stretches of 30 to 60 seconds, which may yield greater improvements in joint range of motion (ACSM 2011, 1344; Feland et al. 2001).

Encourage participants to hold a stretch for only as long as it feels comfortable. In other words, each participant should stop a stretch when he or she feels tired or uncomfortable and then resume the stretch when he or she feels ready, regardless of what the rest of the class is doing. Ideally, end a stretch on a feel-good note (a release, letting go, an "ahhhhhhh" feeling) so that future stretches are more inviting. For a quieter, more relaxing atmosphere, time stretches silently with a clock or stopwatch rather than count aloud.

Repetitions

In general, perform a stretch one to four times. For frail, deconditioned, and new participants, start by leading each stretch one time and gradually build up to more repetitions, when appropriate for the people in your class and if time permits. Additionally, if you are short on time toward the end of class, do each stretch once slowly with concentration. Better yet, schedule enough time at the end of class to

perform each stretch at least twice, or three to four times for optimal flexibility gains.

When repeating a stretch, stretch the muscles in various positions when possible. For example, with the Swan stretch (exercise 7.3), hold the arms at various heights from parallel with the floor to near the sides. Stretching in different positions provides a more complete stretch of the muscle and can improve range of motion of the joints.

 Safety Tip If you are short on time toward the end of class, do each stretch once slowly with concentration.

Speed

Instruct participants to move slowly and smoothly in and out of a stretch for safety and to facilitate the relaxation possibilities while stretching. Coach them to breathe fully as they move gracefully from one repetition of the same stretch to another and between different stretches. The mindful practice of paying attention to the body and breathing can be applied to all exercises, as well as activities of daily living.

Rest Periods

Rest periods may be necessary for frail elders or deconditioned participants, particularly between repetitions of the same stretch. A rest period can be an ideal time to lead an abbreviated posture, breathing, or ROM exercise (see chapter 4), gently shake out the arms or legs that were stretched, or take a drink of water. Performing only one repetition of each stretch is conducive to flowing gracefully from one stretch to the next without a rest period. Conversely, a stretching-only class is conducive to longer rest periods and integrating unabbreviated posture, breathing, or ROM exercises, based on the needs and interest of your participants, between more challenging stretches.

Rest periods between different sides of the same stretch are generally unnecessary. Moreover, for those with memory issues, we recommend that you flow uninterruptedly (remember, slowly and smoothly) from one side to the other to minimize the chance that they will forget which side they just stretched.

Progression and Maintenance

There are numerous ways to move forward with the stretching component for promoting joint ROM and flexibility. After participants have learned good technique and are comfortable with the 12 basic seated stretching exercises, they can progress. Slowly progress your participants by increasing frequency, duration, or repetitions of the stretching exercises; by decreasing rest periods; or by performing the stretches standing. Remember to increase only one variable at a time (as with resistance training and aerobics):

- **Standing exercises**. Participants who are able to stand safely can slowly progress to the standing variations of the basic seated stretching exercises.

- **Frequency**. Increase frequency by one session at a time, up to 7 days per week. Also, encourage participants who are able to stretch on their own to stretch at home, especially on the days that a class with stretching is not offered.

- **Duration**. Hold stretches a little longer, gradually progressing within the recommended range of 10 to 30 seconds, but still keep the neck stretches to 5 seconds or less. You will find that certain stretches are conducive to holding longer than others are. For example, the Swan stretch (exercise 7.3), which requires holding the arms up against gravity, will naturally be held for a shorter time than a stretch that works with gravity, such as exercise 7.6, Side Bends.

- **Repetitions**. Repeat stretches another time, particularly the stretches that participants need more than others. For example, the Swan stretch stretches the chest, which is notoriously tight for most older adults. This tightness can compromise posture, impair balance, and reduce

functional ability. When teaching a stretching-only class, you will have time to progress slowly up to four repetitions, when appropriate.

- **Rest periods**. If you have integrated rest periods between sets of the same stretch or between different stretches, reduce the time of the rest period and eventually eliminate it, when appropriate for your class.

! Safety Tip Always flow slowly and smoothly in and out of stretches to enhance the mood of relaxation and to prevent injury with fast, jerky, or forced movements.

At some point a participant may cease progressing and begin to maintain his or her current degree of flexibility and joint ROM, depending on his or her goals, motivation, physical and mental ability, physician's recommendations, and possibly available equipment that facilitates stretching. A valuable goal is to attain the level of flexibility required for activities of daily living (termed *functional fitness*) that are important to the participant. For example, if a person recovering from a stroke has not achieved her or his goals of being able to reach forward on the affected side and grab an object on the table, focus on progression of upper-body stretches. Conversely, if another has achieved her or his goal of picking dropped objects off the floor without an E-Z Assist Reacher, she or he may be content with maintaining the current lower-body stretching program.

When a participant has reached a goal, reevaluate his or her functional fitness goals related to flexibility before beginning maintenance with the stretching program. You may wish to encourage further progress at this time (when appropriate) based on the guidelines for stretching exercises provided in this section. Individualized stretching programs that involve maintaining with certain stretches and progressing with others can be achieved more easily with one-on-one training, although significant joint ROM and flexibility progress can potentially be attained by a participant in a class setting.

Other Stretching Techniques

Following are a few additional tips to aid you in leading safe, effective, and enjoyable stretching exercises.

- **Wear appropriate clothing**. Recommend that participants wear clothing that does not restrict movement, but do not require trendy fitness attire that may discourage participation.
- **Avoid manual manipulation**. Avoid liability issues by instructing with verbal cues and demonstration only. Do not use manual manipulation or force with participants while they are stretching.
- **Focus on feeling**. For safe and effective stretching, instruct participants to focus on or feel the major muscles that are being stretched.
- **Focus on breath**. For safe and effective stretching, instruct participant to breathe slowly and deeply while holding the stretches and not to hold their breath.
- **Stabilize shoulders**. If participants tend to lift their shoulders while stretching, have them stabilize their shoulders by moving them up, back, and down. Give reminders when needed to release and relax the shoulder throughout the class (and activities of daily living).
- **Avoid hyperextension**. Instruct participants not to hyperextend (overstretch or lock) the knee and elbow joints (a position that can lead to joint irritation or injury) when straightening them during stretches. They should maintain a position of ease (e.g., "ease at the knees"), or softness, in the joints while stretching, not a bent, effortful position.
- **Shake it out, gently**. After a stretch, participants may enjoy gently shaking out the area stretched to release any residual muscle tension. "This is especially important in the beginning stages, since the learning itself may set us up for the stress response" (Scheller 1993, 39).
- **Have fun, and number one, be safe!**

See "AEIOUs of Leading Static Stretching" for an approach to teaching a successful stretching component. Have you observed or experienced firsthand performing stretching consistently and not gaining flexibility? An important objective for you when leading stretching is to guide your participants' minds, as well as their bodies, to release and lengthen the target muscles being stretched. Encourage your participants to follow your cueing carefully to gain flexibility and relaxation benefits. You may photocopy (and perhaps enlarge) "AEIOUs of Leading Static Stretching" to refer to while teaching.

AEIOUs of Leading Static Stretching

Flow smoothly from A thru U:

Announce the name of the stretch and the target body part or muscles.

Elongate the torso (use good seated or standing posture).

Inhale and then exhale, moving slowly from start position to stretch position. With each exhale release more deeply into the stretch, maintaining a neutral spine.

Om.[1] Keep an inner focus on breathing and on feeling and lengthening the target body part or muscles.

Unwind and relax into the stretch for 10 to 30 seconds (except 5 seconds for neck stretches).

Om is considered one of the most important mantras of yoga, used here symbolically for interiorizing the mind.

From E. Best-Martini and K.A. Jones-DiGenova, 2014, *Exercise for frail elders*, 2nd ed. (Champaign, IL: Human Kinetics).

Guidelines for Relaxation Exercises

By the time they reach the cool-down, your participants should be feeling more relaxed than before exercise; exercise is one of the best tools for stress reduction. An effective stretching program also promotes relaxation of mind and body. Adding relaxation exercises to your cool-down can further contribute to a winding down and tranquil mood that complements the stretching component and relieves participants' muscular tension and stress. Following are guidelines for leading relaxation exercises. You will have countless options for being creative with the relaxation portions of your class, within the guidelines of when to lead relaxation exercise during a workout, frequency, duration, repetitions, speed, and other teaching tips. For more information refer to the section "Relaxation and Stress Reduction" in "Suggested Resources."

When to Lead Relaxation Exercises During a Workout

Purposefully use relaxation exercises throughout your class. During the warm-up a short deep-breathing exercise is recommended (see table 4.1) for enhancing mental focus, which can help your participants concentrate better on your instructions and thus avoid injury. Furthermore, you can conduct a fitness class with an emphasis on relaxation, especially in a stretching-only class, by integrating deep breathing and possibly brief guided imagery into the physical activity. For instance, participants can deep-breathe not only during resistance exercises (the standard technique) but also between them to add a relaxation flare. The end of a fitness class can be the best time to focus on the relaxation exercises presented in this chapter.

Frequency

Relaxation exercises can be done 1 to 7 days per week and more than once per day. Because relaxation has proven health benefits, more is generally better, as long as participants are motivated and relaxation exercises are not taking the place of a well-rounded functional fitness program.

Duration

Duration (how much time it takes) for the relaxation exercises can vary as widely as frequency. A relaxation exercise can be as short as 30 to 60 seconds for the three-part deep-breathing exercise in the warm-up or even shorter when used as a rest period with just one slow deep breath between the resistance exercises or stretching exercises. If you have only a minute or less at the end of class, try one or two slow deep breaths and encourage your participants to practice more between classes. In contrast, you can dedicate an entire class to relaxation and stress reduction, and you can teach more than one type of deep breathing and guided imagery exercise. Alternatively, you can have relaxation as a theme of a fitness class by integrating relaxation exercises throughout, when appropriate.

Repetitions

Like duration, the number of times to repeat a relaxation (repetitions) depends on the focus of your class and the time available. During the warm-up and during a short relaxation segment at the end of class, you might do a relaxation exercise just once. On the other hand, breathing exercises can be repeated several times to fill the time available. With a class that focuses on relaxation, you can do relaxation exercises several times. You can also creatively extend an exercise. A tried and true guided imagery technique is to invite participants to go to a favorite, relaxing place in their mind.

Speed

Lead relaxation exercises at a slow pace with a tranquil tone of voice. Never hurry through a relaxation exercise, which can cause a counterproductive stress response. If you start class late, for instance, rather than rushing through three-part deep breathing in the warm-up, you can do one slowly and deliberately. A good goal and habit to develop is to practice deep breathing before arriving to class, early and unhurriedly, to be a model for what you are teaching and to be more effective at promoting a relaxation response.

Other Teaching Tips

Following are a few additional teaching tips for creating a safe and relaxing environment for a successful relaxation component.

- In general, have your participants do the relaxation exercises while seated, not standing, because sitting makes it easier to relax. If your participants practice any of the relaxation exercises at home, let them know that the exercises can also be done while lying down. One advantage of practicing deep breathing and relaxation exercises standing with open eyes is that participants learn that they can relax anywhere, anytime.

- Try to create a quiet, undistracting environment. After participants have learned to relax in silence, they can practice relaxation techniques under normal circumstances, such as while phones are ringing or with the television on in the background.

- Dim the lights for the relaxation exercises, if possible. To prevent falls, turn the lights back to normal before the participants get up.

- Relaxing music can enhance relaxation. Refer to "Media Resources" and "Relaxation and Stress Reduction" in "Suggested Resources."

- You can record the verbal guidance for relaxation exercises involving guided imagery on audiotape for future use.

! Safety Tip If you have dimmed the lights for relaxation, to prevent falls, turn the lights back to normal before the participants get up to leave.

BASIC SEATED COOL-DOWN EXERCISES

The basic seated cool-down focuses on a comprehensive set of 12 stretching exercises and includes relaxation exercises. Before initiating the cool-down exercises, we recommend that you stretch your understanding of the cool-down component by carefully reading the entire chapter and learning the answers to the review questions at the end. Also, if you are a beginner fitness leader or would like to refine your teaching skills, review the three-step instructional process in chapter 3. Begin by teaching the basic seated cool-down exercises first, which eliminate the risk for falling while standing, as you get to know your participants' strengths and current limitations. Then teach the basic standing cool-down exercises. Participants who are able to stand safely can slowly progress to the standing variations of the basic seated cool-down exercises.

Basic Seated Stretching Exercises

The 12 basic seated stretching exercises (refer to table 7.3) are a comprehensive set of 7 upper-body and 5 lower-body functional stretches that target the major muscles of the body. Teach your participants the target body parts, major muscles, and functional benefit of each stretching exercise given in table 7.3. Frail elders and adults with special needs can be motivated by hearing how these exercises can enhance their activities of daily living. In addition, learning the body parts and major muscles targeted by each stretching exercise can be a good memory exercise (see appendix B2, "Muscles of the Human Body"). This knowledge can also help participants focus on feeling the body part or muscles that they are stretching, an important practice for safe and effective stretching. For easy reference, you may make a copy of table 7.3 and appendix B2, which are also useful handouts for participants.

Table 7.3 Basic Stretching Exercises: Seated or Standing[a]

Target body parts and major muscles	Stretch	Functional benefits
UPPER-BODY STRETCHES		
Neck (neck extensors)	7.1 Chin to Chest	Looking down (e.g., dressing, tying shoes, grooming)
Neck (neck rotators and extensors)	7.2 Chin to Shoulder	Turning head (e.g., driving, crossing street)
Chest (pectoralis major) Shoulders (deltoids) Front upper arms (biceps)	[m,s] 7.3 Swan	Posture, using more lung capacity, reaching backward (e.g., personal hygiene, wiping)
Back (latissimus dorsi) Shoulders (deltoids)	7.4 Half Hug	Reaching to opposite side (e.g., passing an item such as salt and pepper, bathing, dressing, cleaning, loading and unloading dishwasher and dryer)
Back of upper arms (triceps) Back (latissimus dorsi)	[m,s] 7.5 Zipper Stretch	Reaching upward and behind back (e.g., scratching back, bathing, hair washing and brushing, dressing, hooking bra, cleaning)
Sides of torso (abdominals)	7.6 Side Bends	Reaching sideways (e.g., cleaning, picking up items, getting in and out of car).
Torso (abdominals, spinal erectors)	[m,s] 7.7 Spinal Twist	Looking behind (e.g., driving, getting in and out of car, passing an item such as a plate, cleaning, loading and unloading dishwasher and dryer)
LOWER-BODY STRETCHES		
Back of thighs (hamstrings) Back (spinal erectors)	[m,s] 7.8 Tib Touches	Posture, walking, grooming (e.g., toe nails, dressing and tying shoes), gardening, housekeeping (e.g., making bed, loading and unloading dishwasher and dryer); improved static and dynamic standing balance
Front thighs (quadriceps) Shins (tibialis anterior)	[s] 7.9 Quad Stretch	Posture, walking; improved static and dynamic standing balance
Inner thighs (hip adductors)	[s] 7.10 Splits	Bathing, getting in and out of car
Outer hips and thighs (hip abductors)	[s] 7.11 Outer-Thigh Stretch	Crossing the legs, dancing requiring cross-over steps
Calves (gastrocnemius, soleus)	[m,s] 7.12 Calf Stretch	Walking (prevents shuffling)

[a]All seated basic stretching exercises can be adapted to standing exercises. See the corresponding standing exercises in the variations and progression options of the illustrated exercises at the end of the chapter. Your participants will receive greater balance benefits with the standing exercises, particularly exercises involving a one-legged stand (indicated by a balance icon).

[m] The five exercises preceded by [m] are recommended for a minimal stretching routine.

[s]The eight exercises preceded by [s] are recommended for a short stretching routine.

From E. Best-Martini and K.A. Jones-DiGenova, 2014, *Exercise for frail elders*, 2nd ed. (Champaign, IL: Human Kinetics).

The number of stretching exercises that you teach in an exercise session and the order in which you teach them can vary. To help you time your cool-down, see table 7.1, Duration of the Segments of a 10- to 15-Minute Cool-Down. If you have only the minimal 10 minutes for the cool-down, start with a shorter stretching routine. Two shorter sets of seated stretching exercises appear in tables 4.3 and 4.4. In table 7.3, the five exercises preceded by *m* are recommended for a minimal stretching routine. The eight exercises preceded by *s* are recommended for a short stretching routine. An easy approach for leading the stretches is to follow the given order of exercises, 7.1 to 7.12, from upper body to lower body. For variety, you can lead the lower-body exercises first and then the upper-body exercises or alternate lower- and upper-body exercises (in an order that you can keep track of), which can be an easier way to start for frail and deconditioned participants. You may copy table 7.3 for easy reference.

Basic Seated Relaxation Exercises

The following relaxation exercises, although versatile, are presented in a recommended order for teaching.

1. Use the three-part deep-breathing exercise (chapter 4) to lead basic deep breathing and teach your participants how to use more of their lung capacity. After learning the basics, the adapted deep-breathing exercise will come more easily and effectively.

2. An ideal time to lead guided imagery is after relaxing with deep breathing.

   a. Start with "Tension Tamers," which is found later in this chapter. First, lead the adapted deep-breathing exercise and then lead a simple, short one-step guided imagery or three-step guided imagery. All the exercises are included on one convenient handout.

   b. "Stressbuster," which is also found later in the chapter, is an excellent alternative.

See "Relaxation and Stress Reduction" in "Suggested Resources" for additional relaxation techniques. For easy reference, you may photocopy the instructions for the three-part deep-breathing exercise (chapter 4), as well as "Tension Tamers" and "Stressbuster."

In a class setting with frail elders, a seated position is the best for relaxation exercises. Seated or lying positions (when appropriate) are more conducive than standing positions to learning to relax and let go. Yet for participants with good standing balance, standing with the eyes open during relaxation exercises can be beneficial to teach that a person can relax anywhere and at any time. Initiate the seated relaxation exercises with participants in good seated posture as they rest their erect torso against the back of a straight-back chair to promote a feeling of letting go. If the chairs that are available to you have an angled back (conducive to slumping), use pillows to prop up participants.

Deep Breathing

Breathing exercises can yield big relaxation benefits and require little time. Ideally, encourage your participants to practice deep breathing throughout the day. Here are two deep-breathing exercises:

1. **Three-part deep-breathing exercise** (Scheller 1993). Instructions for this exercise can be found in chapter 4. Teach this basic breathing exercise before introducing the next one.

2. **Adapted deep-breathing exercise** (Copeland and McKay 2002). General instructions for this breathing exercise are at the top of the sidebar "Tension Tamers." Review the three-part deep-breathing exercise with participants to carry over that basic breathing technique. Then start with an inhale of a slow count of 3,

pause, and then exhale to a slow count of 3. Some participants, with COPD for instance, may need to start with a count of less than 3. Watch participants' responses. When they are comfortable with the count of 4, gradually increase the count of the inhale and the exhale to 8. When participants are ready for more (no hurry), gradually increase the count of the exhale only to 12 or so. A longer exhalation can promote further relaxation and feeling of letting go of tension. Encourage participants to breathe at their own pace, never straining, especially those with COPD.

Guided Imagery

After participants are at ease with the breathing exercises, you have an option of progressing to guided imagery exercises. Guided imagery is a form of autosuggestion or self-hypnosis that uses visual images to elicit a relaxation response. Observe how your participants respond to guided imagery, especially those with moderate to advanced dementia who may not be able to express their interests or fully understand this technique. Use relaxation exercises that elicit a favorable response.

Here are several guided imagery exercises (the first one, "Tension Tamers," includes two exercises):

1. "Tension Tamers" is a multisensory relaxation exercise. Practice reading the script for these exercises aloud with a relaxed voice before reading it to your class. First, lead participants in the adapted deep-breathing exercise and then lead either the one-step guided imagery or three-step guided imagery. If you choose the three-step guided imagery, start with steps 1 and 3. Watch how your class responds. When they are ready for more, add step 2. Be creative (even involve your participants) in conjuring up tranquil settings for step 2.

2. "Stressbuster" (Rossman 2010) is a 12-minute relaxing guided imagery process. Practice reading the script aloud with a calm voice before reading it to your class. Check out Dr. Rossman's website, www.thehealingmind.org, for a free "Stressbuster" imagery link that will let you listen to Dr. Rossman leading you through this 12-minute activity.

Tension Tamers

Guided Imagery With Deep-Breathing Exercise

Adapted Deep-Breathing Exercise

First, guide participants into a comfortable position in good alignment. Next, briefly review "Instructions for Three-Part Deep Breathing" (chapter 4) to remind participants to expand their abdomen, ribs, and chest fully upon inhalation and so on. Then lead this exercise before the guided imagery exercises that follow. With a slow, calm voice, recite the following:

1. *Inhale a deep soothing breath for a count of 3* [Leader slowly counts aloud, "1, 2, 3," and gradually builds up to 8 over time].

2. *Pause for a count of 1.*

3. *Exhale for a count of 3.* [Leader slowly counts aloud, "1, 2, 3," and gradually builds up to 8 over time].

(continued)

Repeat steps 1 through 3, three or more times. Give participants permission to substitute their own words for *soothing*. Also, you can offer alternatives "if they fit for you," such as *relaxing, comforting, uplifting*, and so on. When your class is ready for guided imagery, proceed to "One-Step Guided Imagery" or "Three-Step Guided Imagery."

One-Step Guided Imagery

Continue the deep breathing exercise. Instruct participants to visualize their bodies becoming more relaxed and their minds more alert with each deep breath. With a tranquil voice, say aloud the following:

As you breathe in, imagine your body becoming more relaxed and your mind more alert. As you breathe out, release all tension.

Repeat, slowly, as many times as desired. Give participants permission to substitute their own words for *relaxed*, *alert*, and *tension*. If appropriate for your population, have them continue this exercise independently for a short while.

Three-Step Guided Imagery

With a slow, calm voice recite the following. You have three options; you can lead exercises 1 and 3; 2 and 3; or 1, 2, and 3.

Head-to-Toe Relaxation Imagery

Picture in your mind or just feel a warm, gentle wave of relaxation flowing into your head from above (perhaps rays from the sun, moon . . .). Let the image or feeling of a wave, be your own. It may be a bright, soft, or sparkling light. This wave of relaxation flows slowly through your head down to your chin. Open your eyes and jaw as widely as comfortable, then release. All tension floats away like clouds, leaving a soft, light feeling. Imagine the relaxing wave flowing down your neck, shoulders, and arms, through your elbows, wrists, hands, and fingers. As you wiggle your fingers, all tension flows out your hands, leaving the warmth of relaxation. Feel this comforting wave of relaxation continuing to flow down your torso, one vertebra at a time. You are beginning to feel relaxed all over your body. Now, feel the calming wave flowing down through your hips, thighs, knees, calves, ankles, feet, and toes. As you wiggle your toes, any remaining tension flows out your feet leaving the warmth of relaxation. In the next 15 seconds of silence, enjoy this relaxation. [Leader: Pick an appropriate amount of time, which can increase over time].

Beach Getaway Imagery

Imagine that you are strolling along a beautiful, serene beach. It is a warm, summer day. The sun is glowing behind you, melting away any tension from your head down to your toes. As you exhale fully ("Ahhhhhhhhhhhhhhh"), a gentle ocean breeze touches your face and leaves the taste of saltwater on your lips. With each easy breath, you feel an inner calm. You are more deeply relaxed with each breath. The rhythmic sound of the waves carries any unwanted thoughts away. Your mind is clear and at peace. Keep breathing deeply to the relaxing sounds of the sea.

Conclusion

When you are ready, slowly wiggle your toes and fingers. If your eyes are closed, slowly open them. Take a deep energizing breath. As you continue with your day, keep in mind this relaxing experience that is with you wherever you go.

From E. Best-Martini and K.A. Jones-DiGenova, 2014, *Exercise for frail elders*, 2nd ed. (Champaign, IL: Human Kinetics).

Stressbuster

A 12-Minute Relaxing Guided Imagery Process

Take a deep breath or two and let the 'out' breath be a letting-go kind of breath. Invite your body to feel relaxed, as if it's made out of warm, wet noodles. When you're ready, recall some place you've been in your life where you felt safe, relaxed, and peaceful. If you don't have such a place, perhaps you've seen one in a movie or a magazine, or you can just imagine one right now.

Just let yourself begin to daydream that you are in a safe, beautiful, peaceful place . . . and let yourself notice what you imagine seeing in this safe, beautiful place . . . what colors and shapes, what things you see there. Don't worry about how vividly you see in your mind's eye; just notice what you imagine seeing and accept the way you imagine them. In the same way, notice what you imagine hearing in that beautiful peaceful place. Or is it very quiet? Just notice. Is there an aroma or a quality in the air that you notice? You may or may not and it doesn't really matter. . . . Just notice what you notice in this special peaceful place. Can you tell what time or day or night it is? Can you tell the season of the year? What's the temperature like?

Notice how it feels to be in this safe, beautiful, and peaceful place. Notice how your body feels, and how your face feels. Notice any sense of comfort or peacefulness or relaxation that you may feel there. Take some time to explore and find the spot where you feel most relaxed and at ease in this place, and just let yourself get comfortable there. Take a few minutes just to enjoy being there, with nothing else you need to do. If it feels good to you, imagine that you are soaking up the sense of peacefulness and calmness like a sponge, feeling more and more relaxed and at ease as you enjoy this place of calmness.

Take as long as you want, and when you're ready, let the images go, and gently bring your attention back to the outside world, but if you like, bring back any feeling of peacefulness or calmness that you may feel. When your attention is all the way back, gently stretch, and if your eyes are closed softly open them and look around, bringing back with you anything that seemed interesting or important, including any sense of calmness you may feel.

After the "Stressbuster" guided imagery, you might want to ask your participants, "When you are ready, scan your body again, and see where you would rank yourself on a 0 to 10 scale of tension." Most people find that they feel calmer, more relaxed, and more peaceful after doing this kind of imagery, simply by focusing their imagination in a particular way.

From E. Best-Martini and K.A. Jones-DiGenova, 2014, *Exercise for frail elders*, 2nd ed. (Champaign, IL: Human Kinetics). Adapted, by permission, M. Rossman, 2010, *The worry solution: Using breakthrough brain science to turn anxiety and stress into confidence and happiness* (New York: Crown Archetype), 10-13.

BASIC STANDING COOL-DOWN EXERCISES

The basic standing cool-down, similar to the basic seated cool-down, focuses on stretching and includes relaxation exercises. Refer to chapter 8 to find out more about when to implement standing exercises, benefits of standing exercises, when seated exercises are preferred over standing, and advantages of teaching both the seated and standing exercises simultaneously.

Basic Standing Relaxation Exercises

In general we recommend leading relaxation exercises in a seated position, a safer position than standing for deep breathing in case a participant becomes fatigued, lightheaded, or dizzy. Also, seated or lying positions (when appropriate) are more conducive to learning to relax and let go. But when participants do not have balance issues and you can trust them to sit if needed, it can be beneficial to practice deep breathing and relaxation exercises standing with eyes open to learn that they can relax anywhere, any time. As with all components of a functional fitness program, when standing is a safe and suitable option, give your participants a choice to sit or stand, and encourage them to sit any time during the class when necessary. Before every standing relaxation segment, repeat the general safety precaution, "Stop deep breathing and sit if you feel fatigued, lightheaded, or dizzy."

Basic Standing Stretching and Balance Exercises

Table 7.3 lists the 12 basic stretching exercises that target the major muscles of the body. This comprehensive set of 7 upper-body and 5 lower-body functional exercises can be done seated or standing. Introduce the standing variations (presented in the variations and progression options in the illustrated stretching instruction section) after you get to know your participants' strengths and current limitations while observing them learn the seated exercises. The seated versions eliminate the risk for falling while standing. When a participant has developed good technique with the seated stretching exercises and you have determined that he or she can safely perform standing exercises, encourage him or her to do so for the extra benefits that standing exercises provide. We recommend that anyone who cannot safely stand continue with the seated stretching exercises. Any participant with minor balance problems may perform only those standing exercises that leave a hand available to hold on to a secure support. Standing stretches that require two hands, such as exercise 7.3, Swan; 7.4, Half Hug; and 7.5, Zipper, may be performed only by participants who are steady on their feet.

VARIATIONS AND PROGRESSION

The variations and progression options (VPOs) for each of the 12 basic seated stretching

exercises enable you to be creative and progressive with a functional fitness program to serve the needs of a class full of people from frail to fit. Refer to the illustrated stretching instruction section at the end of this chapter for these options. Introduce one or more of the variations and progression options after your participants have learned the basic seated stretching exercises, with the exception of the few easier options. Some classes may be limited in how far they can progress with stretching (for example, a large class without an assistant in a long-term care setting), yet varying the basic seated stretching exercises can benefit and add to the enjoyment of any class. Then again, other classes may thrive by progressing to all standing stretches (with the option of sitting when needed). Each basic seated stretching exercise has a standing alternative, a beneficial means of progression when a participant can safely stand. Notice this symbol, which comes before the standing exercises with more significant balance benefits, including those with a one-legged stand.

The more you know about the stretching exercises and the more you know about your participants' current abilities and challenges, the more adept you will be at varying and progressing their exercise program. For example, because the pectoralis major muscle (chest) is prone to tightness, especially with progressively poor posture as people age, it can be beneficial to do the Seated Swan (exercise 7.3), which stretches that muscle, along with one variation (to start with, when your class is ready), such as the Seated Swan combined with extending the wrist. For many other ideas for varying and progressing your class, see chapter 8, including "Duration of Cool-Down."

SUMMARY

This chapter gives guidelines, safety precautions, and detailed teaching instructions for leading cool-down stretching and relaxation exercises. Always end your exercise class with a cool-down of 10 minutes at a minimum to ease the transition from exercise to rest and to enhance your participants' flexibility and ability to relax.

For beneficial results, slowly stretch all major muscle groups of the body with good technique 2 to 7 days per week (more days for more gain), performing each stretch up to four times (if participants are able and time permits) for 10 to 30 seconds per static stretch.

Static (held or sustained) stretching is a safe, effective, and convenient method of stretching. Elderly people, especially those who have been inactive, often have diminished flexibility that reduces their ability to perform daily activities independently. Participants who regularly stretch will have greater freedom of movement and enhanced ability to perform activities of daily living.

REVIEW QUESTIONS

1. List three benefits of the cool-down.

2. List three general safety precautions for stretching.

3. Instruct all older adults—particularly stroke survivors, those at risk for stroke, and those with uncontrolled proliferative retinopathy—to keep the head above the _____ when bending forward, because of the danger of increased vascular pressure within the brain and the risk of stroke.

4. A safe modification of the Seated or Standing Tib Touches (exercise 7.8) for a participant with a hip replacement (who you can trust to follow directions) is to do them while seated without leaning forward. The primary objective is to avoid hip _____ of more than 90 degrees to prevent the risk of hip _____.

5. For people with hearing loss, give a clear _____ of the warm-up (and all) exercises. And for people with visual impairment, precisely _____ warm-up (and all) exercises.

6. Match the stretching exercise with the target body parts and major muscles:
    - Seated and standing upper-body stretching exercises
        ___ 7.1 Chin to Chest   a. back upper arms (triceps), back (latissimus dorsi)
        ___ 7.2 Chin to Shoulder   b. neck (neck rotators and extensors)
        ___ 7.3 Swan   c. neck (neck extensors)
        ___ 7.4 Half Hug   d. chest (pectoralis major), shoulders (deltoids), front upper arms (biceps)
        ___ 7.5 Zipper Stretch   e. back (latissimus dorsi), shoulders (deltoid)
        ___ 7.6 Side Bends   f. torso (abdominals, spinal erectors)
        ___ 7.7 Spinal Twist   g. sides of torso (abdominals)
    - Seated and standing lower-body stretching exercises
        ___ 7.8 Tib Touches   h. calves (gastrocnemius, soleus)
        ___ 7.9 Quad Stretch   i. outer hips and thighs (hip abductors)
        ___ 7.10 Seated Splits and   j. back of thighs (hamstrings), back (spinal erectors)
        Standing Half-Splits

(continued)

(continued)

   ___ 7.11 Outer-Thigh Stretch   k. front thighs (quadriceps), shins (tibialis anterior)

   ___ 7.12 Calf Stretch   l. inner thighs (hip adductors)

7. T or F. A safe and effective way to promote balance is to have all participants perform standing stretches that require two hands (both hands are unavailable for holding on for support), such as the Swan, Half Hug, Zipper, and Spinal Twist.

8. _____ _____ is a form of autosuggestion or self-hypnosis that uses visual images to elicit a relaxation response.

ILLUSTRATED INSTRUCTION

Exercises 7.1 through 7.7 are upper-body stretching exercises, and exercises 7.8 through 7.12 are lower-body stretching exercises. The exercise and safety tips and variations and progression options apply to both seated and standing exercises unless otherwise specified. The standing exercises and other variations and progression options that need further expla-nation are accompanied by a photograph and description. Remember you may photocopy "AEIOUs of Leading Static Stretching" to refer to while leading stretching.

Good Seated and Standing Posture

Be sure to refer to the instructions for good seated and standing posture in chapter 4, and remind participants of them often as you do each exercise.

Seated Chin To Chest

TARGET MUSCLES—Neck (neck extensors)

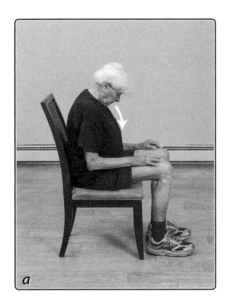

Stretch Position

1. Good seated posture
2. Lower chin toward chest.
3. Feel stretch in the back of the neck.
4. Because this is a neck stretch, hold for less than 5 seconds.

! Exercise and Safety Tips

- Slowly lower the head and slowly lift it back to the starting position.
- Those without balance problems, who do not need to hold on to a chair while standing, can eventually add the interlaced-fingers variation (exercise 7.1B) while standing.

Variations and Progression Options

- *Challenger (Combo):* Combine Chin to Chest with interlaced fingers, pressing downward behind the back. If safe, this can be done seated forward on a chair or, ideally, standing.
- *Standing Chin to Chest.*

Standing Chin to Chest Plus Interlaced Fingers

1. Good standing posture.
2. Hands behind back.
3. Interlace fingers.
4. Press downward.
5. Lower chin toward chest.
6. Feel stretch in the back of the neck.
7. Hold for less than 5 seconds.

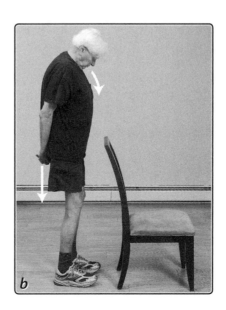

Seated Chin to Shoulder

TARGET MUSCLES—Neck (neck rotators and extensors)

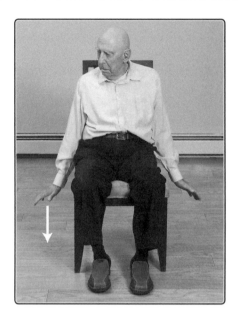

Stretch Position

1. Good seated posture.

2. Arms by the sides.

3. Press palms downward.

4. Turn chin toward shoulder with head slightly angled down diagonally toward shoulder.

5. Feel stretch on the side of the neck.

6. Because this is a neck stretch, hold for less than 5 seconds.

7. Repeat toward the other side.

Exercise and Safety Tips

- If chair arms are in the way when pressing palms downward, hold arms just above the chair arms if comfortable.

- Those without balance problems can eventually add the interlaced-fingers variation while standing.

Variations and Progression Options

- *Neck position:* Stretch one side of the neck and then the other with the head in alignment.

- *Challenger (Combo):* Combine Chin to Shoulder with interlaced fingers, pressing downward behind the back. If safe, this can be done seated forward on a chair or, ideally, standing.

- *Standing Chin to Shoulder.*

Seated Swan

TARGET MUSCLES—Chest (pectoralis major), shoulders (deltoids), front upper arms (biceps)

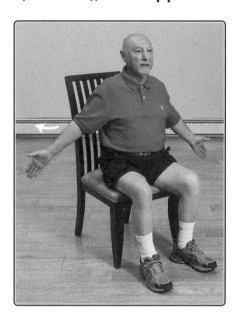

Stretch Position

1. Good seated posture.
2. Palms face forward.
3. Keep shoulders down.
4. Extend arms backward.
5. Feel stretch in the chest and arms.
6. Hold for 10 to 30 seconds.

! Exercise and Safety Tips

- Do not hyperextend (lock) the elbows.

Variations and Progression Options

- *Hand position:* Face palms upward or downward.
- *Challenger (Combo):* Combine the Swan stretch with extending the wrist (fingers toward back of the arm) to stretch the front forearms (forearm flexors).
- *Challenger (Combo):* Combine the Swan stretch with flexing the wrist (fingers toward front of the arm) to stretch the back of the forearms (forearm extensors).
- *Standing Swan.*
- *Props:* Hold a necktie, soft rope, or towel between hands to enhance the Swan stretch.

Seated Half Hug

TARGET MUSCLES—Back (latissimus dorsi), shoulders (deltoids)

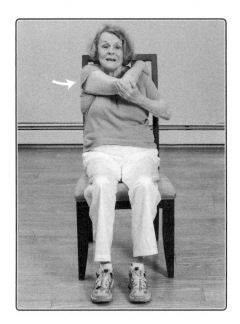

Stretch Position

1. Good seated posture.
2. Place fingertips on top of the opposite shoulder.
3. Place the other hand above the elbow of the opposite arm.
4. Push arm across chest.
5. Feel stretch in the back and shoulder.
6. Hold for 10 to 30 seconds.
7. Repeat with the other arm.

! Exercise and Safety Tips

- Keep shoulders down.

Variations and Progression Options

- *ROM Reward:* Do Shoulder Shrugs (exercise 4.11 in chapter 4) or Shoulder Rotation (exercise 4.9 in chapter 4) after stretching each side.
- *Standing Half Hug.*

Seated Zipper Stretch

TARGET MUSCLES—Back of upper arms (triceps), back (latissimus dorsi)

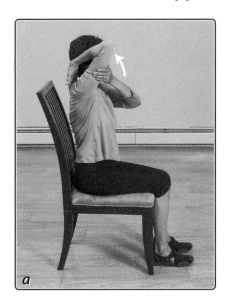

Stretch Position

1. Good seated posture.
2. Place fingertips on top of shoulder on the same side with elbow up and pointing toward the front.
3. Place the other hand on the back of the opposite upper arm.
4. Gently push the arm backward.
5. Feel stretch in the back of the arm.
6. Hold for 10 to 30 seconds.
7. Repeat on the other side.

! Exercise and Safety Tips

- Do not overarch the back.
- Maintain a neutral spine throughout the stretch.

Variations and Progression Options

- *Challenger (Combo):* Combine Zipper stretch (seated or standing) with a gentle side bend (exercise 7.6).
- *Standing Zipper Stretch.*
- *Prop:* Try Zipper Stretch using a towel, belt, or necktie.

Standing Zipper Stretch With Prop

1. Good standing posture.
2. Dangle prop (towel, belt, or necktie) over shoulder and behind back.
3. With the other hand, grasp prop behind back.
4. Gently move the hands closer together along prop.
5. Feel stretch along back of the arm and shoulder.
6. Hold for 10 to 30 seconds.
7. Repeat on the other side.

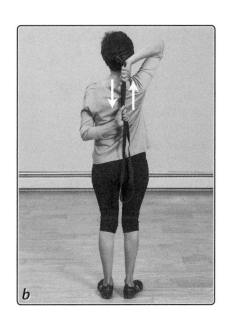

Seated Side Bends

TARGET MUSCLES—Sides of torso (abdominals)

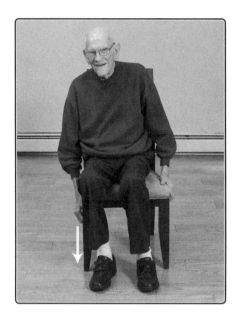

Stretch Position

1. Good seated posture.
2. Hold on to side of chair with one hand.
3. Other hand reaches toward the floor.
4. Feel stretch along the side.
5. Hold for 10 to 30 seconds.
6. Repeat on the other side.

 ## *Exercise and Safety Tips*

- Hold on to the arm or seat of the chair for support during Seated Side Bends.
- Do not bend the neck. Keep the neck in a neutral position.

- Those with osteoporosis should avoid spinal bending and twisting unless the participant has medical clearance for these movements.

Variations and Progression Options

- *Challenger:* Reach with one straight arm overhead and sideward, and then repeat on the other side.

- *Challenger:* Interlace fingers and reach straight arms overhead and sideward, and then repeat on the other side.
- *Standing Side Bends.*

Seated Spinal Twist

TARGET MUSCLES—Torso (abdominals, spinal erectors)

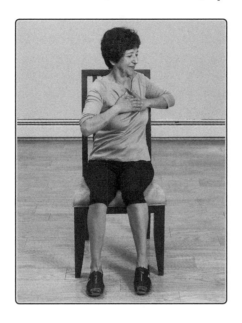

Stretch Position

1. Good seated posture.
2. Place palms on chest.
3. Place one hand on top of the other.
4. Hold elbows out.
5. Twist torso.
6. Feel stretch in the front and back torso.
7. Hold for 10 to 30 seconds.
8. Repeat on the other side.

! *Exercise and Safety Tips*

- Do not twist the neck. Move the head, neck, and shoulders as a unit.
- Keep shoulders down.
- Those with osteoporosis should avoid spinal twisting and bending unless the participant has medical clearance for these movements.

Variations and Progression Options

- *Easier:* Lower elbows if shoulders get tired.
- *Easier (standing):* Spinal Twist holding on with one hand for balance.
- *Hand position:* Place hands in prayer position, resting on sternum (the breast bone).
- *Challenger (standing):* Spinal Twist without holding on.
- *Visualization:* Combine the Spinal Twist with lifting upward and visualizing getting taller with each exhalation.

Seated Tib Touches (Tib for Tibia or Shin Bone)

TARGET MUSCLES—Back of thighs (hamstrings), back (spinal erectors)

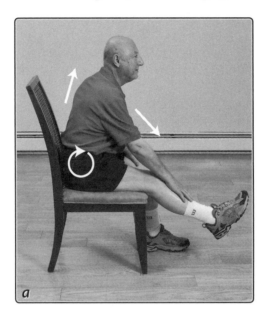

Stretch Position

1. Good seated posture.
2. Place palms on thighs.
3. Straighten one leg.
4. Slide hand down the straight leg.
5. Bend forward at the hips.
6. Feel stretch in back of the thigh.
7. Hold for 10 to 30 seconds.
8. Repeat with the other leg.

Exercise and Safety Tips

- Participants at risk of falling off chair should sit as far back in chair as possible.
- Those with a hip fracture or replacement should avoid bending forward at the hips more than 90 degrees in a seated and standing position.
- Those with osteoporosis (and all participants) should avoid spinal flexion, particularly in combination with stooping.
- Rest one palm on a thigh when leaning forward from the hips.
- Do not twist the torso. The goal is to lengthen the hamstrings, not touch the toes.
- Move the head, neck, and spine as one unit. Do not hang the head.
- Maintain a neutral spine (long and lifted) throughout the stretch.

Variations and Progression Options

- *Easier:* Scoot forward in chair until heel can rest on the floor with leg straight, if safe for participant.
- *Easier (standing):* Start with a slight bend of the leg on the chair (see photograph *b*); gradually straighten the leg.
- *Challenger (Combo):* Combine Seated or Standing Tib Touches with a Calf Stretch, the technique in exercise 7.12*a*.

- *Standing Tib Touches* (involves a one-legged stand).
- *Prop:* When seated, use a towel, strong resistance band, belt, or necktie around the ball of the foot for a calf stretch.
- *Prop:* When seated, use a low stool to prop the foot up.

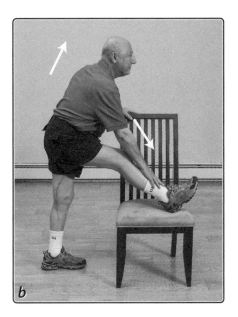

Standing Tib Touches

1. Good standing posture.
2. Place hand on chair back.
3. Place the opposite heel on chair.
4. Slide the free hand down the straight leg.
5. Bend forward at the hips.
6. Feel stretch in the back of the thigh.
7. Hold for 10 to 30 seconds.
8. Repeat with the other leg.

Seated Quad Stretch

TARGET MUSCLES—Front thighs (quadriceps), shins (tibialis anterior)

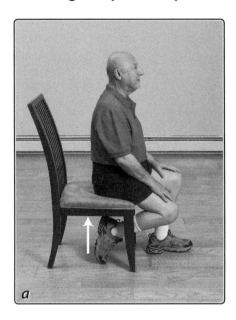

Stretch Position

1. Good seated posture.
2. Place palms on thighs.
3. Place one foot (toes pointed) on the floor under chair.
4. Raise heel toward chair seat.
5. Feel stretch in the front thigh and shin.
6. Hold for 10 to 30 seconds.
7. Repeat with the other leg.

! Exercise and Safety Tips

- Modification: If the front legs of the chairs have bars between them, instruct participants to move forward 4 to 6 inches (10 to 15 cm) in their seats, if they can do so safely. Instruct them to hold on to the sides or arms of their chairs when sitting forward in the chair.

- Participants can hold up the calf in the Standing Quad Stretch in several ways. They can put their fingers in the top of the shoe or in the loop if the shoe has one; a less flexible person can hold on to the pants leg.
- Avoid leaning forward during the Standing Quad Stretch.
- Avoid locking the knee of the standing leg.

Variations and Progression Options

- *Easier (standing):* Rest the shin on the chair seat in the Standing Quad Stretch instead of holding the foot in the hand. Focus on rotating the pelvis backward and point the toe to

facilitate stretching the front thigh and shin, respectively.
- *Standing Quad Stretch (Challenger)* (involves a one-legged stand).

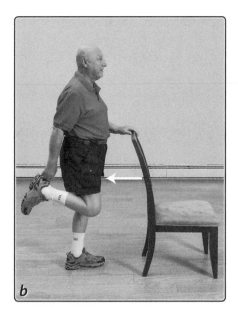

Standing Quad Stretch (Challenger)

1. Good standing posture.
2. Place hand on chair back.
3. Bend the opposite knee (heel toward buttock).
4. With the free hand, hold the calf up (as directed in "Exercise and Safety Tips").
5. Gently pull the thigh and foot backward.
6. Feel stretch in the front thigh and shin.
7. Hold for 10 to 30 seconds.
8. Repeat with the other leg.

Seated Splits

TARGET MUSCLES—Inner thighs (hip adductors)

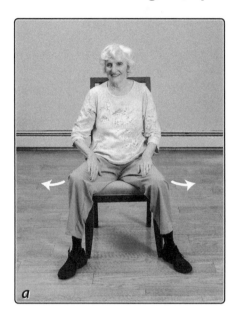

Stretch Position

1. Good seated posture.
2. Place palms on inner thighs.
3. Slide both feet outward.
4. Feel stretch in the inner thighs.
5. Hold for 10 to 30 seconds.

 ## Exercise and Safety Tips

- Keep each foot directly below each knee while doing Seated Splits.
- Press the inner thighs gently outward to enhance the adductor stretch.

- If chairs with arms are used, tell participants to scoot forward in their chairs if they are comfortable doing so. Instruct them to hold on to the sides or arms of their chairs when sitting forward in the chair.

Variations and Progression Options

- *Challenger (Combo):* Combine Seated Splits with a shoulder stretch by grasping under the thighs and bending the elbows until the shoulder stretch is felt (keep the torso erect).

- *Easier (standing):* Place chair in front of participant; participant holds on with both hands.
- *Standing Half-Splits.*

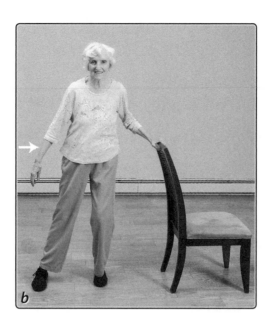

Standing Half-Splits

1. Good standing posture.
2. Place hand on chair back.
3. Move one foot sideward 1.5 to 2 feet (45 to 60 cm).
4. Slightly bend the knee of the other (support) leg.
5. Lean into the support leg.
6. Feel stretch in the inner thigh of the straight leg.
7. Hold for 10 to 30 seconds.
8. Repeat with the other leg.

Seated Outer-Thigh Stretch

TARGET MUSCLES—Outer hips and thighs (hip abductors)

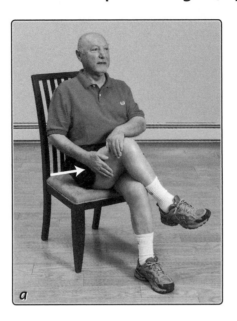

Stretch Position

1. Good seated posture.
2. Cross leg at knees.
3. Place palms on the outer thigh.
4. Feel stretch in the outer hip and thigh.
5. Hold for 10 to 30 seconds.
6. Repeat with the other leg.

Exercise and Safety Tips

- When seated, gently pull the outer thigh inward (bring knee toward opposite shoulder).
- When standing, avoid locking the knees.
- Those with hip fracture or replacement or peripheral vascular disease should not cross their legs. For participants without osteoporosis, teach a seated torso twist with legs together (uncrossed) and both feet together on the floor. Gently twist and lift the torso (not neck) while pulling the outer thigh inward with both hands. Progress, if safe, to Standing Outer-Thigh Stretch.
- Those with osteoporosis should avoid torso twist variations, unless they have medical clearance for twisting movements.

Variations and Progression Options

- *Easier:* Hold legs together and uncrossed in stretch position.
- *Challenger (Seated Torso Twist):* Gently twist and lift the torso (not neck) toward the crossed leg while pulling the outer thigh inward.
- *Standing Outer-Thigh Stretch.*

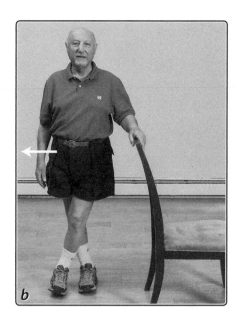

Standing Outer-Thigh Stretch

1. Good standing posture.

2. Place hand on chair back.

3. Cross one leg in front of the other.

4. Lean into the hip of the back leg.

5. Feel stretch in the outer hip and thigh of the back leg.

6. Hold for 10 to 30 seconds.

7. Repeat with the other leg.

Seated Calf Stretch

TARGET MUSCLES—Calves (gastrocnemius, soleus)

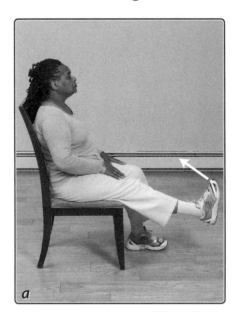

a

Stretch Position

1. Good seated posture.
2. Place palms on thighs.
3. Straighten one leg.
4. Dorsiflex ankle of the straightened leg (move toes toward nose).
5. Feel stretch in back of the calf.
6. Hold for 10 to 30 seconds.
7. Repeat with the other leg.

❗ Exercise and Safety Tips

- Keep the leg being stretched straight; knee soft, not locked.
- Perform the Standing Calf Stretch with the foot straight ahead of the calf that is being stretched.
- Keep the knee above the ankle of the forward standing leg.

Variations and Progression Options

- *Easier:* Scoot forward in chair until the heel of the calf that is being stretched (the straight leg) can rest on the floor, if safe for participant.
- *Standing Calf Stretch.*
- *Prop:* For the Seated Calf Stretch use a towel, strong resistance band, belt, or necktie around the ball of the foot to aid the calf stretch. This is easier when a stool is placed under the foot or with the easier option.

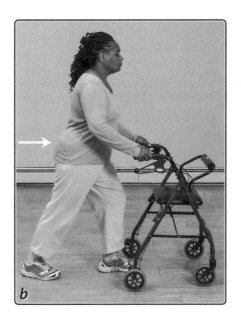

Standing Calf Stretch

1. Good standing posture.
2. Place hands on chair back.
3. Move one foot backward 1.5 to 2 feet (45 to 60 cm).
4. Point toes forward.
5. Slightly bend knee of the forward leg.
6. Lean into that leg.
7. Feel stretch in the calf of the straight leg.
8. Hold for 10 to 30 seconds.
9. Repeat with the other leg.

Putting Your Exercise Program Together

It is not the years in your life
but the life in your years that counts.

—*Adlai Stevenson*

LEARNING OBJECTIVES

After completing this chapter, you will have the tools to

- design, schedule, modify, progress, and maintain a functional fitness program for participants with varying fitness levels and one or more special needs;

- extend a single warm-up, resistance-training, aerobics and dynamic balance, or stretching and relaxation component into an entire class;

- implement a safe exercise session, class, or program that incorporates one or more exercise components—warm-up, resistance training, aerobics, and cool-down; and

- create fun, varied, and progressive exercise routines through the years for new and return participants.

In this chapter you will learn how to put it all together into a safe and effective exercise session, class, or program to promote functional fitness that incorporates one or more exercise components—warm-up, resistance training, aerobic training and dynamic balance activities, and cool-down (stretching and relaxation)—from chapters 4 through 7. You will also gain knowledge of how to design, schedule, modify, and progress (make progressively more challenging) or maintain a smart functional fitness program for frail elders and adults with special needs.

DESIGNING YOUR EXERCISE PROGRAM

A successful exercise program design is based on appropriate precautions to keep participants safe and injury free and evidence-based guidelines for beneficial results. Ideally, exercise prescription for older adults should include aerobic exercise, muscle strengthening exercises, flexibility exercises, and balance training for people at risk for falling or mobility impairment (ACSM 2009b, 1523). For adults with special needs or frailty a primary design objective is to promote functional fitness and restore function as best as possible. You can choose from many options when designing your exercise program, which is an ongoing dynamic process, such as the following:

- Leading one or more exercise components—warm-ups, resistance training, aerobic training and dynamic balance activities, and stretching and relaxation—in one class
- Leading a comprehensive fitness class and program
- Leading a class with a theme such as enhancing balance and fall prevention
- Leading just seated exercises, just standing exercises (with the option of sitting when needed), or seated and standing exercises at the same time
- Leading just upper-body exercises, just lower-body exercises, or both upper- and lower-body exercises
- Using exercise media, such as DVDs

Emphasize the special needs of your participants when designing your exercise program. Participants can achieve current exercise recommendations in many ways; therefore, consider individual preference and enjoyment in the exercise prescription (as far as feasible with a class) (ACSM 2011; Williams 2008). Additionally, tailoring the program for each individual is a long-term investment in adherence (AACVPR 2006, 50).

Exercise Components

You can combine the exercise components in a variety of ways. Table 8.1 shows seven different ways. Class level 1 is the easiest (least physically demanding). Level 7, a comprehensive fitness class, can be the most challenging for the participants to perform and instructor to teach. Levels 3 through 6 are not inherently more difficult than the others, although resistance training or balance activities may need to precede aerobic training with very frail individuals (ACSM 2009b). All levels can be taught at an easier level seated and then gradually made more challenging.

If you are starting an exercise class, we recommend an easier-level class. Level 2, which focuses on warm-up ROM exercises, is an ideal starting point, unless a focus on relaxation (level 1) is more enticing for your population. We offer relaxation and stress reduction as a valuable focus for a class in the right setting. As you get to know your participants and they settle into your class, slowly progress toward the comprehensive fitness class. Choose the class level or focus that works best for you, your class, and your employer.

All classes in table 8.1 include these components:

- A warm-up session, which emphasizes joint range-of-motion (ROM) exercises and includes good posture, deep breathing, and light stretching (fewer stretches, held for a shorter time than during cooldown)
- A relaxation component—at least a short deep-breathing exercise
- An educational component, if only an instructive quotation (use reputable sources; see "Suggested Resources")
- Water breaks to prevent dehydration. Older adults are more susceptible to becoming dehydrated because of age-related decreased thirst mechanism and sensitivity (Bryant and Green 2009, 544; ACSM 2007, 383).

The large X's indicate the focus of each class:

- Level 1 focuses on relaxation exercises.
- Level 2 focuses on warm-up ROM exercises. (Both levels 1 and 2 have the objective of motivating people to come back for more exercise and can include refreshments and a discussion on a fitness-related topic.)
- Level 3 focuses on stretching.
- Level 4 focuses on resistance training.
- Level 5 focuses on balance (both dynamic and static) training.

Table 8.1 Exercise Class Options

Class components	CLASS LEVEL (AND FOCUS OF CLASS)[a]						
	1	2	3	4	5	6	7
EXERCISE							
Warm-up ROM exercises	x	X	x	x	x	x	x
Resistance training				X			x
Aerobic training						X	x
Balance training		x	x	x	X	x	x
Cool-down stretching		x	X	x	x	x	x
Cool-down relaxation exercises	X	x	x	x	x	x	x
MOTIVATIONAL AND OTHER							
Education	x	x	x	x	x	x	x
Healthy snacks	x	x					
Water breaks	x	x	x	x	x	x	x

[a]Large X's indicate the component that is emphasized, the focus of the class. Small x's indicate the components that are included in each exercise class.

- Level 6 focuses on aerobic training (and dynamic balance activities).
- Level 7 is a comprehensive fitness class that includes a warm-up, resistance training, aerobic training, balance training, and cool-down stretching and relaxation exercises.

Remember that although level 1 is the easiest and 7 is the most challenging, levels 2 through 6 are not presented in any order of difficulty—they can be equally challenging and are differentiated by the focus of the session.

Introduce only one new exercise component at a time as you gradually build a functional fitness class or program. A class that focuses on ROM exercises (see table 8.1, level 2), is recommended as an easygoing introduction to an exercise class appropriate for adults with special needs. Remember that you do not have to teach all the exercises in a component on the day that you introduce it. For example, you can start with four resistance exercises the first week and then add one new exercise each week for the following 8 weeks. Initially, do more warm-up ROM exercises. As you increase the resistance exercises, cut back on the ROM component (but always warm up for at least 10 minutes). This easygoing approach to introducing new exercises is helpful for reinforcing good exercise technique and preventing overtraining and injury.

 Safety Tip Introduce only one new exercise class component—warm-up, resistance training, balance, aerobics, or cool-down—at a time to reinforce good exercise technique and prevent overtraining.

Balance Component

Balance training is a vital component of a functional fitness program design for reducing risk and fear of falling, maintaining independence and ability to perform daily tasks, and ultimately, improving quality of life for older adults. Likewise, a beneficial exercise class option is to focus on balance training, both static and dynamic, as shown in table 8.1, class level 5. Notice the small x's in the balance training row for levels 2-4 and 6-7. Those classes (2, ROM; 3, stretching; 4, resistance training; 6, aerobics; and 7, comprehensive fitness class) focus on exercises that can contribute to improving participants' balance when performed regularly and with good technique. The American College of Sports Medicine "Exercise and Physical Activity for Older Adults: Position Stand" (ACSM 2009b, 1520) affirms that physical activity programs that include balance, strength, flexibility, and walking reduce the risk of falls in populations at high risk, such as women with osteoporosis, frail older adults, or people with a history of falls. Exercises that strengthen the postural, or core, muscles—even indirectly, such as heel stands and toe stands (Heyward 2010, 307)—are also advocated for balance training (Rose 2010; Scott 2008). Many of the exercises given in part II of this book provide balance benefits by increasing joint range of motion with ROM and stretching exercises (chapter 4), by strengthening the muscles with resistance training (chapter 5), by increasing flexibility with stretching (chapter 7), and by improving posture (chapter 4). When the aerobic exercises in chapter 6 are performed while standing, they help improve dynamic balance.

An important emphasis of a functional fitness program design—in addition to improving muscular strengthen and endurance, aerobic capacity, and flexibility—is balance training for optimal gains in balance and fall prevention (Bovre 2010; Heyward 2010, 307; Rose 2010; Bryant and Green 2009, 532; Orr et al. 2008; Scott 2008; Shigematsu et al. 2008; Takeshima et al. 2007). Balance training for older adults is recommended at least 2 to 3 days per week (ACSM 2011; Heyward 2010; Bryant and Green 2009). Additionally, teach your participants to apply the fundamental balance principles to their activities of daily living.

The following information in this book will aid you in designing an exercise program or class that includes or focuses on balance:

• In chapter 2 refer to the section "Balance, Core, and Agility Training" and tables 2.2, 2.3, and 2.4, which include balance, core, and agility exercises. Core and agility training are key contributors of balance.

• In chapter 4 refer to "Instructions for Good Seated Posture," an introductory seated balance exercise (Bryant and Green 2009, 534). This exercise is a foundation and prerequisite for progressing to more difficult seated balance exercises, such as sitting erect without back support or practicing good seated posture on an unstable surface (an inflatable disc or stability ball).

• In chapters 4, 5, and 7 (see illustrated instructions sections) the following standing exercises involve a one-legged stand for static balance benefits: 4.3, Hip Rotation; 4.5, Toe Point and Flex and Crane Pose; 4.6, Ankle Rotations (exercises 4.1, 4.2, and 4.4 involve a brief one-legged stand); 5.6 Hip Flexion; 5.7, Hip Abduction and Adduction; 5.8, Knee Flexion; 5.9, Knee Extension; 5.11, Heel Raises; 7.8, Tib Touches; and 7.9, Quad Stretch. The American College of Sports Medicine (2009b, 1511) recommends including progressively difficult balance exercises that gradually reduce the base of support from standing on two legs to standing on one leg. When introducing standing exercises, ease into exercises that involve a one-legged stand, which is much more demanding than standing on two legs.

• In chapter 5 see "Standing Lower-Body Resistance and Balance Exercises" for six steps of facilitating a gradual progression from holding on firmly with two hands to a secure support to safely letting go. These instructions also apply to ROM and aerobic and flexibility exercise, when appropriate. To promote the goal of balance and fall prevention, *2008 Physical Activity Guidelines for Americans* (USDHHS 2008b, 32) advises increasing the difficulty of exercises by progressing from holding on to a stable support (like furniture) while doing the exercises to doing them without support.

• In tables 5.3 and 7.3, see the "Functional benefits" columns for balance benefits of seated and standing resistance training and stretching exercises. Seated stretching and resistance training provide a strong foundation for progressing to the standing exercises and can help participants be more stable on their feet. Because standing exercises can provide significant balance improvements compared with seated exercises, we recommend that you ease any participant who can safely stand into the standing exercises. See "Seated and Standing Exercises" later in this chapter to learn when to implement standing exercises, benefits of standing exercises, when seated exercises are preferred over standing exercises, and advantages of teaching seated and standing exercises simultaneously. Some exercises may have beneficial effects for our target population, but not improve balance, such as hand and wrist ROM exercises.

• In chapter 6 you will find a full and fun aerobics and dynamic balance routine (level 6 class in table 8.1) designed for improving participants' balance while moving in daily activities and for lowering risk for falls.

• In chapters 4 through 7 in the illustrated instructions sections, look for the balance symbol, which comes before exercises with significant balance benefits. These include the dynamic balance exercises (chapter 6) and standing exercises that involve a one-legged stand (chapters 4, 5, and 7).

• In the category "Balance" in "Suggested Resources," you will find books and supplies for developing a class that includes or concentrates on balance.

Comprehensive Fitness Program

A comprehensive fitness class that includes a warm-up, resistance training, aerobics and dynamic balance activities, and a cool-down in one class is not necessarily a goal of an exercise program. But, this format can be ideal when appropriate for groups that meet only three or fewer times per week. Gradually build up to 50 minutes (for beginner or easier level) to 70 minutes (evidence-based minimum duration) of exercise, a duration required for a comprehensive fitness class. Refer to table 8.6 for the timing of a comprehensive fitness class. "If older adults cannot do 150 minutes of moderate-intensity aerobic activity per week because of chronic conditions, it is recommended that they be as physically active as their abilities and conditions allow" (ASCM 2009b, 1511).

Table 8.2 shows a sample weekly schedule for a comprehensive fitness program, including resistance training, aerobics and dynamic balance activities, and stretching exercises in a weekly program, in accordance with minimum evidence-based recommendations for training

Table 8.2 Weekly Schedule for a Comprehensive Fitness Program[a]

Fitness class components	Monday	Tuesday (optional)	Wednesday	Thursday	Friday or Saturday
Warm-up	X	X	X	X	X
Resistance training	X[b]			X	
Aerobics and dynamic balance	X	+	X	+	X
Cool-down and stretch	X	X	X	X	X

[a]Classes are scheduled 4 to 5 days per week; X's show what might be covered each day. If progression is possible from there, the + sign represents adding 2 more days per week of aerobics (1 day at a time) for the recommended minimum 5 days per week (ACSM 2011, 2009b).

[b]As you are easing into a comprehensive program, you can move resistance training to Tuesdays (the optional day) if participants cannot tolerate a comprehensive fitness class.

frequency (ACSM 2011, 2009b), that meets 4 to 5 days per week. Notice that a comprehensive fitness class is offered twice a week, once on Monday and eventually on Thursday after participants adjust to the increase of physical activity. Monday, the most strenuous day, is preceded by 1 or 2 days off and is followed by an optional light workout. To prevent overtraining, avoid having strenuous physical activity 2 days in a row. If the same group of people meet five times per week, one workout (Tuesdays, in this example) can be lighter, such as warm-up and cool-down exercises, until participants are ready for the next step, another day of aerobics.

Seated and Standing Exercises

For fall prevention and ease of getting to know new participants, we recommend teaching the seated warm-up, resistance, aerobic and dynamic balance, and stretching exercises first and then teaching the standing exercises when participants are ready to progress. Encourage participants to tell you how they are feeling so that you can give them individualized recommendations for standing or seated exercises. If you have any doubts about having a participant stand while exercising, use the safer sitting option and consult the participant's physician if appropriate.

In this section you will learn

- when a participant is ready for standing exercises,
- the benefits of standing exercises,
- when seated exercises are preferred over standing ones, and
- the advantages of teaching seated and standing exercises simultaneously.

Progressing From Seated to Standing

When is a participant ready to progress from seated to standing exercises in a class setting? A participant can progress to standing exercises if he or she

- has become proficient with the basic seated exercises, for example, can per-

form seated aerobic and dynamic balance combinations of lower- and upper-body movements well;

- has no balance problems;
- or has minor balance problems but has a competent spotter for one-on-one facilitation or only performs exercises that leave at least one hand free to hold on to a chair or other sturdy support;
- or has major balance problems but has a competent spotter for one-on-one facilitation (although we recommend that upper-body resistance exercises requiring weights in both hands be done while the participant is seated);
- is not frail or at high risk of bone fractures, unless assisted by a competent spotter for one-on-one facilitation; and
- is not feeling fatigued, drowsy, dizzy, or lightheaded, conditions that may affect balance.

Although circumstances such as dehydration, hypertension, or a side effect of medication may cause a person to have one or more symptoms that affect balance, consider that the common symptoms (feeling fatigued, drowsy, dizzy, or lightheaded) may be temporary. Focus on safety while encouraging your participants to progress. Refer to chapter 2 for more possible reasons for balance problems.

Benefits of Standing Exercises

Standing exercises offer remarkable benefits as long as safety is not jeopardized. When standing is a safe and suitable option, give your participants a choice to sit or stand and allow them to sit any time during the class when necessary. Some exercises are more effective or easier standing than seated, especially exercises for which the chair gets in the way. Other benefits of standing exercises include

- improved balance, particularly static standing balance and dynamic balance with standing aerobics and dynamic balance activities;

- improved functional mobility and ability to perform daily activities that require standing;
- maintained or even increased independence;
- improved bone density and reduced risk of falls and bone fractures; and
- added variety in the exercise program.

When participants can stand, integrate seated with standing exercises and give participants regular reminders to listen to their bodies and sit when needed. Encourage them not to sit for too long and to intersperse short bouts of physical activity and standing between periods of sedentary activity (ACSM 2011, 1348). Even for those who come to class regularly and meet current physical activity recommendations, being sedentary is detrimental (ACSM 2011).

When Are Seated Exercises Preferred Over Standing?

Here are some guidelines for you to determine when a participant is better off doing seated exercises:

- When a participant fails to meet any of the previously discussed criteria for determining whether he or she is ready for standing exercises.
- When performing upper-body exercises that use both arms, particularly resistance exercises that require weights in both hands and thus preclude grasping a steady object for support if the participant loses his or her balance.
- When standing exercise requires using one hand to hold on for support and you want to save time by doing upper-body exercises on both sides simultaneously rather than one side at a time.
- When the participant no longer feels steady and balanced when standing.
- When a participant can successfully and safely participate only in chair-seated exercise. For example, for those with Parkinson's disease, an all-seated exercise program is often the only safe option.

Advantages of Teaching Seated and Standing Exercises Simultaneously

By offering seated and standing exercise that can be taught simultaneously, you can accommodate diverse individual needs in a classroom setting, as in these scenarios:

- Some participants can continue to do seated exercises while others progress to the corresponding standing exercises.
- Participants can start with just one standing exercise and gradually progress to more at their own pace.
- If a participant becomes fatigued while doing a standing exercise, he or she can sit and continue with the corresponding seated exercise.
- Participants who have major balance problems can continue to do the seated exercises or gain the benefits of standing if they have a competent assistant to help them with each exercise.
- Participants who have minor balance problems gain the benefits of standing exercises by performing those exercises that leave a hand available to hold on to a stable support.
- Participants who are steady on their feet have the option of performing all standing exercises and sitting for variety or necessity if tired.
- Providing the option to sit or stand, depending on how people feel from day to day, can promote regular attendance.

Upper- and Lower-Body Exercises

The exercises in chapters 4, 5, and 7 are divided into upper- and lower-body exercises. You can teach upper- and lower-body exercises together or separately. For example, if you start with the upper-body exercises, after your class is doing well with them you may add the lower-body exercises. Add them at a comfortable pace, even if just one exercise per class; a basic beginning fitness class for frail elders and adults with special needs can cover warm-up exercises during the first 2 or more weeks of class—the first class may include only upper-body exercises. Add the lower-body exercises over the next few classes.

With aerobic exercise, the lower- and upper-body movements go together. But learning the moves is easier if the lower-body movements are taught first and the upper-body movements are added later. The lower-body movements, the foundation of aerobics, use large muscle groups, which are needed to elevate the heart rate sufficiently to improve cardiovascular endurance. Encourage your participants to go at their own pace with aerobics. For instance, remind them that they may do just lower-body exercise if they start getting tired. Or, if the lower body needs a rest, they may do just upper-body movements. Alternatively, they may do the upper- and lower-body movements at a slower pace than the class.

Exercise Media

Another option for your exercise class is to use an exercise DVD. Use reputable sources that are not too dated. If you are interested in purchasing a DVD or other media appropriate for frail elders and people with special needs, see "Media Resources" in "Suggested Resources."

Table 8.3 delineates the advantages and disadvantages of using exercise media, such as DVDs. Notice that some of the disadvantages can be turned into advantages.

Consider videotaping your class. In your absence, a qualified leader (one who is trained in exercise supervision, knows the conditions and special needs of your participants, and understands all the safety guidelines) can pop in the video and supervise your class as the participants follow your lead.

SCHEDULING YOUR EXERCISE CLASSES

Schedule your exercise program so that your participants receive the greatest benefits. The following sections present guidelines for the frequency and duration of your classes. Focus on safety; increase either frequency (number of times the class is offered per week) or duration (the amount of exercise time per class) one at a time to prevent overtraining. Consider participant feedback, both verbal and nonverbal (what you observe), when increasing the frequency or duration of your class.

Be flexible with participants; for example, allow someone to attend 1 day per week initially if that is all he or she is ready for. The

Table 8.3   Exercise Media

Advantages	Disadvantages
You can videotape your own class to be played in your absence.	Few good-quality videos are available for older adults and those with special needs.
Exposure to a variety of teaching styles can provide new insights.	Videos and other media can be less motivational than a live instructor.
A less highly trained fitness leader can more easily supervise participants while they are following an exercise video.	The class still needs to be carefully supervised while following an exercise video.
A qualified instructor will have more time to modify an exercise for participants when needed during class.	The instructor may not pay as close attention to participants as when he or she is leading in front of the class. For example, those with visual or auditory deficits may not get needed special cues.
Videos and other media can make it possible to offer classes more times per week and provide a more diverse exercise curriculum.	Participants may be less likely to come to class.

publication *2008 Physical Activity Guidelines for Americans* affirm that all adults should avoid inactivity, that some physical activity is better than none, and that adults who participant in any amount of physical activity gain some health benefits. Nonetheless, the guidelines stress that for most health outcomes, additional benefits occur as the amount of physical activity increases with increased intensity, frequency, or duration. The guidelines also emphasize that if older adults cannot do 150 minutes of moderate-intensity aerobic activity per week because of chronic conditions, they should be as physically active as their abilities and conditions allow (ACSM 2009b, 1510; USDHHS 2008b).

Class Frequency

The number of days per week that you schedule a fitness class will depend on whether resistance training or aerobics is included (see table 8.4). You may start with fewer days per week than recommended, even one, and if possible expand your class to meet at least the minimum recommended frequencies. If that is not possible, possibly refer participants to other classes or a home program (when appropriate, such as walking for cardiovascular training) to meet the recommendations. Ideally, spread your classes throughout the week to give participants a longer recovery time between classes, which helps prevent injuries. For example, meeting Monday, Wednesday, and Friday is preferable to meeting Monday, Tuesday, and Wednesday.

After participants have improved their level of fitness, consider offering a comprehensive fitness program. The sample schedule in table

8.2, Weekly Schedule for a Comprehensive Fitness Program, is based on the American College of Sports Medicine's (2011, 2009b) minimum recommended frequencies for resistance and aerobic training. Stretching is offered each workout, more than the minimum recommended two times per week, at the end of the warm-up (see chapter 4) and as an integral part of the cool-down (see chapter 7). Refer to table 8.6 for the timing of a model comprehensive fitness class.

Class Duration

A 1-hour exercise class is a hearty goal for this population. "The intensity and duration of physical activity should be low at the outset for older adults who are highly deconditioned, functionally limited, or have chronic conditions that affect their ability to perform physical tasks" (ACSM 2009b, 1511). Table 8.5 shows four examples of classes lasting 45 to 60 minutes. Notice that each of the four examples has a 5-minute opening and closing, which allows an easygoing start with only 35 minutes of exercise in the 45-minute class. Each class focuses on a different exercise component: warm-up, resistance training, aerobics, or relaxation (cool-down). Table 8.6 puts all the exercise components together into a model comprehensive fitness class that lasts 60 to 80 minutes. The comprehensive fitness class also dedicates 5 minutes to opening and 5 minutes to closing the class. Chapter 3 gives helpful tips for opening and closing your exercise class. Remember to pause for participants to drink water throughout the class. After a class is well established, it can warm the atmosphere to schedule 5 or more minutes for socializing

Table 8.4 Recommended Training Frequencies

Training	Frequency
Resistance training	Two to three times per week on nonconsecutive days.
Aerobic training	Five days per week minimum at a moderate level (start easy and ease into a moderate intensity, if participants are able).
Stretching	Two times per week minimum, although daily is best.

ACSM 2011.

Table 8.5 Four Examples of 45- to 60-Minute Exercise Classes

Model warm-up–only class		Model resistance-training class	
Opening	5 minutes	Opening	5 minutes
Posture exercise	2 minutes	Warm-up	10 minutes
Breathing exercise	3 minutes	Resistance exercises	15–30 minutes
ROM exercises	20–25 minutes	Cool-down	10 minutes
Cool-down	10–20 minutes	Closing	5 minutes
Closing (e.g., cleaning weights)	5 minutes		
Total	45–60 minutes		45–60 minutes
Model aerobics and dynamic balance class		**Model stretching and relaxation class**	
Opening	5 minutes	Opening	5 minutes
Warm-up	10 minutes	Warm-up	10 minutes
Aerobic and dynamic balance exercises	15–30 minutes[a]	Stretching exercises	20–30 minutes
Cool-down	10 minutes	Relaxation exercises	5–10 minutes
Closing	5 minutes	Closing	5 minutes
Total	45–60 minutes		45–60 minutes

Times are approximate.

[a]Aerobics may be better tolerated if it is divided into short bouts (e.g., two to three 10-minute sessions) interspersed with low-level leg movement, such as ROM exercises.

and drinking water. Classes with people who tend to chitchat disruptively can be stylishly channeled to the break: "That sounds like an important topic for the break."

Schedule a set amount of time, such as 45 to 60 minutes, for your exercise class. You can initially do fewer exercises and offer other activities, such as an educational or motivational lecture and discussion and healthy refreshments at the end. Educating people about the benefits of exercise can increase exercise adherence (see "Focus on Education" in chapter 3 and table 3.1). Refreshments can be an extrinsic motivator for people who are resistant to exercise. Healthy snacks at the end of class are also rewarding and can make your class more popular among the less-motivated participants. On the other hand, some may prefer to leave when the exercises are over, so be flexible and leave the choice to each

person. Table 8.7 offers a possible schedule for you to start with. This sample class meets 2 or 3 days per week for 45 to 60 minutes and includes warm-up exercises (posture, deep breathing, ROM, and stretching exercises), an educational component, and healthy refreshments. Beginner classes will need more breaks during exercise as participants build their endurance. Several water breaks are a good habit to establish from the onset. Work with the interests and abilities of your participants as you gradually increase the exercise time and reduce the other activities.

Duration of the Exercise Components

Chapters 4 through 7 give comprehensive sets of warm-up, resistance, aerobic, and stretching exercises. The following sections give specific suggestions for shortening each exercise

Table 8.6   Model Comprehensive Fitness Class

Activity	TIME (MINUTES)[a]	
	Beginner or easier level	Increased aerobic training (ACSM 2011, 2009b)
Opening	5	5
Warm-up	10	10
Resistance training	15	15
Aerobics and dynamic balance	15[b]	25–35[b]
Cool-down	10	10
Closing	5	5
Total class time	60	70–80

[a]Times are approximate.

[b]Including a 5-minute postaerobic cool-down before resistance training (see chapter 7).

If time permits and participants are ready to progress, gradually increase the time for aerobics to meet the minimum evidence-based recommendations. For moderate-intensity aerobics, accumulate at least 30 or up to 60 (for greater benefit) minutes per day in bouts of at least 10 minutes each (ACSM 2011, 1339) to total 150 to 300 minutes per week (ACSM 2009b, 1511).

Table 8.7   Weekly Schedule for Beginning a 45- to 60-minute Exercise Class

Exercise class components	Monday	Wednesday (optional)	Friday
Warm-up: posture, breathing, ROM, and stretching	30–35[a]	30–35	30–35
Education	5–10	5–10	5–10
Healthy refreshments	10–15	10–15	10–15

[a]Suggested times can be adjusted to meet the special needs of your participants.

component or prolonging it to make it more challenging or to fill an entire class. Refer to table 8.5 for timing of the segments (opening, closing, and so on) of classes that concentrate on one component—warm-up, resistance training, aerobics, or cool-down (stretching and relaxation).

Bear in mind that the exercises take longer to lead in the initial learning phase. Practice the exercises before you start the class to establish a good sense of the timing, especially if you are a new fitness leader. The three-step instructional process in chapter 3 can help you learn how to teach the exercises or, if you are an experienced instructor, to refine your teaching.

In general, you can shorten the comprehensive set of 24 ROM, 12 resistance, 12 aerobic and dynamic balance, and 12 stretching exercises by doing fewer exercises or fewer repetitions of each exercise.

Here are some general ways to extend a single warm-up, resistance-training, aerobic-training, or stretching component into an entire class. Initially, teaching all the basic seated exercises of an exercise component might fill an entire class (along with the opening, warm-up, cool-down, and closing for all classes; see table 8.5). When your class is ready for a greater challenge, slowly introduce the following options:

- Repeat some of your participants' favorite exercises.
- Repeat some or all of the basic seated exercises.
- Add variations of some or all of the basic exercises, such as standing exercises.
- Increase the number of repetitions of an exercise.

Many factors influence the duration of an exercise component, such as

- class size,
- number of instructors and assistants,
- participants' need for assistance with equipment and individual exercises,
- instructor's and participants' experience with the exercises, and
- level of fitness and exercise capability of the participants.

Because of these variables, we recommend that you start with teaching just the warm-up exercises (see table 8.5). Expand your exercise class from there, after you are familiar with your participants' needs and current limitations and how long it takes to get through the warm-up.

Duration of Warm-Up

You may shorten or lengthen the duration of the warm-up component (focusing on ROM and including posture, deep breathing, and light stretching exercises, discussed in chapter 4) to fit the special needs of your class, but always warm up for at least 10 minutes before doing any other exercises. Refer to table 4.1 for the general recommended timing of the warm-up posture, deep breathing, ROM, and stretching exercises. If you are leading more than one exercise component in a workout, you need to warm up only at the beginning of class, unless resistance training precedes aerobics. When you teach resistance training before aerobics, stretch briefly (using the minimal five stretching exercises in table 4.3) immediately after resistance training and follow with several minutes of active rhythmic movement (such as slow walking or low-intensity aerobic leg exercises) before moving on to the aerobic workout.

To shorten the warm-up, you can use one of these suggestions (ultimately, it is best to do all 24 ROM exercises):

- Do as many of the 24 ROM exercises as possible in an allotted time. In this case, you can do just the first couple of exercises for each target joint to warm up the entire body.
- Concentrate on the ROM exercises for major joints that move larger muscles, such as hips, knees, ankles, spine, and shoulders (which are more effective for warming up the body than the neck, wrists, and fingers that move smaller muscles).
- Do the upper-body exercises on both sides at the same time. For some exercises learning one side at a time is easier, but after participants learn the exercises do both sides at once for a more effective warm-up.
- Do fewer repetitions of each exercise, such as three or four instead of eight. Use this technique only after participants learn the exercises, because starting with fewer repetitions may not give you enough time to observe and evaluate all participants and give them appropriate feedback with each exercise.

You can extend the warm-up into an entire class by using one or more of these suggestions (see table 8.5):

- Do the upper-body ROM exercises on one side at a time (recommended when participants are learning the exercises).
- Repeat the ROM exercises for a given joint, such as the five shoulder exercises.
- Repeat a movement pattern at each joint, such as circumduction (rotating all the joints that can make a circular pattern) of the hips, ankles, spine (as a unit), shoulders, wrist, and fingers. Do not

circumduct the neck, which can cause neck degeneration or injury.

- Increase the number of sets, of three to eight repetitions, of a ROM exercise.

- Intersperse more sets of a ROM exercise throughout the warm-up. (Seated Up-and-Down Leg March can be a simple and fun one.)

- After participants have learned the basic seated exercises and increased their endurance, combine an upper-body exercise with a lower-body ROM exercise (e.g., Up-and-Down Leg March with Butterfly Wings).

- Also, the other aspects of a warm-up—the initial posture and deep-breathing exercises and final stretching after the

body is warmed up—can be extended with detailed instruction (mainly important initially when learning good technique) and helpful individual feedback when relevant. The three-part deep-breathing exercises and final stretching exercises can be repeated several times, and the stretches can be held longer.

Duration of Resistance Training

You may shorten or lengthen the duration of the resistance training component (chapter 5) to fit the special needs of your class. Remember to include at least a 10-minute warm-up before resistance training and a 10-minute cool-down after resistance training.

For a shorter resistance segment, do just the eight exercises listed in table 8.8, the minimum

Table 8.8 Eight-Exercise Resistance-Training Component: Seated or Standing[a]

Target body parts and muscles	Resistance exercise	Functional benefits
Chest (pectoralis major) Back of upper arms (triceps) Shoulders (deltoids)	5.1 Chest Press	Pushing a door open, pushing up from a lying position
Back (latissimus dorsi, trapezius) Front of upper arms (biceps) Shoulders (deltoids)	5.2 Two-Arm Row	Pulling a door open, posture
Shoulders (deltoids) Back of upper arms (triceps)	5.3 Overhead Press	Lifting (especially overhead)
Front hips and thighs (hip flexors)	5.6 Hip Flexion	Stair climbing, posture; improved static and dynamic standing balance
Outer hips and thighs (hip abductors) Inner thighs (hip adductors)	5.7 Hip Abduction and Adduction	Hip rotation (lateral or medial), pelvic stabilization, posture, walking; improved static and dynamic standing balance
Shins (tibialis anterior)	5.10 Toe Raises	Walking (foot clearance)
Calves (gastrocnemius, soleus)	5.11 Heel Raises	Walking (push off); improved static and dynamic standing balance
Thighs (quadriceps, hamstrings) Buttocks (gluteals)	5.12 Chair Stands (Challenger)	Stand from sitting, stair climbing, walking (forward progression and stability)

[a]All seated basic resistance and balance exercises have a corresponding standing exercise. See the variations and progression options in the illustrated exercises at the end of chapter 5. Your participants will receive greater balance benefits with the standing exercises, particularly exercises involving a one-legged stand (indicated by a balance icon).

From E. Best-Martini and K.A. Jones-DiGenova, 2014, *Exercise for frail elders*, 2nd ed. (Champaign, IL: Human Kinetics).

number of recommended resistance exercises per workout. These eight resistance exercises strengthen the muscles that are notoriously weak for most older adults.

You can extend the duration of a resistance-training component to fill an entire class by

- increasing, gradually, the number of repetitions to 15 maximum or (remember to increase only one, either reps or sets, at a time)
- increasing, gradually, the number of sets to two or three at most (vary how you do the second or third set); refer to the variations and progression options.

Duration of Aerobics

You may shorten or lengthen the duration of the aerobics component (chapter 6) to fit the special needs of your class. Remember to include at least a 10-minute warm-up before aerobics and a 10-minute cool-down after aerobics. For specific duration recommendations for aerobics for promoting cardiovascular endurance see "Duration" in chapter 6.

For a shorter aerobics segment, you can do as many of the 12 aerobic and dynamic balance exercises (or do all 12, each for a shorter time) as possible in an allotted time.

You can increase the aerobics component into an entire class by introducing new variations such as the following:

- Integrate some or all of the additional arm movements (in the variations and progression options).
- Create a pattern by combining two exercises, such as performing three Alternate Toe Touches to Sides (exercise 6.7) and then three Alternate Heel Touches to Sides (exercise 6.8). Repeat the pattern as desired.
- Create a combination with two or more patterns.

Duration of Cool-Down

The cool-down focuses on stretching and includes relaxation exercises, as discussed in

chapter 7. You may shorten or lengthen the duration of the cool-down component to fit the special needs of your class, but always cool-down for at least 10 minutes after aerobics or resistance training. Refer to table 7.1 for the general recommended timing of final stretching after aerobics or resistance training.

If you are short on time toward the end of class, you can do one of the reduced sets of stretches listed in tables 4.3 and 4.4. These shorter sets of stretching exercises include critical stretches for body parts that are notoriously tight for most older adults. In general, do not combine upper- and lower-body stretches to save time. Doing one stretch at a time can be safer and more effective by helping participants focus on the muscles being stretched. Aim to have enough time toward the end of class for a relaxed paced set of the comprehensive 12 stretches (the upper- and lower-body stretches are shown in table 7.3).

You can extend the cool-down component into an entire class by

- increasing the length of time that you hold the stretches up to about 1 minute,
- repeating a stretch up to four times,
- repeating a deep-breathing exercise two or more times, or
- performing more relaxation exercises.

! Safety Tip Gradually and conservatively increase either frequency or duration of your exercise class, one at a time to prevent overtraining.

MODIFYING THE EXERCISES

Not all the basic seated and standing exercises are appropriate for all participants. Refer to participants' medical clearance forms to see whether the physician has made any special exercise recommendations. If you have tried the following suggestions but are still unable to modify an exercise so that a participant can perform it successfully, ask the participant's medical professionals for recommendations for alternative exercises. If your class is large and you do not have an assistant, you can ask a participant (who is able) to come early or stay after class for further individual instruction.

When to Modify an Exercise

You might need to modify an exercise when a participant has one or more of the following:

- Problems performing an exercise
- Problems keeping up with the class
- Special needs
- Strain or pain (also see figures 2.3 and 2.4)

How to Modify an Exercise

You can modify an exercise for a participant in several ways. The *A* through *E* mnemonic that follows can aid you in remembering how to modify an exercise while teaching your class:

- **Adjust the speed of the movement**. Have the participant decrease the speed of movement if he or she is moving faster than the instructor, who needs to be exemplifying good technique. Faster movements increase risk of injury. Support participants in going slower than the pace of the class if that is more comfortable for them.

- **Body position, adjust**. A participant may be performing the exercise in an awkward position or with poor posture. This can be a good time to remind the entire class about good posture.

- **Consult the physician or physical therapist**. Always ask a participant to stop exercising if he or she experiences any pain. If the participant continues to feel pain after trying the suggested modifications, consult with his or her physician, physical therapist, or other health care professional or suggest to the participant or caregiver that he or she consult the appropriate medical professional.

- **Decrease the workload**. Decrease the number of repetitions of the exercise, the number of sets, the amount of weight or resistance (for resistance exercises), or a combination of these.

- **Exercise technique, adjust**. If a participant is not using proper exercise technique, further verbal and visual cues may help. Sometimes gently leading a participant hand over hand (your hand over his or her hand) through a few repetitions of an exercise using proper exercise technique can help. Remember to ask permission before touching a participant. Sometimes the exercise itself needs to be adjusted. Refer to the exercise and safety tips and variations and progression options of the illustrated instruction sections in chapters 4 through 7 for alternate ways of performing every exercise. For example, many of the exercises have an easier option.

Start with one modification to address the most obvious need. For example, if the participant is slouching, facilitate him or her in adjusting body position. If that modification is unsuccessful, try another. Refer to the sections on specific precautions for those with special needs in chapters 4 through 7 to review the recommendations and possible modifications for the participant's special needs.

! Safety Tip Start with one modification to address a participant's most obvious need when she or he is having problems performing an exercise, keeping up with the class, has strain or pain with an exercise, or has other special needs. If that modification is unsuccessful, try another.

PROGRESSING YOUR EXERCISE CLASS

Progression of a successful exercise class is based on tolerance and preference of the participants. A conservative approach is necessary for the most deconditioned and physically limited older adults (ACSM 2009b, 1511). Progression is not necessarily linear; your participants' abilities may vary from day to day, and they may need to go back to an easier level if they have missed classes. On the other hand, exercise progression can be facilitated by gradual increases in intensity, frequency, and duration of training (AACVPR 2006, 84). Some participants need encouragement to progress in their workouts, whereas others need reminders not to push too hard. In this section, you will learn more about when and how to make your class progressively more challenging, including instructions for progressing each exercise component, challenger exercises, and variations and progression options. Remember our KISSS principle—keep it (your class) simple, safe, and slowly progress:

• **Keep it Simple**. We recommend that you start with only one component—an extended warm-up session of posture, breathing, gentle range-of-motion, and stretching exercises. This approach gives your participants a chance to feel successful before they progress to another exercise component. Bear in mind that your class may be some participants' first experience with a fitness program as adults, and they may feel intimidated by receiving too much information early on.

• **Keep it *Safe***. Introducing one exercise component at a time gives participants time to adjust safely to each exercise, and it allows you time to observe and get to know the group. As you learn the strengths and current limitations of your participants, you can appropriately pace the progression of your class.

• **Progress *Slowly***. Slowly introduce new exercises. Gradually make your class more challenging. Because people may start your class at different times, be at different levels of fitness, and progress at different rates, continually encourage them to listen to their bodies, go at their own pace (but not too fast), and rest any time they need to. For instance, if the aerobics pace is too fast for a participant, he or she can do one move for every two that you lead. Discourage competition among participants. Encourage participants to progress safely in their workouts and, most important, to attend class regularly. Regular attendance is key to successful progression.

What are the signs that your participants are ready to progress?

• Their exercise technique is good.

• They have no signs of fatigue. In general, your participants should feel energized or only mildly fatigued at the end of class.

• When you ask them, "Are you ready for a new exercise?" (and so on), they say, "Yes!"

If some are ready to progress while others are not, the ones who are not can take a water break during the new exercises. Encourage them to join in when they are ready.

The rate at which your class progresses and the levels that participants reach depend on several factors, such as

• physicians' recommendations;

• participants' health and fitness goals and motivations;

• stage and severity of participants' special needs and orthopedic and musculoskeletal status;

• the instructor's enthusiasm and skill;

• the size of the class;

• the duration and frequency of the class (and intensity of exercise);

• the frequency, intensity, and duration of exercise that participants participate in outside class;

• participants' level of daily physical activity other than formal exercise (AACVPR 2006, 84); and

• the equipment available.

To begin, let's look at two general modes of progression. For simplicity, safety, and slow progression, use only one mode at a time:

1. Add a fitness component—warm-up, resistance training, aerobics and dynamic balance, or cool-down (stretching and relaxation exercises)—to your class.

2. Add to a fitness component of your class, as in these examples:

   • Add the lower-body exercises after participants have learned the upper-body exercises, or vice versa.

- Add one or more new exercises per class or week and so on, depending on the time available and how quickly participants learn new exercises. When the class is established, the focus changes to varying the exercises rather than adding more. When the class becomes more experienced or advanced, strategically add exercises for interest and progression.
- You can add standing exercises for ambulatory (able to walk) participants after they have learned the seated exercises. If you are working one on one with a nonambulatory client who has physician approval for standing exercises, begin with one standing exercise and gradually increase the number of standing exercises performed. Refer to the section "Seated and Standing Exercises" earlier in this chapter to review when to implement standing exercises, benefits of standing exercises, when seated exercise are preferred over standing exercises, and advantages of teaching seated and standing exercises simultaneously.

! Safety Tip Start a class for frail elders and older adults with special needs with only one component: an extended warm-up session of posture, breathing, gentle range-of-motion, and stretching exercises.

How to Progress the Frequency, Intensity, and Duration of Each Exercise Component

Gradually increase the frequency, intensity, and duration of each exercise component. In general, increase only one parameter (frequency, intensity, or duration) at a time. For example, if you increase the frequency by one session per week, postpone increasing the duration or intensity until participants have adapted to the extra day of exercise. To help you progress your class in resistance training (chapter 5), aerobics (chapter 6), and stretching (chapter 7), review the guidelines in those chapters, which include a progression and maintenance section.

Challenger Exercises

The exercises labeled challenger are intermediate- to advanced-level exercises that many participants have difficulty learning in the beginning of a fitness class. Give your participants an opportunity to feel successful in your exercise class by introducing these more-challenging exercises after they are comfortable with the basic exercises. Participants who attend class regularly will improve their physical fitness and be better able to perform the challengers. For example, the seated Modified Chair Stands and regular Chair Stands are both challenger exercises that are easier after participants have increased their leg strength with the other seated lower-body resistance exercises. When your class is ready for something new, we recommend introducing the challenger exercises (of the basic exercises) first, because they are an integral part of the basic ROM, resistance, and stretching routines. When they are ready for further challenge, the variations and progression options of the illustrated instruction sections of chapters 4 through 7 provide many more challenger exercises. But the aerobic training and dynamic balance activities in chapter 6 are structured differently; you add the upper-body and arm movements introduced in the variations and progression options to increase the intensity and overall challenge of the routine when participants are ready. Therefore, chapter 6 does not have challenger exercises.

Variations and Progression Options

The variations and progression options enable you to design a creative and progressive fitness program and adapt it to meet the needs of one person or a class full of people from frail to fit.

Chapters 4 through 7 offer variations and progression options (VPOs) for each of the basic seated 24 ROM exercises, 12 resistance-training exercises, 12 aerobic and dynamic balance exercises, and 12 stretching exercises. Each basic seated exercise has a standing alternative—a key option for varying and progressing an exercise program. Standing exercises offer participants the greatest benefits in functional mobility and increased independence.

When your class is ready for a greater challenge, after they have learned all the basic seated exercises for the components that you are teaching (and the easier option, when appropriate), teach VPOs of one or more of the basic exercises. Although there are countless possibilities with the VPOs, you might introduce one new one each class, each week, or each month, depending on the interest and abilities of the participants, your comfort level, and the time available and focus of the class. For instance, if you are leading a warm-up–only class, it can be fun for the participants and easy for you to add a ROM VPO regularly.

Although participants may have a huge potential for progression from their current level to an elite level of functional fitness, you will find that the path of progression may vary widely among participants and classes. For instance, a large class without an assistant in a long-term care setting will be more limited in potential for progression than a smaller class with an assistant. In any case, varying the basic seated exercises can benefit and add to the enjoyment of any class. Then again, other classes may thrive by progressing to all standing exercises (with the option of sitting when needed). Keep in mind that some people will thrive on regular change, whereas others, such as those with Alzheimer's disease and related dementias, may prefer consistency, minimal variation, and slow and steady progress.

MAINTAINING FITNESS RESULTS

An effective exercise program is dynamic, regularly changing to meet participants' needs.

Even a program designed to maintain exercise at a current level is not static. If a participant gets ill, for instance, he or she should resume exercise at an easier level and slowly progress to his or her maintenance level. Whether progressing or maintaining their exercise, participants have day-to-day variations in their ability for physical activity that may allow them to do a little more than usual or may require them to integrate rest into the workout or decrease the workload (number of repetitions of the exercise, number of sets, amount of weight or resistance [for resistance exercises], or a combination of these). In general, however, the frequency, intensity, and duration of the exercise prescription used at the conclusion of the progression phase remain unchanged during the maintenance phase. Naturally, if a participant increases frequency, intensity, or duration during the maintenance phase, he or she will gain additional health and fitness benefits (AACVPR 2006).

Whether a participant is ready to stop progressing and start maintaining his or her exercise program depends on several factors, including his or her short- and long-term goals, motivation, physical and mental ability, physician's recommendations, and equipment available. Reevaluate short-term and long-term goals before entering the maintenance stage (see "Goal Setting" in chapter 2).

Some participants in an exercise class may be maintaining their exercise levels, but others may be progressing. In addition, some may be maintaining one component of exercise (e.g., resistance training) and progressing in another (e.g., aerobic training). Some participants cannot progress very far and thus reach the maintenance phase earlier than others do. For example, if you have any concern that a participant with Alzheimer's or related dementia may injure him- or herself by dropping a free weight, progress may be limited to a 1-pound (.45 kg) free weight. When participants are maintaining a current level of fitness, focus on varying their exercises. The numerous variation options in the illustrated instruction sections of chapters 4 through 7 make that easy.

SUMMARY

One size does not fit all when teaching a fitness class to frail elders and adults with special needs. This chapter provided information about designing, scheduling, progressing, modifying, and maintaining a personalized functional fitness class or program. After learning the objectives of chapters 1 through 8, you will have powerful tools as an exercise leader to guide people from frail to fit toward their best functional fitness possible. You will be equipped to teach safe and effective exercise to all adults, including adults with special needs ranging from an occasional joint with minor arthritis to the complex condition of frailty. We encourage you to be a dynamic teacher and a lifelong learner, an attribute necessary for the evolving adult fitness and wellness fields. We wish you the best in guiding the people in your class toward better functional fitness and quality of life.

REVIEW QUESTIONS

1. Which of the following are options for you to choose from when designing your exercise program? (*Circle only one.*)
    a. leading one or more exercise components—warm-up, resistance training, aerobics, and cool-down—in one class
    b. a comprehensive fitness class or program
    c. leading just seated exercises, just standing exercises, or seated and standing exercises at the same time
    d. leading both upper- and lower-body exercises or initially just upper-body or just lower-body exercises
    e. using exercise media, such as DVDs
    f. all of the above
    g. *a, b, c,* and *d* only

2. T or F. With frail elders and adults with special needs, introduce only one new exercise component—warm-up, resistance training, aerobics, or cool-down—at a time. If true, why? If false, why not? _____

3. Which of the following is a benefit of standing exercises? (*Circle only one.*)
    a. improved balance, particularly static standing balance
    b. improved ability to perform daily activities that require standing
    c. improved bone density and reduced risk of falls and bone fractures
    d. added exercise variety to your exercise program
    e. all of the above
    f. *a, b,* and *c* only

4. If you were teaching a 60-minute resistance-training class, each segment of the class would be approximately how long?

Activity	Time (minutes)
Opening	_____
Warm-up	_____
Resistance training	_____
Cool-down	_____
Closing	_____

5. List four ways to extend a single warm-up, resistance-training, aerobic, or stretching component into an entire class:

   a. _____

   b. _____

   c. _____

   d. _____

6. List and briefly describe five ways to modify an exercise (use the *A* to *E* mnemonic):

   a. _____

   b. _____

   c. _____

   d. _____

   e. _____

7. The variations and progression options enable you to design a creative and progressive fitness program and adapt it to meet participants' _____.

8. Which of the following factors determine whether a participant is ready to stop progressing and start maintaining in one or more exercise components of his or her exercise program? *(Circle only one.)*

   a. short- and long-term goals

   b. motivation

   c. physical and mental ability

   d. physician's and physical therapist's recommendations

   e. equipment available

   f. all of the above

   g. *a, c,* and *d* only

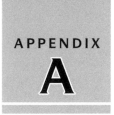

APPENDIX

A

Health and Fitness Appraisal

Physical Activity Readiness
Questionnaire - PAR-Q
(revised 2002)

PAR-Q & YOU

(A Questionnaire for People Aged 15 to 69)

Regular physical activity is fun and healthy, and increasingly more people are starting to become more active every day. Being more active is very safe for most people. However, some people should check with their doctor before they start becoming much more physically active.

If you are planning to become much more physically active than you are now, start by answering the seven questions in the box below. If you are between the ages of 15 and 69, the PAR-Q will tell you if you should check with your doctor before you start. If you are over 69 years of age, and you are not used to being very active, check with your doctor.

Common sense is your best guide when you answer these questions. Please read the questions carefully and answer each one honestly: check YES or NO.

YES	NO		
☐	☐	1.	**Has your doctor ever said that you have a heart condition <u>and</u> that you should only do physical activity recommended by a doctor?**
☐	☐	2.	**Do you feel pain in your chest when you do physical activity?**
☐	☐	3.	**In the past month, have you had chest pain when you were not doing physical activity?**
☐	☐	4.	**Do you lose your balance because of dizziness or do you ever lose consciousness?**
☐	☐	5.	**Do you have a bone or joint problem (for example, back, knee or hip) that could be made worse by a change in your physical activity?**
☐	☐	6.	**Is your doctor currently prescribing drugs (for example, water pills) for your blood pressure or heart condition?**
☐	☐	7.	**Do you know of <u>any other reason</u> why you should not do physical activity?**

If you answered

YES to one or more questions

Talk with your doctor by phone or in person BEFORE you start becoming much more physically active or BEFORE you have a fitness appraisal. Tell your doctor about the PAR-Q and which questions you answered YES.

- You may be able to do any activity you want — as long as you start slowly and build up gradually. Or, you may need to restrict your activities to those which are safe for you. Talk with your doctor about the kinds of activities you wish to participate in and follow his/her advice.
- Find out which community programs are safe and helpful for you.

NO to all questions

If you answered NO honestly to <u>all</u> PAR-Q questions, you can be reasonably sure that you can:
- start becoming much more physically active – begin slowly and build up gradually. This is the safest and easiest way to go.
- take part in a fitness appraisal – this is an excellent way to determine your basic fitness so that you can plan the best way for you to live actively. It is also highly recommended that you have your blood pressure evaluated. If your reading is over 144/94, talk with your doctor before you start becoming much more physically active.

DELAY BECOMING MUCH MORE ACTIVE:
- if you are not feeling well because of a temporary illness such as a cold or a fever – wait until you feel better; or
- if you are or may be pregnant – talk to your doctor before you start becoming more active.

PLEASE NOTE: If your health changes so that you then answer YES to any of the above questions, tell your fitness or health professional. Ask whether you should change your physical activity plan.

<u>Informed Use of the PAR-Q</u>: The Canadian Society for Exercise Physiology, Health Canada, and their agents assume no liability for persons who undertake physical activity, and if in doubt after completing this questionnaire, consult your doctor prior to physical activity.

No changes permitted. You are encouraged to photocopy the PAR-Q but only if you use the entire form.

NOTE: If the PAR-Q is being given to a person before he or she participates in a physical activity program or a fitness appraisal, this section may be used for legal or administrative purposes.

"I have read, understood and completed this questionnaire. Any questions I had were answered to my full satisfaction."

NAME _____

SIGNATURE _____ DATE _____

SIGNATURE OF PARENT _____ WITNESS _____
or GUARDIAN (for participants under the age of majority)

Note: This physical activity clearance is valid for a maximum of 12 months from the date it is completed and becomes invalid if your condition changes so that you would answer YES to any of the seven questions.

 CSEP | SCPE
THE HEALTH STANDARD IN EXERCISE SCIENCE AND PERSONAL TRAINING

© Canadian Society for Exercise Physiology www.csep.ca/forms

STATEMENT OF MEDICAL CLEARANCE FOR EXERCISE

Participant's name: _____

Address: _____

Date of birth: _____

Diagnosis: _____

Physician's name: _____

Address: _____

Telephone number: _____

☐ Yes. My patient _____ has no current unstable medical problems that are a contraindication to participating in an exercise or resistance-training program. I approve of and support his or her participation in this progressive strength, balance, and flexibility-training exercise program.

Comments: _____

_____

_____

☐ No. My patient _____ is not eligible to participate in the exercise program due to his or her current medical status.

Comments: _____

_____

_____

Please indicate any special recommendations or specific comments:

_____

_____

_____

_____

_____   _____

Physician's signature   Date

From E. Best-Martini and K.A. Jones-DiGenova, 2014, *Exercise for frail elders*, 2nd ed. (Champaign, IL: Human Kinetics).

COVER LETTER TO PHYSICIAN

(For use with the medical clearance form, appendix A2.)

_____ [*Date*]

Dear Dr. _____,

Your patient, _____, is interested in participating in an exercise class, which may include resistance training, at _____ [*name of facility*]. The goals of this program are to improve muscular strength, balance, and functional fitness in older adults.

We are enclosing a statement of medical clearance for exercise and request that you indicate your patient's eligibility for this program. Please be sure to include any specific exercise recommendations or adaptations to address your patient's needs.

If you have any questions regarding this exercise program or your patient's participation, please contact me at _____ [*Phone numbers*].

Thank you very much.

Sincerely,

_____ [*Name*]

_____ [*Title*]

MEDICAL HISTORY AND RISK FACTOR QUESTIONNAIRE

Date: _____

Name: _____ Age: _____

Emergency contact and phone number: _____

Medical history: Have you ever had, or do you currently have, any of the following?

- ☐ Abnormal EKG
- ☐ Anemia
- ☐ Arthritis
- ☐ Asthma
- ☐ Cancer
- ☐ Cardiac problems
- ☐ Chest pains
- ☐ Diabetes
- ☐ Emphysema
- ☐ Fainting
- ☐ High blood pressure
- ☐ High cholesterol
- ☐ Hypoglycemia
- ☐ Irregular heart beats
- ☐ Memory loss
- ☐ Osteoporosis
- ☐ Parkinson's disease
- ☐ Phlebitis
- ☐ Pulmonary disorder
- ☐ Shortness of breath
- ☐ Stroke (CVA)
- ☐ Injury to
    - ☐ shoulder
    - ☐ wrist
    - ☐ back
    - ☐ hip
    - ☐ knee
    - ☐ other: _____

(continued)

Medical History and Risk Factor Questionnaire *(continued)*

Do you take any medications? If so, please list all of them. _____

_____

_____

_____

_____

Are you experiencing any pain? ☐ NO ☐ YES   If yes, where is the pain felt?

_____

_____

Do you have any movement limitations? ☐ NO ☐ YES   If yes, please describe.

_____

_____

Are you currently receiving physical, occupational, or speech therapy? ☐ NO ☐ YES   If yes, what type and for what reason?

_____

_____

Do you consider yourself active, moderately active, slightly active, or sedentary (inactive)? (Circle one.)

Active   Moderately active   Slightly active   Sedentary (inactive)

Describe how often, how intensely (light, moderate, hard), and how long you exercise. What type of exercise do you do? _____

_____

List one fitness goal that you would like to achieve:

_____

_____

Are there any physical movements that you would like to be able to do more easily (for example, scratching your back, picking something up off the floor)? If so, please list them.

_____

_____

Thanks for your time and information!

EXERCISE PROGRAM INFORMED CONSENT

The risks and benefits of this exercise program have been reviewed and explained to me. I understand and confirm that I will choose the level of activity that will not harm me. In consideration of my participation in this exercise program, I hereby release

_____ [*name of facility*], its officers, employees, or agents from any liability for my personal injury or otherwise, arising out of or in any way connected to my participation in this exercise program.

Name: _____ Date: _____

Phone numbers: _____

Signature: _____

FITNESS LEADER'S LOG

Name: _____

Diagnosis from physician: _____

Medications: _____

Physician's or physical therapist's special recommendations: _____

_____

Exercise clearance forms completed: ☐ Informed consent ☐ Questionnaire ☐ Medical clearance form
☐ PAR-Q

Contact person and phone number: _____

Comments	Date	Fitness and modified goals

From E. Best-Martini and K.A. Jones-DiGenova, 2014, *Exercise for frail elders*, 2nd ed. (Champaign, IL: Human Kinetics).

Teaching Aids and Educational Handouts

BENEFITS OF PHYSICAL ACTIVITY FOR OLDER PERSONS

Physiological Benefits

Immediate Benefits

- **Glucose levels**: Physical activity helps regulate blood glucose levels.
- **Catecholamine activity**: Both adrenaline and noradrenaline levels are stimulated by physical activity.
- **Improved sleep**: Physical activity has been shown to enhance sleep quality and quantity in individuals of all ages.

Long-Term Effects

- **Aerobic and cardiovascular endurance**: Substantial improvements in almost all aspects of cardiovascular functioning have been observed following appropriate physical training.

- **Resistive training and muscle strengthening**: People of all ages can benefit from muscle-strengthening exercises. Resistance training can have a significant effect on the maintenance of independence in old age.
- **Flexibility**: Exercise that stimulates movement throughout the range of motion assists in the preservation and restoration of flexibility.
- **Balance and coordination**: Regular activity helps prevent or postpone the age-associated declines in balance and coordination that are a major risk factor for falls.
- **Velocity of movement**: Behavioral slowing is a characteristic of advancing age. People who are regularly active can often postpone these age-related declines.

Psychological Benefits

Immediate Benefits

- **Relaxation**: Appropriate physical activity enhances relaxation.
- **Reduces stress and anxiety**: Evidence shows that regular physical activity can reduce stress and anxiety.
- **Enhanced mood state**: Numerous people report improvement in mood state following appropriate physical activity.

Long-Term Effects

- **General well-being**: Improvements in almost all aspects of psychological functioning have been observed following periods of extended physical activity.

- **Improved mental health**: Regular exercise can make an important contribution in the treatment of several mental illnesses, including depression and anxiety neurosis.
- **Cognitive improvements**: Regular physical activity may help postpone age-related declines in central nervous system processing speed and improve reaction time.
- **Motor control and performance**: Regular activity helps prevent or postpone the age-associated declines in both fine and gross motor performance.
- **Skills acquisition**: New skills can be learned and existing skills refined by all people regardless of age.

From E. Best-Martini and K.A. Jones-DiGenova, 2014, *Exercise for frail elders*, 2nd ed. (Champaign, IL: Human Kinetics). Adapted from World Health Organization, 1997, "The Heidelberg guidelines for promoting physical activity among older persons." *Journal of Aging and Physical Activity* 5(1):2-8. The WHO guidelines have been placed in the public domain and can be freely copied and distributed.

MUSCLES OF THE HUMAN BODY

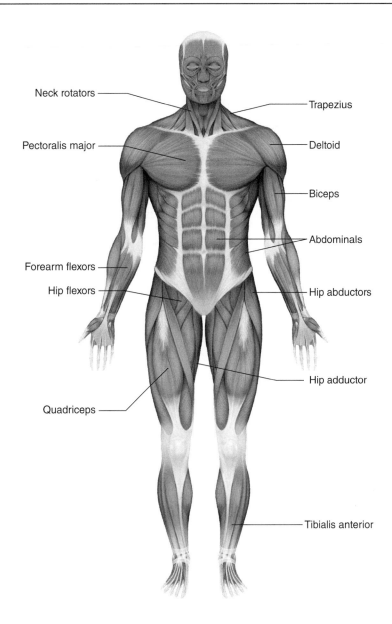

Neck rotators — Trapezius

Pectoralis major — Deltoid

Biceps

Abdominals

Forearm flexors

Hip flexors — Hip abductors

Hip adductor

Quadriceps

Tibialis anterior

From E. Best-Martini and K.A. Jones-DiGenova, 2014, *Exercise for frail elders*, 2nd ed. (Champaign, IL: Human Kinetics).

(continued)

Muscles of the Human Body   *(continued)*

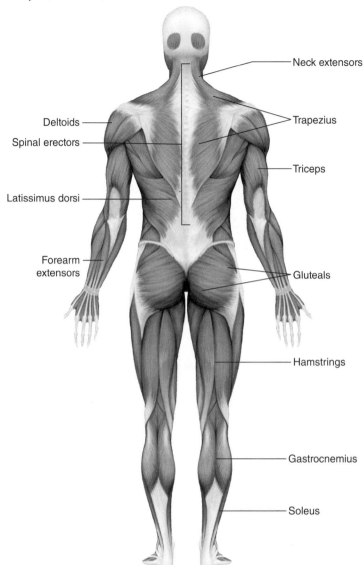

Neck extensors

Deltoids

Spinal erectors

Latissimus dorsi

Forearm extensors

Trapezius

Triceps

Gluteals

Hamstrings

Gastrocnemius

Soleus

CUEING FOR SAFE AND CONSTRUCTIVE BIOMECHANICS DURING EXERCISE AND ACTIVITIES OF DAILY LIVING (ADL)

Body part or joint	General cueing for safe and constructive biomechanics
Feet	Place the feet a comfortable distance apart (between hips and shoulders) and symmetrical. The weight of the body should be evenly distributed on the feet, front to back and side to side.
Knees	Keep the knees soft (not bent) and not locked while standing and during a straight-leg position of an exercise or ADL. Keep the knees behind the toes with squats or Modified Chair Stand exercises or squatting or lunging outside class.
Hips and pelvis	Slowly tilt the pelvis forward and then backward (staying within a comfortable ROM and not collapsing the torso). Continue until you find a neutral spine. (Refer to exercise 4.21 for instructions for Pelvic Tilt.)
Vertebral column[a]	Maintain a neutral spine, the natural curves of the spine, except when an exercise requires spinal movement, such as Pelvic Tilt and Back Arch (Challenger). In general, emphasize spinal extension and deemphasize spinal flexion (commonly known as slumping).
Neck	Maintain the natural cervical curve with the chin parallel with the floor, except when an exercise requires neck movement, such as Chin to Chest ROM (exercise 4.19) and Chin to Chest stretch (exercise 7.1). Do not circumduct, or roll, the neck (more commonly known as head rolls).
Shoulders	Set or stabilize the shoulders. Move them up, back, and down and keep the shoulders gently down (away from the ears), except when an exercise requires shoulder elevation, such as Shoulder Shrugs and Shoulder Rotation. This relaxation tip is helpful throughout the day.
Elbows	Keep the elbows soft (not bent) and not locked, during a straight-arm position of an exercise or ADL.
Wrists	Maintain a neutral or straight wrist ("wrist of steel") with each resistance exercise, except forearm exercises that require wrist movement. Computer typing is a typical ADL for which neutral wrists are beneficial.
Hands	Do not grip resistance devices or other objects with ADL too tightly. Keep hands as relaxed as possible and practical.

[a]See figure 4.2, the natural curves of the spine, and instructions for seated and standing posture exercises in chapter 4. A primary objective of the posture exercises is to find the natural curves of the spine—a neutral spine.

From E. Best-Martini and K.A. Jones-DiGenova, 2014, *Exercise for frail elders*, 2nd ed. (Champaign, IL: Human Kinetics).

EXERCISE EQUIPMENT

Type of equipment	Exercise component	Special needs and adaptations	Where to get, how to use, and other considerations
Ankle and wrist weights	Resistance training	Wrist weights are better than hand weights for beginner frail elders, adults with arthritis in their hands, and those with hemiparesis or hemiplegia from a stroke.	The weight is worn on the wrist and does not need to be held in the hand.
Balls, small rubber (5–10 inches, or 13–25 cm, in diameter)	Warm-ups Resistance training	Balls develop coordination and increase hand strength. They are helpful before using dumbbells. Smaller balls can be held by those having contractures in their hands.	Start the warm-up with one ball per participant, to be used for hand exercises. Participants can also pass the balls around the circle.
Balance balls (large for sitting) (small for holding)	Balance	Balls can be used with a stand to provide safety for the seated participant.	Have participants sit on large ball and shift weight from one side to the other. They can hold a small ball and move it from side to side while balancing on the ball.
Balance disc	Balance	Some participants may need chairs with arms.	Sit on for part or all of seated exercise class.
Beanbags (large)	Warm-ups Resistance training Stretching	Beanbags can improve body awareness, posture, and balance of all participants, especially those with stroke or neurological disorders resulting in loss of sensation. They are good for proprioception (awareness of posture and changes of equilibrium during exercises).	Large beanbags, for sitting on the floor, are recommended only with physician or physical therapist approval.
Box lids	Warm-ups Resistance training Stretching	Box lids are helpful for people whose legs cannot touch the floor when seated.	Place in front of the chair so that the participant can exercise with the feet firmly planted.
Cans (food) of different sizes	Resistance training	Cans can be used instead of dumbbells.	Use with caution if the participant has arthritis in the hands or cannot hold can firmly.
Chairs	All	A chair with a vertical, straight back can aid the participant in achieving proper posture.	
Dowels, wooden (2–4 feet, or 60–120 cm, long)	ROM Resistance training	The length depends on the ROM of participants.	Use a light dowel for ROM exercises.
Dumbbells (also called free weights or hand weights)	Resistance training	For those who have problems holding on to a dumbbell, weights with handles can be easier to hold (see ankle and wrist weights).	Cast-iron dumbbells are the least expensive type of free weights. They are commonly available in the United States in weights of 1, 2, 3, 5, 8, 10, 12, and 15 pounds (.45, .9, 1.4, 2.3, 3.6, 4.5, 5.4, 6.8 kg) (and more).

Type of equipment	Exercise component	Special needs and adaptations	Where to get, how to use, and other considerations
			Neoprene and vinyl-covered weights typically come in weights from 1 to 12 pounds in 1-pound increments, and each weight is a different color—a fun extrinsic motivator, but they are significantly more expensive than cast-iron weights.
Handkerchiefs, scarves	Warm-ups Stretching Aerobics Balance	Handkerchiefs and scarves are good for visual stimulation. To inspire liveliness and fun during aerobics, participants can hold an end of the hankie or scarf with one hand and wave it about (changing hands occasionally).	Good visual reminders to use full ROM movements. **Seated**: Sit tall without touching the back of the chair. Throw the scarf into the air and catch it, keeping good seated posture. **Standing**: Throw the scarf up and catch it while keeping good standing posture. (Having a scarf in each hand provides more of a challenge.)
Microphone	Warm-ups Aerobics Resistance training Stretching	A microphone allows those with hearing loss to hear the instructor.	A cordless microphone is ideal, because the fitness leader can move around and be heard clearly by all in the class.
Mirrors	Warm-ups Aerobics Resistance training Stretching	Participants who have had a stroke are often unaware of the affected side of their bodies. A mirror helps bring both sides together for them. Be aware that some participants with dementia do not feel comfortable with their reflection in a mirror.	A mirror on a wall or door enables participants to watch their technique.
Paper plates	Resistance training Balance	Paper plate are useful for those with arthritis.	Create gentle air resistance by holding them during exercises. Have participants place the plate on their head with the chin up and hold the pose. Place the plate upside down for more stability and ease.
Parachutes	ROM	Some parachutes have handles, and others do not. Be aware of participants who have limited ROM or who cannot hold on to the parachute for long.	Use for group and team play.
Pinwheels	Breathing exercises Relaxation	These multisensory tools are helpful for those with COPD or with dementia or vision loss.	Useful for breathing exercises and for visual stimulation.

(continued)

Exercise Equipment   *(continued)*

Type of equipment	Exercise component	Special needs and adaptations	Where to get, how to use, and other considerations
Plastic water bottles (20 ounces [600 ml] or less), filled with water, pennies, or sand	Resistance training	Frail participants should start with .5-pound (.2 kg) weights.	If the water bottles are sealed, drink the water after resistance training.
Puttylike substances	Resistance training	This item is good for participants who have arthritis in the hands or hemiparesis or hemiplegia from a stroke.	Good for hand contractures and hand exercises.
Resistance bands	Resistance training Stretching	Resistance bands are ideal for participants at risk of dropping hand weights. Bands or tubes with handles can be easier to hold for people with arthritis in their hands or hemiparesis or hemiplegia from a stroke. Avoid placing bands or tubes around the legs and feet of those with diabetes, especially those with neuropathy.	Store in a dark, dry, cool place. Inspect them before using for holes or tears; discard damaged ones. Sharp objects (e.g., long fingernails and rings) can damage bands. Use firmer bands or tubes as a stretching prop. You can make handles with a loop and a knot in longer bands and tubes. For more information, see "Suggested Resources."
Riverstones	Balance	Colorful props are good for seated and standing exercises.	**Seated**: Place one in front of a chair. Place the feet on a riverstone, press down, and then shift weight from one foot to the other. See www.flaghouse.com.
Ropes (soft)	Stretching	Ropes are helpful for those with limited ROM and flexibility.	Soft ropes can be used for upper- and lower-extremity exercises. Longer ropes work better for participants with limited ROM.
Socks, filled with beans or rice	Resistance training	Socks are useful for frail participants or those with dementia or arthritis in the hands.	Participants who are at risk of dropping hand weights can feel success by progressing from learning the resistance exercise with body weight to using hand weights in the form of filled socks.
Sponges (large and small)	Warm-ups Resistance training	Sponges have enough give to them that a frail participant can feel the effect of their motion on the sponge.	Large sponges can be squeezed between the knees as an isometric exercise, if this is safe for a participant. Smaller sponges can be used for hand and under-the-arm exercises.
Spot markers	Warm-ups Aerobics Balance	These are good for seated and standing exercises.	These plastic round disks are placed on floor and used as visual props (www.flaghouse.com).
Towels	Warm-ups Aerobics Resistance training	Towels are helpful to extend the reach of those with limited ROM and flexibility. A folded towel can be placed under the feet of those whose legs do not touch the floor when seated.	Towels can be used for upper- and lower-extremity exercises. Longer towels work better for participants with limited ROM. Shorter towels are better for hand exercises.

A cart with wheels is recommended for storing and transporting exercise supplies.

From E. Best-Martini and K.A. Jones-DiGenova, 2014, *Exercise for frail elders*, 2nd ed. (Champaign, IL: Human Kinetics).

FITNESS TRAINING LOG

Name: _____

- The eight exercises marked by an asterisk are recommended for a shorter program.
- Use blank spaces for writing in alternative exercises or variations.
- Strengthen abdominal (postural) muscles by performing these exercises with the abs gently contracted, while gradually building up to sitting erect and not leaning against the back of the chair.
- Always warm up before and cool down after aerobics and dynamic balance or resistance training. Happy exercising!

Resistance training and aerobics and dynamic balance		Date		Date		Date		Date		Date		Date		Date		Date		Date		Date	
Body region	Resistance exercise	W	R	W	R	W	R	W	R	W	R	W	R	W	R	W	R	W	R	W	R
Chest Arms Shoulders	*5.1 Chest Press																				
Back Arms Shoulders	*5.2 Two-Arm Row																				
Shoulders Arms	*5.3 Overhead Press																				
Upper arms	5.4 Biceps Curl																				
	5.5 Triceps Extension[C]																				
Hip Upper leg	*5.6 Hip Flexion																				
	*5.7 Hip Abduction and Hip Adduction																				
	5.8 Knee Flexion																				
	5.9 Knee Extension																				
	*5.12 Modified Chair Stands[C]																				
Lower leg	*5.10 Toe Raises																				
	*5.11 Heel Raises																				
Aerobics and dynamic balance (minutes)																					
Notes:																					

Key: [C] = challenger exercise; W = weight; R = repetitions.

From E. Best-Martini and K.A. Jones-DiGenova, 2014, *Exercise for frail elders*, 2nd ed. (Champaign, IL: Human Kinetics).

APPENDIX
C

Professional Development

PROFESSIONAL ETHICS FOR GROUP FITNESS TRAINERS
IDEA Code of Ethics

As a member of IDEA Health & Fitness Association, I will be guided by the best interests of the client and will practice within the scope of my education and knowledge. I will maintain the education and experience necessary to appropriately teach classes, will behave in a positive and constructive manner, and will use truth, fairness, and integrity to guide all my professional decisions and relationships.

Ethical Practice Guidelines for Group Fitness Trainers

1. Always be guided by the best interests of the group, while acknowledging individuals.

a. Remember that a group fitness instructor's primary obligation is to the group as a whole, taking class level and class description into account.

b. Strive to provide options and realistic goals that take individual variations into account.

c. Offer modifications for all levels of fitness and experience (i.e., demonstrate easy and more challenging options).

d. Recommend products or services only if they will benefit a client's health and well-being, not because they will benefit you or your employer financially or occupationally.

2. Provide a safe exercise environment.

a. Prioritize all movement choices by (1) safety, (2) effectiveness, and (3) creativity. Do not allow creativity to compromise safety.

b. Use good judgment in exercise selection. Assess all class moves according to risk versus reward, making sure rewards and benefits always outweigh risks.

c. Adhere to safe guidelines for music speed in all classes.

d. Follow guidelines for maximum music volume. IDEA recommends that "music intensity during group exercise classes should measure no more than 90 decibels (dB). Since the instructor's voice needs to be about 10dB louder than the music in order to be heard, the instructor's voice should measure no more than 100dB."

e. Consider whether exercises that can be properly monitored in a one-to-one setting are appropriate in a group environment.

3. Obtain the education and training necessary to lead group exercise.

a. Continuously strive to keep abreast of the latest research and exercise techniques essential to providing effective and safe classes.

b. Maintain certifications and continuing education.

c. Obtain specific training for teaching specialty classes or instructing special populations. Teach a class such as kickboxing or yoga only after mastering the skill and understanding the important aspects of the class. Instruct a special population, like older adults or perinatal women, only after studying the specific needs of the group.

d. Work within the scope of your knowledge and skill. When necessary, refer participants to professionals with appropriate training and expertise beyond your realm of knowledge.

(continued)

Professional Ethics for Group Fitness Trainers   *(continued)*

4. Use truth, fairness, and integrity to guide all professional decisions and relationships.

   a. In all professional and business relationships, clearly demonstrate and support honesty, integrity, and trustworthiness.

   b. Speak in a positive manner about fellow instructors, other staff, participants, and competitive facilities and organizations, or say nothing at all.

   c. When disagreements or conflicts occur, focus on behavior, factual evidence, and nonderogatory forms of communication, not on judgmental statements, hearsay, the placing of blame, or other destructive responses.

   d. Accurately represent your certifications, training, and education.

   e. Do not discriminate based on race, creed, color, gender, age, physical handicap, or nationality.

5. Maintain appropriate professional boundaries.

   a. Never exploit—sexually, economically, or otherwise—a professional relationship with a supervisor, an employee, a colleague, or a client.

   b. Use physical touching appropriately during training sessions, as a means of correcting alignment or focusing a client's concentration on the targeted area. Immediately discontinue the use of touch at a client's request or if the client displays signs of discomfort.

   c. Avoid sexually oriented banter and inappropriate physical contact.

6. Uphold a professional image through conduct and appearance.

   a. Model behavior that values physical ability, function, and health over appearance.

   b. Demonstrate healthy behaviors and attitudes about bodies (including your own). Avoid smoking, substance abuse, and unhealthy exercise and eating habits.

   c. Encourage healthful eating for yourself and others.

   d. Dress in a manner that allows you to perform your job while increasing the comfort level of class participants. Be more conservative in dress, decorum, and speech when the class standard is unclear.

   e. Establish a mood in class that encourages and supports individual effort and all levels of expertise.

ANSWERS TO REVIEW QUESTIONS

Chapter 1

1. Nine possible answers:
   - overview of aging and physical activity
   - psychological, sociocultural, and physiological aspects of physical activity and older adults
   - screening, assessment, and goal setting
   - program design and management
   - program design for older adults with stable medical conditions
   - teaching skills
   - leadership, communication, and marketing skills
   - client safety and first aid
   - ethics and professional conduct

2. f

3. Nine possible characteristics of dementia:
   - short attention span
   - overreaction to situations
   - difficulty communicating
   - spatial or perceptual problems
   - apraxia
   - need for visual and tactile cues
   - balance problems
   - anxiety and depression
   - misunderstanding or overstimulation

4. osteoarthritis

5. Emphysema, chronic bronchitis, asthma

6. d

7. Definitions of the following symptoms of Parkinson's disease:
   a. bradykinesia—slow movements
   b. festination—acceleration or abbreviation of walking movements
   c. dyskinesia—uncontrolled movements
   d. ataxia—shaking movements of limbs

8. f

Chapter 2

1. (a) Intrinsic goals come from within the individual and are self-directed motivators—for example, "I want to walk a mile a day to build up my endurance." (b) Extrinsic goals are external motivators such as pursing training to achieve a certification that will be good for my profession.

2. A fitness goal that is realistic, specific, measurable, and time based: Participant will be able to lift 2-pound (.9 kg) weights with shoulder lifts within 2 months.

(continued)

Answers to Review Questions   *(continued)*

3. Participant will be able to lift 2-pound (.9 kg) weights with shoulder lift within 2 months unless symptoms of rheumatoid arthritis are present. If symptoms are present, participant will use only the body as resistance.

4. Functional fitness is the ability to perform activities of daily living such as pushing, pulling, lifting, squatting, balancing, sitting, and standing erect.

5. Nine symptoms:
   - unconsciousness
   - difficulty breathing
   - persistent chest pain or pressure
   - severe bleeding
   - seizures
   - severe headache
   - slurred speech
   - broken bones
   - spinal injuries

6. c

7. Four components to an effective exercise program and their benefits:
   a. warm-ups—increase internal body temperature
   b. resistance training—build muscular strength
   c. aerobics—improve cardiorespiratory endurance
   d. cool-down—improve flexibility and relaxation

8. Physically elite, physically fit, physically independent, physically frail, physically dependent

9. Physical, emotional, creative expressive, cultural, vocational, cognitive, social, spiritual, and environmental wellness

Chapter 3

1. Setup
   - Arrange chairs and allow space for wheelchairs within a circle.
   - Avoid seating people facing a glare from the window.
   - Seat participants so that everyone can see the leader.
   - Identify a space to store walkers.

2. Music may be too distracting, may drown out instructions, may overstimulate.

3. Steps of the instructional process:
   - Demonstrate and describe exercise.
   - Observe and evaluate each participant.
   - Give group and individual feedback.

4. T

5. expressive, receptive, global

6. Cognitive

7. Use gestures, check that the participant is wearing glasses, seat the participant near the leader, offer large print instructions.

Chapter 4

1. f
2. neck
3. vertebral
4. e
5. neutral
6. mental focus
7. 10
8. e

Chapter 5

1. The benefits of a well-rounded resistance-training program include the following:
   - Improved posture
   - Improved balance
   - Preventing or even reversing the usual decline in strength
   - Improved ability to perform daily activities that require strength
2. Counting aloud, practicing optimal breathing.
3. This knowledge can help participants focus on the body part or muscles they are strengthening.
4. The exercises are matched as follows:

   d. 5.1 Chest Press
   e. 5.2 Two-Arm Row
   b. 5.3 Overhead Press
   c. 5.4 Biceps Curl
   a. 5.5 Triceps Extension

   l. 5.6 Hip Flexion
   f. 5.7 Hip Abduction and Adduction
   g. 5.8 Knee Flexion
   k. 5.9 Knee Extension
   j. 5.10 Toe Raises
   h. 5.11 Heel Raises
   i. 5.12 Chair Stands

5. Remember the mnemonic ABCD
   - *a*bnormal heart rhythm
   - shortness of *b*reath
   - *c*hest discomfort (or pain)
   - *d*izziness
6. 4, no
7. g
8. 12

Chapter 6

1. The five keys are:

   a. Individualization: Personalizing training to match the individual participant's health and fitness status, skill level, and training tolerance.

   b. Integration of training variables: Employing intensity, frequency, and duration in a way that permits gradual, progressive training.

(continued)

Answers to Review Questions   *(continued)*

  c. Inclusion of essential components: Ensuring that an aerobics segment includes an initial warm-up period, the aerobic exercises, and a cool-down period.

  d. Safety awareness: Following established safety guidelines to help keep aerobics participants injury-free.

  e. Creativity: Including enjoyable features such as music, variety, and fun in order to foster a stimulating, motivational environment.

2. T

3. F

4. Alternate energetic training periods with easy training periods, accumulate the desired duration by performing short bouts of exercise throughout the day, or work at an intensity near the lower end of the desirable range.

5. e

6. frequency, duration

7. static

Chapter 7

1. Benefits of the cool-down:
   - facilitates the transition between exercise and rest
   - promotes flexibility and relaxation
   - slowly lowers the heart rate
   - promotes cardiorespiratory endurance

2. General safety precautions for stretching:
   - Do not move a joint beyond its strain-free and pain-free range of motion.
   - Avoid hyperextending (locking) any joints, particularly the elbow and knee.
   - Avoid exercises with two feet off the floor, which can strain the lower back.
   - Continually encourage your participants to maintain good posture and breathing (no breath holding).

3. heart

4. flexion, dislocation

5. demonstration, describe

6. The exercises are matched as follows:

   c. 7.1 Chin to Chest

   b. 7.2 Chin to Shoulder

   d. 7.3 Swan

   e. 7.4 Half Hug

   a. 7.5 Zipper Stretch

   g. 7.6 Side Bends

   f. 7.7 Spinal Twist

   j. 7.8 Tib Touches

   k. 7.9 Quad Stretch

   l. 7.10 Seated Splits and Standing Half-Splits

   i. 7.11 Outer-Thigh Stretch

   h. 7.12 Calf Stretch

7. F

8. Guided imagery

Chapter 8

1. f

2. T. Why? Helpful for reinforcing good exercise technique and preventing overtraining and injury.

3. e

4. Approximate length for each segment of a 60-minute resistance-training class:

Activity	Time (minutes)
Opening	5
Warm-up	10
Resistance training	30
Cool-down	10
Closing	5

5. Four ways to extend a single warm-up, resistance-training, aerobic, or stretching component into an entire class:

   a. Repeat some of your participants' favorite exercises.

   b. Repeat some or all of the basic exercises.

   c. Add variations of some or all of the exercises.

   d. Increase the number of repetitions of an exercise.

6. Five ways five ways to modify an exercise using the **A** to **E** mnemonic:

   a. **A**djust the speed of the movement.

   b. **B**ody position, adjust.

   c. **C**onsult the physician or physical therapist.

   d. **D**ecrease the workload.

   e. **E**xercise technique, adjust.

7. needs (or synonym of needs)

8. f

Day, L., B. Fildes, I. Gordon, M. Fitzharris, H. Flamer, and S. Lord. 2002. Randomized factorial trial of falls prevention among older people living in their own homes. *BMJ* 325 (7356): 128. www.bmj.com/content/325/7356/128.full.

Decoster L.C., J. Cleland, C. Altieri, and P. Russell. 2005. The effects of hamstring stretching on range of motion: a systematic literature review. *Journal of Orthopaedic and Sports Physical Therapy* 35 (6): 377–387.

Delavier, F. 2003. *Women's strength training anatomy*. Champaign, IL: Human Kinetics.

Delavier, F. 2006. *Strength training anatomy*, 2nd ed. Champaign, IL: Human Kinetics.

Delavier, F. 2012. *Core training anatomy*. Champaign, IL: Human Kinetics.

de Vos, N.J., N.A. Singh, D.A. Ross, T.M. Stavrinos, R. Orr, and M.A. Fiatarone-Singh. 2005. Optimal load for increasing muscle power during explosive resistance training in older adults. *Journals of Gerontology Series A: Biological Sciences and Medical Sciences* 60 (5): 638–647.

Diamond, J. 1996. *Exercises for airplanes (and other confined spaces)*. New York: Excalibur.

Dunn, A.L., M.H. Trivedi, and H.A. O'Neal. 2001. Physical activity dose-response effects on outcomes of depression and anxiety. *Medicine and Science in Sports and Exercise* 33 (6): S587–S597.

Ecclestone, N.A., and C.J. Jones. 2004. The international curriculum guidelines for preparing physical activity instructors of older adults. *Journal of Aging and Physical Activity* 12, 5.

Ehsani, A.A. 1987. Cardiovascular adaptations to endurance exercise training in ischemic heart disease. *Exercise and Sport Sciences Review* 15: 53–66.

Evans, W.J. 1999. Exercise training guidelines for the elderly. *Medicine and Science in Sports and Exercise* 31 (1): 12–17.

Feigenbaum, M.S., and M.L. Pollock. 1999. Prescription of resistance training for health and disease. *Medicine and Science in Sports and Exercise* 31 (1): 38–45.

Feland, J.B., J.W. Myrer, S.S. Schulthies, G.W. Fellingham, and G.W. Measom. 2001. The effect of duration of stretching of the hamstring muscle group for increasing range of motion in people aged 65 years or older. *Physical Therapy* 81 (5): 1110–1117. http://ptjournal.apta.org/content/81/5/1110.full.pdf+html.

Fiatarone, M. et al. 1994. Exercise training and nutritional supplementation for physical frailty in very elderly people. *New England Journal of Medicine* 330: 1769–75.

Frontera, W.R., D. Slovik, and D. Dawson. 2006. *Exercise in rehabilitation medicine*, 2nd ed. Champaign, IL: Human Kinetics.

Garber, C.E., B. Blissmer, M.R. Deschenes, B.A. Franklin, M.J. Lamonte, I. Lee, D.C. Nieman, and D.P. Swain. 2011. Quantity and quality of exercise for developing and maintaining cardiorespiratory, musculoskeletal, and neuromotor fitness in apparently healthy adults: Guidance for prescribing exercise. *Medicine and Science in Sports and Exercise* 43: 7 (July): 1334–1359.

Gardner, M.M., M.C. Robertson, and A.J. Campbell. 2000. Exercise in preventing falls and fall related injuries in older people: A review of randomized controlled trials. *British Journal of Sports Medicine* 34: 7–17.

Gregg, E.W., M.A. Pereira, and C.J. Caspersen. 2000. Physical activity, falls and fractures among older adults: A review of the epidemiologic evidence. *Journal of the American Geriatrics Society* 48: 883–893.

Gordon, N., M. Gulanick, F. Costa, et al. 2004. Physical activity and exercise recommendations for stroke survivors: An American Heart Association scientific statement from the Council on Clinical Cardiology, Subcommittee on Exercise, Cardiac Rehabilitation, and Prevention; the Council on Cardiovascular Nursing; the Council on Nutrition, Physical Activity, and Metabolism; and the stroke council. *Circulation* 109 (16): 2031–2041. http://circ.ahajournals.org/content/109/16/2031.full.

Hall, C.M., and L.T. Brody. 2010. *Therapeutic exercise: Moving toward function*, 3rd ed. Philadelphia: Lippincott Williams and Wilkins.

Haskell, W.L. 2001. What to look for in assessing responsiveness to exercise in a health context. *Medicine and Science in Sports and Exercise* 33 (6): S454–S458.

Hawley, J.A., and J.R. Zierath. 2008. *Physical activity and type 2 diabetes*. Champaign, IL: Human Kinetics.

Health Care Financing Administration. 1999. *HCFA's quality indicators and new survey pro-*

cedures. State Operations Manual Provider Certification (Transmittal No. 10, July 1999). Washington, DC: Health Care Financing Administration.

Healy, G.N., D.W. Dunstan, J. Salmon E. Cerin, et al. 2008. Breaks in sedentary time: beneficial association with metabolic risk. *Diabetes Care* 31 (4): 661–666.

Healy, G.N., D.W. Dunstan, J. Salmon, P.Z. Zimmet, and N. Owen. 2008. Television time and continuous metabolic risk in physically active adults. *Medicine and Science in Sports and Exercise* 40 (4): 639–645.

Hess, J.A., and M. Woollacott. 2005. Effect of high-intensity strength-training on functional measures of balance ability in balance-impaired older adults. *Journal of Manipulative and Physiological Therapeutics* 28: 582–590.

Heyward, V.H. 2010. *Advanced fitness assessment and exercise prescription*, 6th ed. Champaign, IL: Human Kinetics.

Houglum, P.A. 2010. *Therapeutic exercise for musculoskeletal injuries*, 3rd ed. Champaign, IL: Human Kinetics.

Hyatt, G. 2010. *Exercise and diabetes*, 4th ed. Tucson, AZ: Desert Southwest Fitness.

Hyatt, G., and K.P. Nelson. 2012. *Exercise and arthritis*, 5th ed. Tucson, AZ: Desert Southwest Fitness.

International Council on Active Aging (ICAA). 2008. Blueprint for wellness. *Journal on Active Aging* 7 (2): 66–75.

International Council on Active Aging (ICAA). 2010a. Environmental wellness. *Journal on Active Aging* 9 (1): 8, 24–33.

International Council on Active Aging (ICAA). 2010b. The value of wellness. *Journal on Active Aging* 9 (4): 40–46.

International Council on Active Aging (ICAA). 2011. Industry news: HHS announces new health "roadmap and compass." *Journal on Active Aging* 9 (1): 18.

Jones, C.J., and D.J. Rose, eds. 2005. *Physical activity instruction of older adults*. Champaign, IL: Human Kinetics.

Kaiser Permanente. 2010. *Healthwise handbook*. Boise, ID: Healthwise.

Kalkstein, S. 2009. *Fortify your frame comprehensive exercise program*. Davie, FL: Keep the Beat.

Kaplanek, B.A. 2011. *Pilates for hip and knee syndromes and arthroplasties*. Champaign, IL: Human Kinetics.

Karinkanta, S., A. Heinonen, H. Sievanen, R. Uusi-Rasi, M. Pasanen, K Ojala, M. Fogelholm, and P. Kannus. 2007. A multi-component exercise regimen to prevent functional decline and bone fragility in home-dwelling elderly women: Randomized, controlled trail. *Osteoporosis International* 18 (4): 453–62.

Kelley, D.E., and B.H. Goodpaster. 2001. Effects of exercise on glucose homeostasis in type 2 diabetes mellitus. *Medicine and Science in Sports and Exercise* 33 (6): S495–S501.

Kesaniemi, Y.A., E. Danforth, Jr., M.D. Jensen, P.G. Kopelman, P. Lefebvre, and B.A. Reeder. 2001. Dose-response issues concerning physical activity and health: An evidence-based symposium. *Medicine and Science in Sports and Exercise* 33 (6): S351–S358.

Kouzes, J., and B. Posner. 2008. *The leadership challenge*, 4th ed. San Francisco: Jossey Bass.

Levine, P.G. 2009. *Stronger after stroke*. New York: Demos Medical.

Lorig, K., H. Holman, D. Sobel, D. Laurent, V. Gonzalez, and M. Minor. 2000. *Living a healthy life with chronic conditions: Self-management of heart disease, arthritis, diabetes, asthma, bronchitis, emphysema and others*, 2nd ed. Palo Alto, CA: Bull.

Marks, R., J.P. Allegrante, C.R. MacKenzie, and J.M. Lane. 2003. Hip fractures among the elderly: Causes, consequences and control. *Ageing Research Reviews* 2 (1): 57–93.

Mazzeo, R.S. 2001. Exercise prescription for the elderly: Current recommendations. *Sports Medicine* 31 (11): 809–818.

McArdle, W.D., F.I. Katch, and V.L. Katch. 2011. *Essentials of exercise physiology*, 4th ed. Baltimore: Lippincott Williams and Wilkins.

McCartney, N. 1999. Acute responses to resistance training and safety. *Medicine and Science in Sports and Exercise* 31 (1): 31–37.

MedicineNet. 2011. *Fitness: Exercise for a healthy heart*. www.medicinenet.com/fitness_exercise_for_a_healthy_heart/page2.htm.

Minne, H.W., and M. Pfeifer. 2005. *Invest in your bones. Move it or lose it*. Nyon, Switzerland: International Osteoporosis Foundation. www.iofbonehealth.org/sites/default/files/PDFs/WOD%20Reports/move_it_or_lose_it_en.pdf.

Miszko, T.A., M.E. Cress, J.M. Slade, C.J. Covey, S.K. Agrawal, and C.E. Doerr. 2003. Effect of strength and power training on physical function in community-dwelling older adults. *Journals of Gerontology Series A: Biological Sciences and Medical Sciences* 58 (2): 171–175.

Montague, J. *Whole person wellness for vital living.* 2011. American Senior Fitness Association. ASFA Archives, www.seniorfitness.net.

National Center on Physical Activity and Disability (NCPAD). 2009a. *Disability/condition: Multiple sclerosis and exercise.* www.ncpad.org/disability/fact_sheet.php?sheet=186&view=all.

———. 2009b. *Disability/condition: Parkinson's disease and exercise.* www.ncpad.org/disability/fact_sheet.php?sheet=59&view=all#4.

National Institute on Aging. 2000. *Older Americans.* Washington, DC: United States Department of Health and Human Services.

National Institutes of Health, Arthritis and Musculoskeletal and Skin Disease. 2011. Washington, DC: National Institutes of Health.

National Institutes of Health. 2002. Physical activity and cardiovascular health. *NIH Consensus Statement Online 101/101* 13 (3): 1–33. http://consensus.nih.gov/.

National Institute of Neurological Disorders and Stroke (NINDS). 2011. www.ninds.nih.gov/disorders/stroke/knowstroke.htm.

Nelson, M.E., W.J. Rejeski, S.N. Blair, P.W. Duncan, J.O. Judge, A.C. King, C.A. Macera, and C. Castaneda-Sceppa. 2007. Physical activity and public health in older adults: Recommendation from the American College of Sports and the American Heart Association. *Circulation* 116 (9): 1094–1105.

Nelson, M.E., and S. Wernick. 2000. *Strong women stay young,* rev. ed. New York: Bantam Books.

O'Connor, G.T., J.E. Buring, S. Yusuf, S.Z. Goldhaber, E.M. Olmstead, R.S. Paffenbarger, and C.H. Hennekens. 1989. An overview of randomized trials of rehabilitation with exercise after myocardial infarction. *Circulation* 80: 234–244.

Orr, R., N.J. de Vos, N.A. Singh, D.A. Ross, T.M. Stavrinos, and M.A. Fiatarone-Singh. 2006. Power training improves balance in healthy older adults. *The Journals of Gerontology Series A: Biological Sciences and Medical Sciences* 61 (1): 78–85.

Orr, R., J Raymond, and M. Fiatarone-Singh. 2008. Efficacy of progressive resistance training on balance performance in older adults.

A systematic review of randomized controlled trials. *Sports Medicine* 38 (4): 317–342.

Owen, N., G.N. Healy, C.E. Matthews, and D.W. Dunstan. 2010. Too much sitting: The population health science of sedentary behavior. *Exercise and Sport Science Reviews* 38 (3): 105–113.

Peterson, T.J. 2004. *SrFit: The personal trainer's resource for senior fitness.* Tonganoxie, KS: American Academy of Health and Fitness.

Picone, R.E. 2000. Improving functional flexibility. In *Maximize your training: Insights from leading strength and fitness professionals,* ed. M. Brzycki. Lincolnwood, IL: Masters Press.

Province, M.A., E.C. Hadley, M.C. Hornbrook, L.A. Lipsitz, J.P. Miller, C.D. Mulrow, M.G. Ory, R.W. Sattin, M.E. Tinetti, and S.L. Wolf. 1995. The effects of exercise on falls in elderly patients. A preplanned meta-analysis of the FICSIT trails. Frailty and injuries: Cooperative studies of intervention techniques. *JAMA* 273 (17): 1341–1347.

Pryse-Phillips, W. 1989. Infarction of the medulla and cervical cord after fitness exercises. *Stroke* 20: 292–294.

Rahl, R.L. 2010. *Physical activity and health guidelines.* Champaign, IL: Human Kinetics.

Reid, K.F., and R.A. Fielding. 2012. Skeletal muscle power: A critical determinant of physical functioning in older adults. *Exercise and Sport Sciences Reviews* 40 (1) 4–12.

Rickli, R.E., and J. Jones. 2013. *Senior fitness test manual.* Champaign, IL: Human Kinetics.

Rose, D.J. 2002. Promoting functional independence among "at risk" and physically frail older adults through community-based fall-risk-reduction programs. *Journal of Aging Physical Activity* 10 (2): 207–225. http://hhd.fullerton.edu/csa/Research/documents/Rose2002PromotingFunctionalIndependence_000.pdf.

Rose, D.J. 2010. *FallProof!: A comprehensive balance and mobility training program,* 2nd ed. Champaign, IL: Human Kinetics.

Rossman, M. 2010. *The worry solution: Using breakthrough brain science to turn anxiety and stress into confidence and happiness.* New York: Crown Archetype.

Rowe, R.L., and J.W. Kahn. 1998. *Successful aging.* New York: Dell.

Said, C.M., P.A. Goldie, A.E. Patla, E. Culham, W.A. Sparrow, and M.E. Morris. 2008. Balance during obstacle crossing following stroke. *Gait & Posture* 27 (1): 23–30.

Sayers, S.P. 2005. Resistance training in older adults: The importance of muscle power and speed of movement. *American Journal of Recreation Therapy* 4 (1): 21–26.

Scheller, M.D. 1993. *Growing older feeling better in body, mind and spirit*. Palo Alto, CA: Bull.

Schift, D. 2011. *Safe simple and effective exercises for seniors and the elderly*. www.eldergym.com.

Scott, S. 2008. *Able bodies balance training*. Champaign, IL: Human Kinetics.

Shigematsu, R., T. Okura, M. Nakagaichi, K. Tanaka, T. Sakai, S. Kitazumi, and T. Rantanen. 2008. Square-stepping exercise and fall risk factors in older adults: A single-blind, randomized controlled trial. *Journals of Gerontology Series A: Biological Sciences and Medical Sciences* 63 (1): 76–82.

Signorile, J.F. 2011. *Bending the aging curve*. Champaign, IL: Human Kinetics.

Singh, N., K. Clements, and M. Fiatarone. 1997. A randomized controlled trial of progressive resistance training in depressed elders. *Journals of Gerontology Series A: Biological Sciences and Medical Sciences* 52A (1): M27–M35.

Singh, N.A., K.M. Clements, and M.A. Singh. 2001. The efficacy of exercise as a long-term antidepressant in elderly subjects: a randomized controlled trial. *Journals of Gerontology Series A: Biological Sciences and Medical Sciences* 56 (8): M497–M504.

Spirduso, W., K. Francis, and P. Macrae. 2005. *Physical dimensions of aging*, 2nd ed. Champaign, IL: Human Kinetics.

St. Louis Psychologists and Counseling Information and Referral. 2011. *Depression and the elderly: United States and abroad*. www.psychtreatment.com.

Stroke Association. 2011. *Spot a stroke*. http://strokeassociation.org/STROKEORG/WarningSigns/Stroke-Warning-Signs-and-Symptoms_UCM_308528_SubHomePage.jsp.

Sullivan, D.H., P.T. Wall, J.R. Bariola, M.M. Bopp, and Y.M. Frost. 2001. Progressive resistance muscle strength training of hospitalized frail elderly. *American Journal of Physical Medicine and Rehabilitation* 80 (7): 503–509.

Swart, D.L., M.L. Pollock, and W.F. Brechue. 1996. Aerobic exercise for older participants. In *Exercise programming for older adults*, ed. J. Clark. New York: Haworth.

Takeshima, N., N.L. Rogers, M.E. Rogers, M.M. Islam, D. Koizumi, and S. Lee. 2007. Functional fitness gain varies in older adults depending on exercise mode. *Medicine and Science in Sports and Exercise* 39 (11): 2036–2043.

Taylor, A.W., and M.J. Johnson. 2008. *Physiology of exercise and healthy aging*. Champaign, IL: Human Kinetics.

Tennant, K.F. 2011. *Assessment of fatigue in older adults: The facit fatigue scale (version 4). Try this: Best practices in nursing care to older adults*. Hartford Institute for Geriatric Nursing, New York University, College of Nursing. Issue # 30.

Thompson, P.D., B.A. Franklin, G.J. Balady, S.N. Blair, D. Corrado, M. Estes III, J.E. Fulton, N.F. Gordon, W.L. Haskell, M.S. Link, B.J. Maron, M.A. Mittleman, A. Pelliccia, N.K. Wenger, S.N. Willich, and F. Costa. 2007. Exercise and acute cardiovascular events placing the risks into perspective: A scientific statement from the American Heart Association Council on Nutrition, Physical Activity, and Metabolism and the Council on Clinical Cardiology. *Circulation* 115 (17): 2358–2368.

University of Michigan: U.M. University Health Service. 2011. *Exercise*. www.uhs.umich.edu/exercise.

U.S. Department of Health and Human Services (USDHHS). 2002. *Physical activity and older adults: Benefits and strategies*. Agency for Healthcare Research and Quality and the Centers for Disease Control. www.ahrq.gov/legacy/ppip/activity.htm.

U.S. Department of Health and Human Services (USDHHS). 2008a. *Healthy people 2010*, 2nd ed. With *Understanding and improving health and objectives for improving health*. 2 vols. Washington, DC: U.S. Government Printing Office.

U.S. Department of Health and Human Services (USDHHS). 2008b. *2008 Physical activity guidelines for Americans*. Washington, DC: U.S. Department of Health and Human Services. www.health.gov/paguidelines.

U.S. Department of Health and Human Services (USDHSS). 2010a. *Healthy people 2020*. Washington, DC: U.S. Government Printing Office. www.cdc.gov/nchs/healthy_people/hp2020.htm.

U.S. Department of Health and Human Services (USDHHS). 2010b. *The Surgeon General's vision for a healthy and fit nation*. Rockville (MD): HHS, Public Health Service, Office of the Surgeon General. Also available from: URL: www.surgeongeneral.gov/library/obesityvision/obesityvision2010.pdf.

U.S. Surgeon General. 1996. *Physical activity and health: A report of the surgeon general*. Atlanta, GA: U.S. Department of Health and Human Services, Centers for Disease Control and Prevention, National Center for Chronic Disease Prevention and Health Promotion.

Venes, D. 2009. *Taber's cyclopedic medical dictionary*, 21st ed. Philadelphia: Davis.

Vincent, K.R., and R.W. Braith. 2002. Resistance exercise and bone turnover in elderly men and women. *Medicine and Science in Sports and Exercise* 34 (1): 17–23.

Vitti, K.A., C.M. Bayles, W.J. Carender, J.M. Prendergast, and F.J. D'Amico. 1993. A low-level strength training exercise program for frail elderly adults living in an extended attention facility. *Aging, Clinical and Experimental Research* 5 (5): 363–369.

Wagenaar, D., Colenda, C.C., Kreft, M., Sawade, J., Gardiner, J., and Poverejan, E. 2003. Treating depression in nursing homes: Practice guidelines in the real world. *Journal of the American Osteopathic Association* 103(10): 465-469.

Wescott, W.L., and T.R. Baechle. 2007. *Strength training past 50*, 2nd ed. Champaign, IL: Human Kinetics.

Williams, D.M. 2008. Exercise, affect, and adherence: An integrated model and a case for self-paced exercise. *Journal of Sport and Exercise Psychology* 30 (5): 471–496.

Williamson, P. 2011. *Exercise for special populations*. Philadelphia: Wolters Kluwer Health/ Lippincott Williams and Wilkins.

Williford, H.N., J.B. East, F.H. Smith, and L.A. Burry. 1986. Evaluation of warm-up for improvement in flexibility. *American Journal of Sports Medicine* 14: 316–319.

World Health Organization. 1997. The Heidelberg guidelines for promoting physical activity among older persons. *Journal of Aging and Physical Activity* 5 (1): 2–8.

World Health Organization. 2013. *Definitions: emergencies*. www.who.int/hac/about/definitions.

Suggested Resources

Books, Manuals, Other Printed Material

Balance

American College of Sports Medicine. 2011. *Selecting and effectively using balance training for older adults.* Brochure. www.acsm.org.

Bovre, S. 2010. *Balance training: A program for improving balance in older adults,* 3rd ed. Tucson, AZ: Desert Southwest Fitness. 800-873-6759.

Jones, C.J., and D.J. Rose, eds. 2005. *Physical activity instruction of older adults.* Champaign, IL: Human Kinetics.

Perkins-Carpenter, B. 2006. *How to prevent falls: Better balance, independence and energy in 6 simple steps.* Penfield, NY: Senior Fitness Productions.

Rose, D.J. 2010. *FallProof!: A comprehensive balance and mobility training program,* 2nd ed. Champaign, IL: Human Kinetics.

Scott, S. 2008. *Able bodies balance training.* Champaign, IL: Human Kinetics.

Continuing Education

American Senior Fitness Association. 2014a (updated yearly, since 1994). *Long term care fitness leader training manual,* New Smyrna Beach, FL: American Senior Fitness Association. 888-689-6791 or (international) 386-423-6634. www.seniorfitness.org.

———. 2014b. (updated yearly, since 1994). *Senior fitness instructor training manual,* New Smyrna Beach, FL: American Senior Fitness Association.

———. 2014c. (updated yearly, since 1996). *Senior personal trainer training manual,* New Smyrna Beach, FL: American Senior Fitness Association.

Arkin, S. 2005. *Language-enriched exercise for clients with Alzheimer's disease.* Tucson, AZ: Desert Southwest Fitness. 800-873-6759.

Bovre, S. 2010. *Balance training: A program for improving balance in older adults,* 3rd ed. Tucson, AZ: Desert Southwest Fitness. 800-873-6759.

Fitness, Wellness, and Special Needs

American Association of Cardiovascular and Pulmonary Rehabilitation (AACVPR). 2004. *Guidelines for cardiac rehabilitation and secondary prevention programs,* 4th ed. Champaign IL: Human Kinetics.

———. 2006. *Cardiac rehabilitation resource manual.* Champaign, IL: Human Kinetics.

———. 2011. *Guidelines for pulmonary rehabilitation programs,* 4th ed. Champaign, IL: Human Kinetics.

American College of Sports Medicine (ACSM). 2009. *Exercise management for persons with chronic diseases and disabilities,* 3rd ed. Champaign, IL: Human Kinetics.

———. 2011. *Selecting and effectively using a stationary bicycle.* Brochure. www.acsm.org.

American College of Sports Medicine (ACSM) and the American Heart Association. 2011. *Selecting and effectively using a walking program.* Brochure. www.acsm.org.

Boelen, M. P. 2009. *Health professionals' guide to physical management of Parkinson's disease.* Champaign, IL: Human Kinetics.

Buettner, L., and S. Fitzsimmons. 2008. *Dementia practice guideline for recreational therapy: Treatment of disturbing behaviors.* Hattiesburg, MS: ATRA (American Therapeutic Recreation Association).

Buettner, L., and D. Greenstein. 2000. *Simple pleasures—A multi level sensorimotor intervention for nursing home residents with dementia.* Hattiesburg, MS: ATRA (American Therapeutic Recreation Association).

Clark, J. 2012. *Seniorcise: A simple guide to fitness for the elderly and disabled,* 3rd ed. New Smyrna Beach, FL: American Senior Fitness Association.

Frontera, W., D. Slovick, and D. Dawson. 2006. *Exercise in rehabilitation medicine.* Champaign, IL: Human Kinetics.

Hawley, J.A., and J.R. Zierath. 2008. *Physical activity and type 2 diabetes.* Champaign, IL: Human Kinetics.

Kalkstein, S. 2009. *Fortify your frame comprehensive exercise program.* 14 SW 110th Way,

Davie, FL 33324. Keep the Beat, Inc. www.fortifyyourframe.com.

Knopf, K. 2006. *Weights for 50+*. Berkeley, CA: Ulysses Press.

Knopf, K. 2010a. *Healthy shoulder handbook*. Berkeley, CA: Ulysses Press.

Knopf, K. 2010b. *Healthy hip handbook*. Berkeley, CA: Ulysses Press.

Levine, P.G. 2009. *Stronger after stroke*. New York: Demos Medical.

National Institutes of Health and the National Institute on Aging. 2011. *Exercise: A guide from the National Institute on Aging*. Bethesda, MD: National Institutes of Health/National Institute on Aging. Free publication. 800-222-2225.

Rikli, R.E., and C. Jessie Jones. 2013. *Senior fitness test manual*, 2nd ed. Champaign, IL: Human Kinetics.

Schleck, L.A., ed. 2000. *Staying strong: A senior's guide to a more active and independent life*. Minneapolis, MN: Fairview Press. 800-544-8207.

Schroeder, J. 2004. *Strength programs for frail and well elderly*. Hasbrouck Heights, NJ: Flaghouse.

Sharkey, B.J. 2007. *Fitness and health*, 6th ed. Champaign, IL: Human Kinetics.

Signorile, J.F. 2011. *Bending the aging curve*. Champaign, IL: Human Kinetics.

Spirduso, W., K. Francis, and P. Macrae. 2005. *Physical dimensions of aging*, 2nd ed. Champaign, IL: Human Kinetics.

Van Norman, Kay. 2010. *Exercise and wellness for older adults*, 2nd ed. Champaign, IL: Human Kinetics.

Inspirational

Clark, E. 1995. *Growing old is not for sissies II: Portraits of senior athletes*. San Francisco: Pomegranate Artbooks.

Erickson, Erik, J. Erickson, and H. Kivnick. 1986. *Vital involvement in old age*. New York: Norton.

Ferrin, K. 2005. *What's age got to do with it? Secret to aging in extraordinary ways*. San Diego, CA: Alti.

Rowe, J.W., and R.L. Kahn. 1998. *Successful aging*. New York: Dell.

Reference

Berkow, R., M.H. Beers, R.M. Bogin, and A.J. Fletcher, eds. 2011. *Merck manual of medical information*, 19th ed. New York: Simon and Schuster.

Delavier, Frederic. 2006. *Strength training anatomy*, 3rd ed. Champaign, IL: Human Kinetics.

Dirckx, J.H., ed. 2011. *Stedman's concise medical dictionary for the health professions*, illus. 7th ed. Baltimore: Lippincott Williams and Wilkins.

Kapit, W., and L.M. Elson. 2001. *The anatomy coloring book*, 3rd ed. Reading, MA: Addison-Wesley.

Nelson, Arnold, and J. Kokkonen. 2007. *Stretching anatomy*. Champaign, IL: Human Kinetics.

Porter, H., and J. Burlingame. 2006. *Recreational therapy handbook of practice ICF-based diagnosis and treatment*. Enumclaw, WA; Idyll Arbor.

Sieg, K.W., and S.P. Adams. 2009. *Illustrated essentials of musculoskeletal anatomy*, 5th ed. Gainesville, FL: Megabooks.

Relaxation and Stress Reduction

Dworkis, S. 1997. *Recovery yoga: A practical guide for chronically ill, injured, and post-operative people*. New York: Three Rivers.

Kabat-Zinn, J. 1990. *Full catastrophe living (program of the Stress Reduction Clinic at University of Massachusetts Medical Center)*. New York: Dell. Mindfullnesscds.com.

Korb-Khalsa, K.L., and E.A Leutenberg. 2000. *Life management skills VII*. Beachwood, OH: Wellness Reproductions.

Rossman, M. 2010. *The worry solution: Using breakthrough brain science to turn anxiety and stress into confidence and happiness*. New York: Crown Archetype. www.worrysolution.com or www.thehealingmind.org.

Resistance Bands and Isometric Exercises

American College of Sports Medicine. 2011. *Selecting and effectively using rubber band resistance exercise*. Brochure. www.acsm.org.

Corning Creager, C. 1998. *Therapeutic exercises using resistive bands*. Berthoud, CO: Executive Physical Therapy. 800-367-7393.

O'Driscoll, E. 2005. *The complete book of isometrics: The anywhere, anytime fitness book*. New York: Hatherleigh Press (a division of Random House). 800-733-3000.

Journals and Newsletters

Creative forecasting. A monthly newsletter for activity and recreation professionals. P.O. Box

7789, Colorado Springs, CO 80937-7789. 719-633-3174. cfi@cfactive.com. "Let's Get Moving" column written by Betsy Best-Martini.

Experience! Free senior health and fitness newsletter. American Senior Fitness Association, P.O. Box 2575, New Smyrna Beach, FL 32170. 888-689-6791 or (international) 386-423-6634. www.seniorfitness.org.

Journal of aging and physical activity. Champaign, IL: Human Kinetics. 800-747-4457. www.HumanKinetics.com.

Journal on active aging. Comprehensive and inspirational journal about wellness and active aging. International Council on Active Aging. www.icaa.cc.

Professional Certifications and Trainings

American Senior Fitness Association Advanced Qualification Professional Training: Lonterm care fitness leader; senior personal trainer; senior fitness instructor
American Senior Fitness Association
P.O. Box 2575
New Smyrna Beach, FL 32170
888-689-6791 or (international) 386-423-6634
www.seniorfitness.org

Exercise for Adults With Special Needs Instructor
College of Marin
835 College Avenue
Kentfield, CA 94904
415-453-6130, betsybest@comcast.net
415-897-BFIT (2348), kjones@mycom.marin.edu

Arthritis Foundation Exercise Program Instructor
www.arthritis.org
(800) 283-7800

Several courses focusing on special needs
DSW Fitness
www.dswfitness.com

Professional Liability Insurance

ACE-Certified Fitness Professional Insurance Program
www.insurepersonaltrainers.com, www.fitnesspak.com.

International Dance Exercise Association (IDEA)
FWI Fitness and Wellness Insurance
www.ideafit.com/fitness-insurance
800-999-4332, ext. 7

Professional Organizations and Foundations

Fitness and Wellness

Aerobics and Fitness Association of America
www.afaa.com

American Alliance for Health, Physical Education, Recreation and Dance (AAHPERD)
www.aahperd.org

American College of Sports Medicine (ACSM)
www.acsm.org

American Council on Exercise (ACE)
www.acefitness.com

American Therapeutic Recreation Association
www.atra-online.com

Centers for Disease Control and Prevention (CDC)
www.cdc.gov

Cooper Institute for Aerobics Research
www.cooperinst.org

Desert Southwest Fitness, Inc.
www.dswfitness.com

Human Kinetics (Publisher)
www.HumanKinetics.com

International Curriculum Guidelines for Preparing Physical Activity Instructors of Older Adults
www.humankinetics.com/aacc-policies-and-guidelines/aacc-policies-and-guidelines/international-curriculum-guidelines-for-preparing-physical-activity-instructors-of-older-adults

International Dance Exercise Association (IDEA)
www.ideafit.com

National Association of Activity Professionals
www.naap.info

National Center for Physical Activity and Disability (NCPAD)
ncpad@uic.edu
www.ncpad.org

National Strength and Conditioning Association (NSCA)
www.nsca-lift.org

Older Adults

National Strength Professionals Association (NSPA)
www.nspainc.com

U.S. Department of Health and Human Services (USDHHS)
U.S. Office of Disease Prevention and Health Promotion, Healthy People 2020
www.health.gov/healthypeople

Older Adults

American Association of Retired Persons (AARP)
www.aarp.org

American Senior Fitness Association (SFA)
www.seniorfitness.org

American Society on Aging
www.asaging.org

50-Plusfitness Association
www.50plus.org

International Coalition for Aging and Physical Activity (ICAPA)
Wojtek Chodzko-Zajko, PhD
www.humankinetics.com/icapa

International Council on Active Aging (ICAA)
www.icaa.cc

Keiser Institute on Aging
Keiser Corporation
http://kioa.keiser.com/

National Center for Assisted Living
www.ncal.org

National Institute on Aging
www.nia.nih.gov

Special Needs

Alzheimer's Disease and Related Dementias
Alzheimer's Association
www.alz.org

Arthritis
Arthritis Foundation
www.arthritis.org

Cerebrovascular Accident (Stroke)
American Stroke Association
www.strokeassociation.org

Chronic Obstructive Pulmonary Disease
American Lung Association
www.lung.org

Coronary Artery Disease, Heart Disease, and Hypertension
American Heart Association
www.americanheart.org

Depression
St. Louis Psychologists and Counseling Information and Referral
www.psychtreatment.com

Diabetes
American Diabetes Association
www.diabetes.org

Hearing Loss Association of America
www.hearingloss.org

Hip Fracture or Replacement and Knee Replacement
Mayo Clinic
www.mayoclinic.com/health/hip-replacement/MY00235
www.mayoclinic.com/health/knee-replacement/MY00091

Multiple Sclerosis
Multiple Sclerosis Foundation
www.msfocus.org

Osteoporosis
Foundation for Osteoporosis Research and Education (FORE)
info@fore.org
www.fore.org

Parkinson's Disease
American Parkinson Disease Association, Inc.
www.apdaparkinson.org

Sensory Losses
National Association for Visually Handicapped
www.navh.org

Resources and Supplies

Balance Supplies

Adventure Buddies, Poles for Balance and Mobility
www.PolesForMobility.com

Balance discs, foam pads, balance boards, stability balls
www.performbetter.com
(888) 556-7462

Color discs and balance discs (for balance exercises)
www.flaghouse.com, www.enasco.com

Riverstones (for balance exercises)
www.flaghouse.com, www.gonge.com

Scarves (for balance and flexibility)
www.enasco.com

Sensory and balance supply catalog
www.adultsensoryactivities.com

Soundsteps (make sounds when touched—
good for seated and standing)
www.flaghouse.com

Catalogs

Briggs
www.BriggsCorp.com
800-247-2343

Flaghouse
www.flaghouse.com
800-265-6900

Nasco
www.eNASCO.com
800-558-9595

Seabay
www.seabaygame.com
800-568-0188

S&S Primelife
www.ssww.com
800-243-9232

Posters

RPE (Rating of Perceived Exertion) poster
featuring facial expressions to represent
intensity levels
Young Enterprises, Inc.
800-765-3975
www.youngposters.com

Stretching and Resistance Bands

MatsMatsMats
Good stretching mats and bands
www.matsmatsmats.com

Evidence-Based Older Adult Exercise Programs

Healthways Silver Sneakers
www.silversneakers.com
800-295-4993 or 888-423-4632

OTAGA Exercise Program (New Zealand)
info@laterlifetraining.co.uk

Project Enhance
projectenhance.org
206-448-5725

Conductorcise
www.conductorcise.com
914-244-3803

www.ebrsr.com.
This site has stroke rehab evidence-based research.

www.eldergym.com
This site, created by a physical therapist, has excellent exercises, videos, and resources.

www.exerciseismedicine.org
This site was created by a collaborative venture between ACSM and AMA.

Media Resources

Balance

Rose, Debra. 2008. *FallProof at home, level 1, 2, 3.* Instructional DVDs including warm-up, balance, strengthening, and flexibility. Fall Prevention Center of Excellence. www.stopfalls.org.

Fitness

Go4Life from the National Institute on Aging at NIH (DVD). Routine that includes strength, balance, and flexibility. Free. http://go4life.nia.nih.gov/.

Schmidt, Kathy. 2013. *Be healthy be fit senior series.* San Leandro, CA: Three Palms Studios. 650-346-4444, (DVDs that are fun and functional, including seated and standing options.)

Stolove, J. 2011. Del Mar, CA: Chair Dancing International. 800-551-4386, www.chair-dancingfitness.com.

Tahoe Forest Hospital. 1998. *Fitness forever: The exercise program for healthy aging!* Fitness Forever, P.O. Box 981316, Park City, UT 84098-1316, 877-654-EVER. www.lifespanfitness.com

Wilson, Mary Ann. Spokane, WA: Sit and Be Fit. 509-448-9438, www.sitandbefit.org.

Special conditions workout DVDs:
Arthritis workout (2008), *Fibromyalgia workout* (2005), *COPD workout* (2010), *Diabetes workout* (2006), *Osteoporosis workout* (2005), *Parkinson's workout* (2006), *Neuro rehab workout* (2010)

Prevention workout DVDs:
Balance & fall prevention (2009), *Brain fitness workout* (2010), *Relax to heal* (2011), *Prevent DVT [Deep Vein Thrombosis] workout* (2010)

Music

Ken Alan Associates
323-653-5040

Musicflex
718-738-6839

Power Productions
800-777-2328

Sports Music, Inc
800-878-4764

Relaxation and Stress Reduction, Including Mindfulness and Meditation

Stress Reduction CDs
www.mindfulnesscds.com

Emmett. E. Miller, MD
www.lightseed.com

Center for Mindfulness
www.umassmed.edu/cfm/index.aspx

Martin Rossman, MD
Guided imagery resources for sleep, pain
relief, preparing for surgery and more
www.drrossman.info, www.thehealing-
mind.org, and www.worrysolution.com

Wilson, Mary Ann. 2011. *Relax to heal* (DVD).
Spokane, WA: Sit and Be Fit. 509-448-9438.
www.sitandbefit.org.

Index

Note: Page numbers followed with an italicized *f* or *t* indicates that a figure or table will be found on those pages, respectively.

and resistance training 142
  safety precautions 90, 183, 222
free weights 292
frequency
  in aerobic training 186-187
  of exercise classes 267
  for resistance training 148
  for stretching 227-228

G
gastrocnemius 290
gastrocnemius exercises. *See* calf exercises
gerokinesiology 4
glucose levels 288
gluteals 290
gluteals exercises. *See* buttocks exercises
goals
  of balance and fall prevention 262
  group 60
  setting 36-37
guided imagery 235-236
guidelines
  for aerobic training 184-190, 185*t*
  ethical practice for trainers 297-298
  for feedback 93
  joint range-of-motion 94-95
  posture-awareness 92-93, 92*t*
  for relaxation exercises 231-232
  for resistance training 145-152, 147*t*
  for safety 42-43
  safety checklist 42
  for stretching 92*t*, 95
  for stretching exercises 224-230, 225*t*
  for three-part breathing 92*t*, 94-95
  for warm-ups 92-95, 92*t*

H
half hug exercise 244
hamstrings 290
hamstrings exercises. *See* thigh exercises
handkerchiefs 293
hand weights 292
hands, cues for 291
hands open and closed exercise 125
head injury, traumatic 17-18, 31*t*
head-to-toe relaxation imagery 236
health, definition of 4-5
Healthy People 2010 33
heel lifts 197-198
heel raises exercise 174
heel touches to front exercise 205-206
heel touches to sides exercise 209-210
hemorrhagic stroke 10
high blood pressure 15
hip abductors 288

hip adductors exercises. *See* thigh exercises
hip and thigh exercises
  hip abduction and adduction 167-168
  hip flexion 166
  hip rotation 110-111
  out-and-in leg march 109
  outer-thigh stretch 252-253
  up-and-down leg march 108
hip flexion exercise 166
hip flexors 288
hip fracture
  described 15
  and resistance training 142
  safety precautions 183, 222-223
  teaching tips for 26*t*
  warm-up exercises 90-91
hips, cues for 291
hyperglycemia 14
hypertension
  described 15
  and resistance training 142-143
  safety precautions 183, 223
  teaching tips for 26*t*
  warm-up exercises 91
hypoglycemia 14

I
IDEA code of ethics 297-298
image, professional 298
informed consent form 40, 285
Institute for Health and Aging 17
instruction guides. *See* exercises
integrity 298
International Council on Active Aging 34
International Curriculum Guidelines 4
ischemic stroke 10

J
joint range-of-motion guidelines 94-95
Journal of Aging and Physical Activity (Ecclestone) 4

K
knee exercises
  best foot forward and backward 112
  extension 171-172
  flexion 169-170
  lifts 215-216
knee replacement 15
knees, cues for 291
kyphosis 16

L
large-group safety checklist 47
latissimus dorsi exercises. *See* back exercises
latissimus dorsi muscles 290

left-side CVA 10
leg march exercises 108-109
lower-body exercises
  range-of-motion 108-117
  resistance 166-176
  stretching 248-257

M
maintaining boundaries 298
manic-depressive illness 13
marching in place exercise 201-202
media, exercise 266, 266*t*
medical clearance 40
Medical History and Risk Factor Questionnaire 40, 43, 283-284
medications 7
mental health, improved 288
microphones 293
mirrors 293
mobility and transfer issues 68-69
mood, described 13
mood state, enhanced 288
motor control and performance 288
motivation 35-36
movement, velocity of 288
multiple sclerosis
  described 15-16
  and resistance training 144
  safety precautions 183, 223
  teaching tips for 27*t*
  warm-up exercises 91
muscles
  core body 52
  of the human body 289-290
muscle strengthening 288
music, during exercise classes 65-67
myocardial ischemia 13
myths about resistance training 138, 139*t*

N
National Blueprint 33
National Institute of Neurological Disorders and Stroke 11
neck, cues for 291
neck exercises
  chin to chest 241
  chin to shoulder 242
neck extensors 290
neck rotators and extensors 288. *See also* neck exercises

O
osteoarthritis 9
osteoporosis 91
  described 16-17
  and resistance training 144
  safety precautions 16, 183, 223
  teaching tips for 28*t*
out-and-in leg march exercise 109
outer-thigh stretch exercise 252-253
overexertion 13
overhead press exercise 163

About the Authors

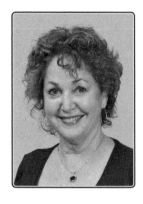

Elizabeth (Betsy) Best-Martini, MS, CTRS, is a certified recreational therapist specializing in the field of fitness, aging, wellness, and long-term care. Best-Martini is the owner of Recreation Consultation, a firm that provides training and recreational therapy consultation to retirement communities, skilled nursing settings, subacute settings, and residential and assisted care facilities in northern California. Her practice also includes Fit For Life one-to-one personal training for adults and older adults.

Best-Martini specializes in working with adults with special needs and brings more than 30 years as a rehabilitation therapist to this work. In addition to consulting, she lectures and provides training across the United States and in Canada. She also teaches a weekly seated strength training class in an assisted living setting.

Best-Martini is an instructor at the College of Marin in Kentfield, California, where she teaches courses in strength, flexibility, and balance for adults and older adults. She trains new fitness instructors in the Exercise for Adults with Special Needs Fitness Instructor Training and Certification course through the American Senior Fitness Association. In addition, she facilitates the Activity Coordinator Training course, which certifies students through the Department of Public Health to become activity coordinators working with older adults and frail elders.

She has authored two other texts, *Long-Term Care for Activity Professionals, Social Services Professionals, and Recreational Therapists, Sixth Edition,* and *Quality Assurance for Activity Programs.* Best-Martini also writes a column focusing on fitness and wellness programs for older adults in *Creative Forecasting,* a national newsletter for activity professionals and recreational therapists.

In 2006 and 2008, Best-Martini received the American Therapeutic Recreation Association (ATRA) Member of the Year Award. She was awarded the 1998 Distinguished Merit Award from the Northern California Council of Activity Coordinators (NCCAC) and the Pete Croughan Award for her volunteer efforts with the nonprofit organization, Love Is The Answer (LITA). She also served on the Visionary Advisory Board for the International Council on Active Aging (ICAA).

In her free time, Best-Martini can be found gardening, hiking, exercising, and spending time with her husband, family, and many pets. She lives in Fairfax, California.

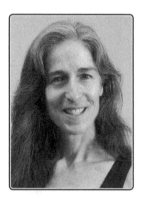

Kim A. Jones-DiGenova, MA, received her master's degree in physical education (exercise physiology) and the Distinguished Achievement in a Major Field Award from San Francisco State University. She is a physical education instructor at the College of Marin in Kentfield, California, where she teaches courses on strength and fitness training for older adults. She also serves as a health and fitness consultant and personal trainer in the San Francisco and San Rafael metropolitan areas.

Jones-DiGenova has been working in the fitness field since 1971. She is an ACSM-certified health fitness specialist; SFA-certified senior personal trainer, senior fitness instructor, and long-term care fitness leader; Arthritis Foundation exercise program instructor; and YMCA strength training instructor trainer. She is the Northern California academic administrator for the American Senior Fitness Association and has developed and implemented resistance training programs in several convalescent, retirement, and senior facilities throughout California. Jones-DiGenova has also assisted handicapable adults with weight training, aerobic exercise, and stress reduction at the Recreation Center for the Handicapped in San Francisco. In addition to her work on *Exercise for Frail Elders*, Jones-DiGenova is a regular contributor to national and local newsletters.

Jones-DiGenova resides in Novato, California. She enjoys spending time with family and friends and reading. She stays active by walking, hiking, swimming, weight training, and practicing yoga. She has swum from the Golden Gate Bridge to the San Francisco–Oakland Bay Bridge and has successfully escaped from Alcatraz many times.

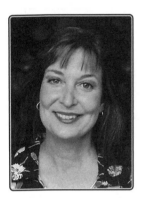

Janie Clark, MA, is president of the American Senior Fitness Association (SFA), the international organization for fitness professionals who serve older adults. She earned a master's degree in exercise physiology and wellness manage-ment from the University of Central Florida, with an emphasis in older adult health and fitness.

Clark is a contributing author of *Physical Activity Instruction of Older Adults* and *Exercise for Older Adults: ACE's Guide for Fitness Professionals*. She is the author of *Brain Fitness for Older Adults: How to Incorporate Cognitive Fitness Into Physical Activity Programming; Quality-of-Life Fitness; Seniorcise: A Simple Guide to Fitness for the Elderly and Disabled; Full Life Fitness: A Complete Exercise Program for Mature Adults;* and *Exercise Programming for Older Adults*. She has authored hundreds of articles for periodicals, including the *Journal of Aging and Physical Activity; Activities, Adaptation & Aging Journal; ACE Certified News;* and *Modern Maturity.*

Janie served on the National AFib Support Team sponsored by Sanofi-Aventis pharmaceutical corporation to provide patients and health care professionals with current information on atrial fibrillation. She also served as a reviewer for the LifeSpan project, which developed functional fitness tests for older adults, and as a member of the Coalition to Develop National Curriculum Standards for Senior Fitness Professionals.

Clark resides in Florida with her husband, son, and ever-growing menagerie of cats, dogs, and other furry creatures.

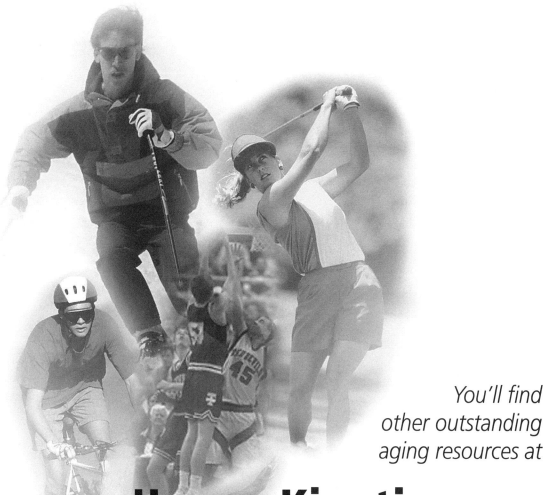

You'll find
other outstanding
aging resources at

www.HumanKinetics.com

In the U.S. call

1-800-747-4457

Australia..08 8372 0999
Canada 1-800-465-7301
Europe..+44 (0) 113 255 5665
New Zealand..0800 222 062

HUMAN KINETICS
The Information Leader in Physical Activity & Health
P.O. Box 5076 • Champaign, IL 61825-5076 USA